Perioperative Care of the Elderly Patient

Perioperative Care of the Elderly Patient

Edited by

Sheila Ryan Barnett

Vice-Chair of Perioperative Medicine, Department of Anesthesia, Critical Care and Pain Medicine, Beth Israel Deaconess Medical Center, Associate Professor of Anesthesia, Harvard Medical School, Boston, MA, USA

Sara E. Neves

Instructor of Anesthesia, Harvard Medical School, Department of Anesthesia, Critical Care and Pain Medicine, Beth Israel Deaconess Medical Center, Boston, MA, USA

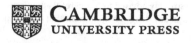

CAMBRIDGE
UNIVERSITY PRESS

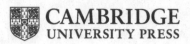

CAMBRIDGE
UNIVERSITY PRESS

Shaftesbury Road, Cambridge CB2 8EA, United Kingdom

One Liberty Plaza, 20th Floor, New York, NY 10006, USA

477 Williamstown Road, Port Melbourne, VIC 3207, Australia

314–321, 3rd Floor, Plot 3, Splendor Forum, Jasola District Centre, New Delhi – 110025, India

103 Penang Road, #05–06/07, Visioncrest Commercial, Singapore 238467

Cambridge University Press is part of Cambridge University Press & Assessment,
a department of the University of Cambridge.

We share the University's mission to contribute to society through the pursuit of
education, learning and research at the highest international levels of excellence.

www.cambridge.org
Information on this title: www.cambridge.org/9781107576292

© Cambridge University Press & Assessment 2018

First published 2018

A catalogue record for this publication is available from the British Library

Library of Congress Cataloging-in-Publication data
Names: Barnett, Sheila Ryan, editor. | Neves, Sara E., editor.
Title: Perioperative care of the elderly patient / edited by Sheila Ryan
    Barnett, Sara E. Neves.
Description: Cambridge, United Kingdom ; New York : Cambridge
    University Press, [2017] | Includes bibliographical references
    and index.
Identifiers: LCCN 2017035930 | ISBN 9781107576292 (pbk.)
Subjects: | MESH: Perioperative Care | Aged
Classification: LCC RD49 | NLM WO 950 | DDC 617.9/192—dc23
    LC record available at https://lccn.loc.gov/2017035930

ISBN   978-1-107-57629-2   Paperback

....

I would specifically like to thank my co-editor Sara
Neves, an anesthesiology intensivist, who represents
the next generation of perioperative champions. I look
forward to continued collaborations over shared elderly
patients and new "gero-centric" endeavors.

I would also like to thank my colleagues, many of whom
co-authored chapters, for their interest and support of all
things "geriatric" in our emerging perioperative world.

Finally, to my family: John, Elizabeth and Gannon –
thank you for your patience and enthusiasm for my
work endeavors and the humor and love you bring into
my life.

Sheila Ryan Barnett

I would like to dedicate this book to my parents, whose
love and support have guided me throughout my life.
I also want to thank my husband and two daughters for
their love and patience in allowing me to contribute to
this important work.

Sara E. Neves

Contents

Section 4 – Postoperative Issues

Contributors

Anthony J. Baldea MD
Assistant Professor, Trauma, Surgical
Critical Care and Burns, Loyola University
Medical Center, Maywood, IL, USA

Sheila Ryan Barnett MD
Associate Professor, Harvard Medical
School, Department of Anesthesiology,
Critical Care and Pain Medicine, Vice
Chair for Perioperative Medicine, Beth
Israel Deaconess Medical Center, Boston,
MA, USA

Gwendolyn L. Boyd MD
Chief, Department of Anesthesiology,
UAB Callahan Eye Foundation Hospital,
Birmingham, AL, USA

Kristine E. W. Breyer MD
Assistant Professor, Department of
Anesthesia, UCSF School of Medicine,
San Francisco, CA, USA

Charles H. Brown IV MD MS
Assistant Professor, Division of
Cardiac Anesthesia, Department of
Anesthesiology and Critical Care
Medicine, Johns Hopkins University,
Baltimore, MD, USA

Mary K. Buss MD MPH
Assistant Professor, Harvard Medical
School, Director, Ambulatory Palliative
Care, Beth Israel Deaconess Medical
Center, Boston, MA, USA

Angela Georgia Catic MD
Assistant Professor, Director Geriatric
Medicine Fellowship, Baylor College
of Medicine, Medical Director, Geriatric PA
Residency Program, Michael E. DeBakey
VA Medical Center, Houston, TX, USA

Stephanie Cintora MD
Assistant Professor, Department of
Anesthesiology, University of Massachusetts
Medical School, UMass Memorial Medical
Center, Worcester, MA, USA

Elifce Cosar MD
Clinical Vice-Chair, University of
Massachusetts Medical School,
UMass Memorial Medical Center,
Worcester, MA, USA

Carol Ann B. Diachun MD MSEd
Professor, Department of Anesthesiology,
University of Florida, Jacksonville, FL, USA

Jeffrey B. Dobyns DO
Associate Professor, Department of
Anesthesiology and Perioperative
Medicine, University of Alabama School
of Medicine, Birmingham, AL, USA

George A. Dumas MD
Assistant Professor, Department of
Anesthesiology and Perioperative
Medicine, University of Alabama School
of Medicine, Birmingham, AL, USA

Elizabeth Fouts-Palmer MD
Instructor in Anesthesiology, Weill
Cornell Medical College, Cornell
University, New York, NY, USA

Christopher G. Hughes MD
Associate Professor, Division of Critical
Care, Department of Anesthesiology,
Vanderbilt University School of Medicine,
Nashville, TN, USA

James M. Hunter, Jr. MD
Associate Professor, Division of Critical
Care and Perioperative Medicine,
Department of Anesthesiology, University
of Alabama, Birmingham, AL, USA

Dae Hyun Kim MD MPH ScD
Assistant Professor, Division of
Gerontology, Department of Medicine,
Beth Israel Deaconess Medical Center,
Harvard Medical School, Boston, MA, USA

Abirami Kumaresan MD
Department of Anesthesia, Critical Care
and Pain Medicine, Beth Israel Deaconess
Medical Center, Boston, MA, USA

Lisa Kunze MD PhD
Assistant Professor Anesthesiology,
Harvard Medical School, Department of
Anesthesiology, Critical Care and Pain
Medicine, Beth Israel Deaconess Medical
Center, Boston, MA, USA

Michael C. Lewis MBBS
Chair and Professor, Department of
Anesthesiology, University of Florida
College of Medicine, Jacksonville, FL, USA

Fred A. Luchette MD
Vice-Chair of VA Affairs and Professor of
Surgery, Department of Surgery, Stritch
School of Medicine, Loyola University of
Chicago, Maywood, IL, USA

Robina Matyal MD
Associate Professor Anesthesiology,
Harvard Medical School, Department of
Anesthesiology, Critical Care and Pain
Medicine, Beth Israel Deaconess Medical
Center, Boston, MA, USA

Ellen P. McCarthy PhD, MPH
Associate Professor, Medicine,
Assistant Dean of Development and
Diversity, Harvard Medical School,
Division of General Medicine and
Primary Care, Beth Israel Deaconess
Medical Center, Boston, MA, USA

Jason L. McKeown MD
Division of Gerontology, Geriatrics
and Palliative Care, Department of
Anesthesiology and Perioperative
Medicine, University of Alabama,
Birmingham, AL, USA

John D. Mitchell MD
Associate Professor, Harvard Medical
School, Residency Program Director,
Department of Anesthesiology, Critical
Care and Pain Medicine, Beth Israel
Deaconess Medical Center,
Boston, MA, USA

Mario E. Montealegre MD
Resident, Department of Anesthesiology,
Critical Care and Pain Medicine, Beth
Israel Deaconess Medical Center, Boston,
MA, USA

Sara E. Neves
Instructor in Anesthesiology, Harvard
Medical School, Department of
Anesthesiology, Critical Care and Pain
Medicine, Beth Israel Deaconess Medical
Center, Boston, MA, USA

Rita S. Patel MD
Department of Anesthesiology,
University of Florida College of Medicine,
Jacksonville, FL, USA

Shachi C. Patel MD
Medical Director, Delmarva Pain and
Spine Center, Newark, DE, USA

Varun Rimmalapudi MD
University of Florida, Jacksonville,
FL, USA

Rabya S. Saraf BA
Department of Anesthesia, Critical Care
and Pain Medicine, Beth Israel Deaconess
Medical Center, Boston, MA, USA

Shahzad Shaefi MD
Instructor in Anaesthesia, Beth Israel
Deaconess Medical Center, Harvard
Medical School, Boston, MA, USA

Gail A. Van Norman MD
Professor, Anesthesiology and Pain
Medicine, Adjunct Professor, Bioethics,
University of Washington,
Seattle, WA, USA

Anasuya Vasudevan MD MBBS
Department of Anesthesiology, Geisinger
Commonwealth School of Medicine,
Danville, PA, USA

Thomas R. Vetter MD MPH
Director of Perioperative Care, Professor,
Department of Surgery and Perioperative
Care, Dell Medical School, University of
Texas at Austin, Austin, TX, USA

Marissa Wagner Mery MD
Anesthesiologist, Department of
Anesthesiology, Baylor College of
Medicine, Houston, TX, USA

Cynthia E. Weber MD
Department of Surgery, Loyola University
Medical Center, Maywood, IL, USA

Preface

The steady rise of older patients represents one of the biggest economic and societal challenges facing health care, leading to an increased demand for a deeper understanding of the impact of aging in the perioperative period. Although some disease states, like dementia, can be considered a classic "geriatric" condition, others, such as heart disease, hypertension, degenerative osteoarthritis, cataracts and complex pain syndromes, are not unique to the elderly, but still contribute significantly to the disease burden of this demographic. Despite a higher morbidity and mortality risk, elderly patients frequently need to undergo invasive procedures and surgery, and this can raise questions about what constitutes appropriate perioperative care. For example, which geriatric patient needs preoperative functional and/or frailty assessment, what is a meaningful recovery in the patient with dementia and how does one address the ethics of performing procedures near the end of life? These questions frequently require interdisciplinary collaboration amongst multiple perioperative providers, including surgeons, anesthesiologists, cardiologists, geriatricians and hospitalists. In this text we have attempted to highlight perioperative areas of vulnerability for the older patient undergoing anesthesia and surgery.

From the patient's perspective, the surgical event is often the central event during a hospitalization or illness; however, for most patients surgery and anesthesia represent just one part of the continuum of perioperative care. It is not surprising then that perioperative medicine is assuming an increasingly important role in surgery and anesthesia, and interdisciplinary communication and sharing of expertise amongst multiple specialists is needed to optimize outcomes for frail and complex older patients. The elements of perioperative care – from the preoperative preparation, the choice for surgery and informed consent, the anesthetic options and surgery itself, and the postoperative period – contribute to a successful outcome for the patient. In this book, we attempt to bring together these perioperative issues by discussing multiple "geriatric" issues, such as evaluations for frailty, the types of dementia and how they may be characterized. How should we address issues of competence and decision-making? What is the role of palliative care for an 80-year-old patient needing surgery? What is the impact of noninvasive cardiac surgery versus traditional surgical approaches? These are a few of the important issues that face clinicians daily as they care for sick older patients – admitted from home or through the emergency unit. We hope that this book will increase awareness of issues pertaining to the elderly in the perioperative period and even lead to the generation of more questions and curiosity about the older patient.

When I started in geriatric medicine over 20 years ago it was rare to personally encounter an anesthesiologist, pain medicine was not yet established as a specialty and critical care was still a small subspecialty. So when I retrained to pursue a career in anesthesiology my goal was to improve the care of older patients undergoing anesthesia and surgery. Early on I realized communication and collaboration would be the cornerstone of "geriatric anesthesiology" and I, along with many like-minded colleagues, have dedicated our careers to educating, researching and mentoring others in this area. However, even as our field evolves, I believe that the successful development of "perioperative medicine" – which incorporates expertise from multiple specialists like geriatricians, anesthesiologists, intensivists and surgeons – is the best way forward for our elders and the future of medicine. A major motivation for this text for me was a desire to establish the importance of a perioperative approach when caring for the older patient.

Background

Preoperative Assessment of the Elderly

Sara E. Neves and Sheila Ryan Barnett

Key Points

- Preoperative assessment of the elderly patient includes performing an accurate estimation of the functional reserve of organ systems, distinguishing the impact of age versus the effect of disease processes on organ function, providing a realistic risk assessment and making appropriate recommendations regarding optimization of the patient's condition.
- Diminished organ reserve can be unpredictable and even significant limitations may only become apparent during stressful events.
- Major perioperative complications and in-hospital mortality are high in the elderly; the rate of perioperative morbidity increases progressively with each decade of life and in-hospital mortality is significantly higher in patients 80 years of age or older, especially after major and emergency surgery.
- Individuals aged over 65 years have, on average, three or four medical diseases, often limiting function and increasing morbidity.
- Polypharmacy is a major issue in this population. Many older patients are on multiple medications that may impact the administration of anesthesia.
- It is important to obtain information on advance directives, health care proxy agents, and the patient's wishes regarding advanced life support in advance of the day of surgery.

Introduction

Among the steadily increasing population of surgical patients aged 65 years and older, the fastest growing sector is individuals 85 years or older. Major perioperative complications and in-hospital mortality are high in the elderly; moreover, age has been stated as an independent risk factor for postoperative complications per the American Heart Association 2007 guidelines. The rate of perioperative morbidity increases progressively with each decade of life (4.3% of patients 59 years of age or younger, 5.7% in patients 60 to 69 years of age, 9.6% in patients 70 to 79 years of age and 12.5% in patients 80 years of age or older). In-hospital mortality is also significantly higher in patients 80 years of age or older than in those younger than 80 years of age (0.7% versus 2.6%, respectively). Major and emergent surgeries carry the highest morbidity and mortality rates in the elderly; for example, emergency abdominal surgery results in a 9.7% mortality for patients over 80 years of age and thoracotomy has a 17% mortality for those over 70 years of age. It is estimated that 50% of all Americans over 65 years will undergo a surgery before

Table 1.1 ASA physical status

ASA I: healthy patient; no organic pathology

ASA II: systemic disease that is well controlled, either by the condition that is being treated or by another pathologic process (e.g. controlled hypertension, acute sinusitis, treated hypothyroidism)

ASA III: severe systemic disturbance from any cause or causes (e.g. complicated or uncontrolled diabetes mellitus)

ASA IV: extreme systemic disturbance that is a constant threat to life (e.g. end-stage renal failure on hemodialysis, severe trauma)

ASA V: condition in which the patient will not survive without surgery (e.g. dissecting aortic aneurysm)

ASA VI: a person who is brain-dead who is presenting for organ donation

death; a working knowledge of geriatric physiology is therefore essential for all practicing anesthesiologists. Thorough preoperative assessment of the elderly patient includes performing an accurate estimate of the functional reserve of organ systems, distinguishing the impact of age versus the effect of disease processes on organ function, providing a realistic risk assessment associated with the procedure and making appropriate recommendations regarding optimization of the patient's condition.[1,2,3]

Preoperative Assessment of Physiologic Status

Risk Assessment Tools

One of the goals of the preoperative assessment is to identify high-risk individuals and suggest treatment strategies that may reduce morbidity and mortality. Assessment of perioperative risk includes an assessment of baseline physical status, functional reserve of organ systems, co-morbid conditions, including their severity and optimization, and the surgery-specific risk. This composite risk profile should be shared with all the physicians involved in the care of the individual, as well as the patient and relevant family members before proceeding with the surgery. A standardized risk assessment can help delineate which elderly patients can tolerate minor surgery as an outpatient, which will need overnight admission and which elderly patients will need a modified approach to surgery.

The ASA Physical Status (ASA PS) Classification (Table 1.1) is universally used to stratify patients preoperatively. The classification takes into consideration the preoperative systemic co-morbid illnesses and their impact on daily function. However, the ASA PS has some significant limitations. It does not take into consideration the age of the patient or the underlying functional and physiological reserves and it does not include the inherent risk associated with the surgical procedure in the estimation of a risk profile. The ASA classification system does provide a useful way for health care providers from multiple disciplines to communicate the severity of illness of an individual or group of patients.

Organ System-Specific Risk Assessment

Neurologic System

A standard neurologic history and physical should be obtained, focusing on the presence of any neurologic disease, such as cerebrovascular ischemia, seizures, neurologic malignancy, spinal cord disease, neuromuscular problems or other conditions. Physical exam should include basic strength, sensory and cranial nerve exams. The preoperative evaluation is an opportunity to carefully assess and document the diagnosis, medications currently prescribed and status of current symptomatology. Patients with a history of cerebrovascular disease may be at increased risk of aspiration (impaired swallowing reflex) and may have a contraindication to succinylcholine administration (extremity weakness and hyperkalemic response to succinylcholine).

However, in the elderly population there should be a particular focus paid to neurologic conditions more prevalent in this patient population. An evaluation of preoperative cognitive function and identification of risk factors for postoperative delirium can be valuable not only in the preoperative workup, but also in evaluation of any cognitive dysfunction postoperatively. An easy-to-perform Mini-Cog[4] evaluation, and discussion of patient's cognitive function with family, can help elucidate these problems and determine need for referral to a geriatrician or neurologist for further workup. Risk factors for postoperative delirium include severe illness, uncontrolled pain, dehydration and malnutrition, hearing or vision impairment, dementia or other cognitive impairment, age greater than 70 and use of psychoactive medications. Techniques to mitigate these risk factors, such as avoidance of benzodiazepines, limiting narcotics and reorienting techniques should be used in patients at increased risk, and probably in any geriatric patient undergoing surgery.

The presence of depression can increase morbidity in surgical patients, and geriatric patients may have atypical presentations or have depressive symptoms attributed to other co-morbidities, leading to a delay in diagnosis. Geriatric patients can be screened for depression by using the Patient Health Questionnaire (PHQ-2), though this test has not been validated in the extremely frail or debilitated patient.[4]

It is important to screen all patients, but specifically geriatric patients, for decision-making capacity. There is no age cutoff at which patients lose decision-making capacity; as long as the patient can exhibit the four legal criteria for capacity – appreciation, reasoning, understanding and expressing a choice – then they can make their own decisions regarding their health. Even in the competent patient, however, it is helpful to involve the family (with the patient's consent) in the expectations for major surgery and the perioperative period.

Cardiovascular System

Cardiovascular complications represent the primary source of perioperative complications in elderly patients. Pre-existing cardiac conditions such as coronary artery disease, hypertension and abnormal left ventricular function put the patient at risk for a postoperative cardiac event. The incidence of cardiovascular complications is higher in the elderly population by virtue of increased prevalence of coronary artery disease, hypertension and diabetes in this population. This risk is compounded by the various age-related changes that occur in the cardiovascular system, which limit the patient's ability to compensate for the stress of illness and surgery.[5,6]

The decision to send a patient for further cardiac evaluation is complex and includes consideration of patient co-morbidities as well as the level of risk of the planned procedure. The American College of Cardiology and the American Heart Association have published guidelines for preoperative evaluation and risk assessment of patients undergoing noncardiac surgery. These guidelines formulate a composite risk of perioperative

Table 1.2 Cardiac risk stratification for noncardiac surgical procedures

Major Surgical Risk: reported cardiac risk often more than 5%
Aortic and other major vascular surgery
Large intra-abdominal procedures

Intermediate Surgical Risk: reported cardiac risk generally 1% to 5%
Intraperitoneal and intrathoracic surgery
Carotid endarterectomy
Head and neck surgery
Orthopedic surgery
Prostate surgery

Low Surgical Risk: reported cardiac risk generally less than 1%
Endoscopic procedures
Superficial procedure
Cataract surgery
Breast surgery
Ambulatory surgery

cardiac events based on the preoperative history of cardiovascular events and risk factors. Recommendations have been formulated based on the acuity of surgical procedure and severity of the disease process. The surgical procedures have been classified into major, intermediate and minor risk procedures, based on the likelihood for postoperative morbidity and mortality associated with them (Table 1.2).

Major Risk Factors

Major risk factors for perioperative cardiac events are active cardiac conditions including: acute coronary syndromes, decompensated heart failure, significant arrhythmias (ventricular tachycardia/ventricular fibrillation) and severe valvular disease. These risk factors may warrant cancellation of nonemergent or life-saving surgery due to the significant risk of a perioperative adverse cardiac event or even death. Further medical or surgical management of these conditions should occur before proceeding with surgery. However, if the surgery is truly emergent, the risks and benefits of proceeding should be carefully weighed and discussed with the surgeon, patient and family.

Intermediate Risk Factors

The Revised Cardiac Risk Indices have been included in the intermediate risk factors.

These are ischemic heart disease, compensated congestive heart failure, cerebrovascular disease, insulin-dependent diabetes mellitus and a serum creatinine greater than 2 mg/dl. The incidence of postoperative cardiac complications increase from 0.4% to 11%, depending on the number of predictors (one, two or more than three) present.

Minor Risk Factors

Minor predictors are recognized markers for cardiovascular disease that have not been proven to increase perioperative risk independently; for example, advanced age (greater than 70 years), abnormal ECG (LV hypertrophy, left bundle-branch block, ST-T abnormalities), rhythm other than sinus and uncontrolled systemic hypertension. The presence of multiple minor predictors might lead to a higher suspicion of CAD, but is not incorporated into the recommendations for treatment (Table 1.3).

Table 1.3 Cardiac risk factors

Major
- Acute coronary syndromes: unstable or severe angina, recent MI
- Decompensated congestive heart failure: NYHA functional class IV
- Significant arrhythmias: complete heart block, symptomatic ventricular arrhythmias, supraventricular arrhythmias with uncontrolled ventricular rate
- Severe valvular disease: severe aortic stenosis, symptomatic mitral stenosis

Intermediate
- Ischemic heart disease
- Compensated congestive heart failure
- Cerebrovascular disease
- Insulin-dependent diabetes mellitus
- Serum creatinine >2 mg/dl

Minor
- Advanced age (greater than 70 years)
- Abnormal ECG (left bundle-branch block, ST-T abnormalities)
- Rhythm other than sinus
- Uncontrolled systemic hypertension

Table 1.4 Estimation of exercise tolerance

1 MET	Eating, dressing, using toilet
2–3 METs	Walking around house
	Walking a block on level ground at regular pace
4 METs	Light housework (laundry, dishes)
5–9 METs	Running a short distance
	Heavy housework (scrubbing floors, moving furniture)
	Moderate exercise (dancing, golf)
10 METs or more	Strenuous sports (tennis, swimming, skiing, long-distance running)

Exercise Tolerance

Functional status has been shown to be a reliable predictor for perioperative and long-term cardiac complications. For a patient without active or major cardiac conditions an assessment of the patient's functional status is a critical step in the testing algorithm. Functional capacity can be expressed as metabolic equivalents (METs). A MET represents the resting or basal oxygen consumption (VO_2), 1 MET is the equivalent of an expenditure of 3.5 ml/kg/min. The MET of common activities and exercise are shown in Table 1.4. According to these guidelines, if the patient's functional status is good (greater than 4 METS), even higher-risk procedures may be undertaken without further cardiac noninvasive testing (Table 1.4).

When it is not possible to establish the functional capacity of a patient with significant clinical risk factors for coronary artery disease or of those undergoing high-risk surgery, noninvasive cardiac testing may be required. The rationale for further evaluation should also be determined by the impact of the test results on the plan of care for that particular surgery.

The stepwise algorithm for preoperative assessment of a patient for noncardiac surgery is summarized in the flow chart in Figure 1.1.[7]

The ACC/AHA guidelines for perioperative use of beta-blockers state that preoperative beta-blockers are indicated in patients who are currently on beta-blockade therapy or who have a history of coronary artery disease or significant risk factors for ischemic heart disease, and are undergoing intermediate-risk or vascular surgery. Statin therapy should be started preoperatively in patients with known cardiac ischemia, vascular disease or elevated low-density lipoprotein levels.

Pulmonary System

Pulmonary reserve decreases with age, and it can often be difficult to separate age-related changes from those secondary to disease and environmental factors. The influences of prior smoking and environmental exposures are particularly difficult to distinguish from senescence.

The major changes that occur with aging can be broadly attributed to the following factors: blunting of the central nervous system reflexes, a decrease in the compliance of the thoracic wall, a decrease in alveolar gas exchange surface and a generalized deconditioning of chest wall musculature. Functionally this translates into increased work of breathing and an increased predisposition to hypoxemia. Overall there is a decrease in the maximal breathing capacity.[6,8]

Several risk factors predict postoperative pulmonary complications, including the presence of COPD, functional dependence, tobacco use and signs of preoperative illness such as an altered mental status, sepsis, hypoalbuminemia, unintentional weight loss, elevated serum creatinine and congestive heart failure. A detailed history of the patient's functional capacity and 6-minute walk test may be helpful to establish a baseline pulmonary function. Smokers should be counseled on cessation of smoking at least 6 weeks prior to surgery and preoperative breathing exercises should be recommended. Additional imaging, such as a chest x-ray, can be useful to establish a baseline severity of lung disease such as COPD. Pulmonary function tests should not be ordered routinely, but in order to help predict postoperative pulmonary function. Preoperative room air arterial blood gas can establish a level of pre-existing hypercapnia or hypoxemia.

As with patients of any age, an airway history should be attained during the preoperative evaluation. A prior intubation or course in the intensive care unit may result in residual damage such as tracheal stenosis. A history of a difficult intubation should prompt an attempt to obtain prior medical records.[6]

Gastrointestinal System

The gastrointestinal system ages largely intact. There is no strong evidence to suggest significant changes in motility or digestion in the aging patient. Furthermore, the large physiologic reserve of the liver and pancreas means that the function of these organs is relatively preserved. However, elderly patients may have an impaired swallowing reflex and be at increased risk of aspiration. Atrophic gastritis occurs more frequently in the elderly, leading to impaired absorption of B12, calcium carbonate and iron, contributing to anemia and osteoporosis. It is important to note pre-existing gastrointestinal pathology, namely to determine aspiration risk with induction.[9,10]

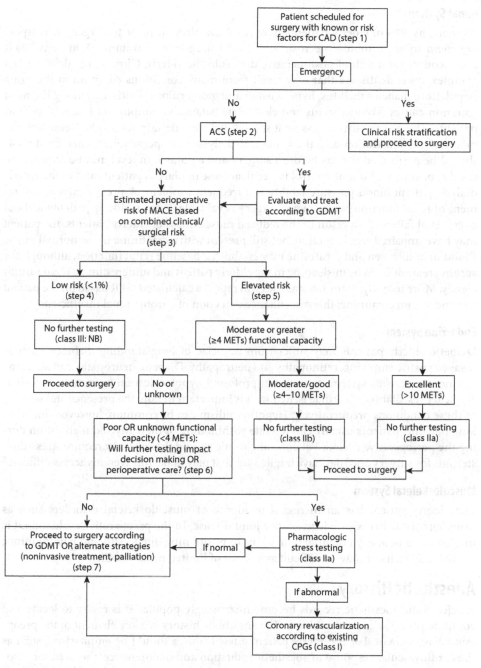

Figure 1.1 Preoperative cardiac assessment for patients undergoing noncardiac surgery.

Reproduced from: Fleisher LA, Fleischmann KE, Auerbach AD, et al. 2014 ACC/AHA guideline on perioperative cardiovascular evaluation and management of patients undergoing noncardiac surgery: a report of the American College of Cardiology/ American Heart Association Task Force on Practice Guidelines. *Circulation* 2014; 130:e278–e333.

Renal System

As many as 30% of elderly patients have renal impairment prior to surgery, predisposing them to acute tubular necrosis after major surgery and trauma. Acute renal failure accounts for a fifth of postoperative deaths in the elderly. Chronic renal failure is a complex systemic disease that may result from many conditions common in the aging population; diabetes mellitus, hypertension and glomerulonephritis are among the most common causes. Volume status and electrolyte balance are important issues in dialysis patients. The preoperative assessment should include a description of the frequency, the mode of administration and the timing of dialysis perioperatively. Generally dialysis should be performed the day before a surgery and a potassium level may be required on the day of surgery. Volume control is a critical issue in dialysis patients and in the elderly dialysis patient blood pressure lability is a frequent problem. A preoperative measurement of renal function before major surgery is valuable, even in elderly patients without overt renal failure. As a result of the reduced muscle mass of elderly patients, the patient may have impaired renal function, but still present with a creatinine in the normal range. Blood urea nitrogen and creatinine may establish a baseline renal function, although the serum creatinine can be misleading in the elderly patient and underestimate renal insufficiency. More recently, many laboratories will report a calculated GFR based on the patient age and serum creatinine; this can enhance detection of chronic renal insufficiency.[6,8]

Endocrine System

Diabetic elderly patients may suffer from sequelae of long-standing diabetes, such as delayed gastric emptying, retinopathy and neuropathy. Diabetic neuropathy can affect the autonomic nervous system, resulting in profound hypotension on induction, as well as atypical presentation of cardiac ischemia. It is important to note the presence and severity of these conditions preoperatively. Hypothyroidism can be common; however, due to its long half-life, patients usually can tolerate withholding of their thyroid medication during the perioperative period. Patients on chronic steroid therapy may require stress-dose steroids for surgery and may have fragile skin that may make intravenous access difficult.[5]

Musculoskeletal System

The elderly patient has an increased incidence of musculoskeletal disorders such as osteoporosis, arthritis and degenerative joint disease. In the preoperative evaluation it is important to note any potential limitations of positioning due to stiff and painful joints; airway management may be difficult as a result of limited neck mobility.

Anesthetic History

As electronic anesthetic records become increasingly popular it is easier to locate and compare previous anesthetic charts. The anesthetic history is a key element of the preoperative assessment. For an elderly patient a few features should be emphasized, such as the cardiovascular response to anesthetic induction and maintenance, the need for vasopressors during a case, the volume tolerated and the overall lability of the blood pressure. It is also important to obtain information from the patient and their family regarding emergence and previous postoperative and postanesthetic complications, such as delirium, postoperative pulmonary complications and perioperative cardiac events. This type of assessment can lead to positive recommendations regarding blood pressure expectations, pain control and medication dosing.

Table 1.5 Suggested preoperative medication regimen

Medications to continue

Antiarrhythmics

Antiepileptics

Anti-Parkinson medications

Anxiolytics

Antireflux medications (proton-pump inhibitor, H2 blocker)

Steroids

Chronic pain medications

Anticholinesterase inhibitors to treat for myasthenia gravis

Some level of basal insulin in type 1 diabetes mellitus

Consider some amount of long-acting insulin in patients with high insulin requirements

Antiplatelet agents in patients with recent cardiac stents (consultation with surgeon and cardiologist generally required)

Medications to hold

Diuretics, antihypertensives

Oral hypoglycemic agents

Antidepressants (MAO-inhibitors)

Holding anticoagulant/antiplatelet medications should be done in close communication with the surgeon and with the physician who prescribed the medication

Medications

Polypharmacy is a major concern in the elderly population. Significant effort should be made to obtain a complete and accurate list of medications – including both prescription and over-the-counter medications. Asking patients to bring in all of their medications, or calling a patient's pharmacy directly may result in a more accurate list, as elderly patients may not recall specific names and doses. An accurate preoperative medication list is helpful in the postoperative setting when patients are admitted as inpatients following surgery. Typical medication regimens for the morning of surgery are listed in Table 1.5. Nonessential medications should usually be held and initiation of new medications immediately preoperatively should be limited.[8]

Laboratory Evaluation

Although older patients frequently have multiple co-morbid illnesses, preoperative laboratory testing should be directed by the type of surgery planned and the patient's current medical status, regardless of age. Similarly, advanced age alone is not an indication for extensive preoperative testing. Routine screening can lead to excessive cost as well as potential morbidity for further investigation of false positive results.

Hemoglobin, Hematocrit

A measurement of blood count is usually indicated in elderly patients undergoing any type of surgery, especially patients with a history of or concern for anemia. Elevated hemoglobin in a very old patient is unusual and may indicate hemoconcentration from dehydration or an underlying hematological disorder.

Coagulation Studies

Patients on anticoagulants such as warfarin should have coagulation studies drawn and/ or generally repeated on the morning of the surgery if warfarin has been discontinued, so that normal coagulation parameters can be documented. Other indications for preoperative coagulation studies include significant liver disease, known coagulopathies or for surgeries in which small changes in coagulation parameters can have significant consequences.

Electrolytes and Blood Chemistry

Elderly ambulatory patients with mild to moderate systemic disease such as hypertension do not need routine electrolytes. However, renal function tests such as BUN, creatinine and electrolytes are usually indicated in elderly patients having significant surgery. A creatinine clearance should also be measured. Note that elderly patients have significantly reduced muscle mass, so a "normal" creatinine level of 0.9 in an elderly patient may in fact indicate significant baseline renal disease. Electrolytes should be measured in patients with renal disease or congestive heart failure, or who are on electrolyte-modifying medications such as diuretics. Serum albumin levels are helpful in patients undergoing major surgery; low serum albumin levels have been shown to be a predictor of poor outcome in older patients and can signal a baseline level of malnutrition.[11]

Electrocardiograms

A preoperative ECG should be done in patients with cardiac risk factors or a history of cardiac disease and in those undergoing intermediate or vascular surgery. Occult cardiac disease is very common in older patients; however, many institutions are moving away from using age-based criteria for ECG screening in healthy elderly patients undergoing surgery. A prior ECG within 3–6 months of the surgery in the absence of ongoing symptoms or changes in cardiac status is generally acceptable.

Chest Radiographs

Chest x-rays should be ordered preoperatively in patients older than 70 years who have chronic cardiopulmonary disease. Those who have been stable should have had a chest x-ray within the previous 6 months; those who have had changes in their clinical condition should have the x-ray repeated closer to the surgery date. Patients who will have planned postoperative mechanical ventilation or admission to the intensive care unit may benefit from a preoperative baseline chest x-ray; however, several studies have demonstrated that widespread routine chest x-rays can often lead led to significant morbidity, but rarely discover unexpected findings resulting in a change in management.

Type and Screen

These should be drawn prior to surgeries with the potential for significant blood loss. The presence of antibodies may make it difficult and time-consuming to find compatible products.

As with all preoperative testing, requests for laboratory studies or further investigations should be directed by the history and a physical examination that includes a functional assessment. Further testing beyond the history and physical will be determined by the risk associated with the surgical procedure and the baseline co-morbidities of the patient. For instance, a patient with significant cardiac morbidity coming in for a low-risk cataract surgery may not need further cardiac evaluation, whereas a patient with lesser cardiac risk factors coming in for high-risk surgery will need a comprehensive cardiac evaluation.[12]

Special Considerations in the Elderly

The preoperative evaluation in patients with complicated medical histories can be very difficult in patients with baseline dementia and memory loss, and every effort should be made to obtain prior medical records and contact the primary care physician taking care of the patient. Preoperative depression and alcohol abuse are relatively common and not always admitted by the patient or family, but will increase the risk of delirium in the postoperative period.

In addition to a high incidence of co-morbidities, the overall health status of the aged patient may also significantly influence the choice of anesthetic technique. For instance, chronic pain, agitation and dementia may prohibit the patient from lying still during the procedure, making a plan for deep sedation unfeasible even though the procedure may be minor. The preoperative visit helps to identify medical or socioeconomic conditions that could cause a delay or cancellation of the procedure on the day of surgery. The early identification of patients requiring further investigations or those with social issues may help with advance planning and room scheduling. For instance a patient with minimal social and family support should be admitted postoperatively after a minor procedure.[2,5]

During the course of the preoperative evaluation it may become obvious that a patient may not be able to provide informed consent for the procedure due to a variety of reasons. In that case a health care proxy who is determined by the patient may have to be contacted.

Outside Facilities

The preoperative assessment of institutionalized patients can be especially challenging. It may be difficult or impractical to require these patients to come to a hospital or facility for a preoperative visit. In these instances a remote preoperative screen can be conducted. If possible, the facility physician should provide a brief history and physical, and the results of any laboratory testing done recently. These can be reviewed by the anesthesiology team who may decide if more testing is indicated. The preoperative examination can be completed the day of the surgery. Arrangements for consent from a legal guardian or family member should be made in advance to prevent delays on the day of surgery.[13]

Advanced Directives

Recent data suggest that half of patients over the age of 60 will require decisions about treatment in the final days of life, with the majority of those patients lacking decision-making capacity at that time. It is therefore important that we encourage patients of all ages, but especially the elderly, to make decisions regarding personal goals and treatment preferences, as well as formally designate a health care proxy agent who will represent those preferences should the patient be unable to do so. Clarification on the types of advance directives is listed in Table 1.6.

Table 1.6 Types of advance directives

Health Care Proxy: legal document in which a patient assigns a person to legally make health care decisions on behalf of the patient, should the patient become incapable of doing so

Durable Power of Attorney: legal document in which an individual assigns another person to legally make decisions (in any situation, not just health-care-related) on behalf of the individual, in the event the individual is incapable of doing so

Legal Guardian: person who has the legal authority to care for the personal and property interests of an individual; usually an assignment made by the court

Living Will: legal document that specifies medical treatments that the patient would or would not want used to prolong life. This can include decisions about cardiopulmonary resuscitation, enteral feeding, mechanical ventilation, pain management and organ donation

Do Not Resuscitate (DNR): medical order instructing providers not to perform CPR if a patient's cardiac activity ceases

Do Not Intubate (DNI): medical order instructing providers not to intubate the patient or place the patient on mechanical ventilation

It is a common misconception that "do not resuscitate/do not intubate" (DNR/DNI) orders are automatically reversed for patients going to the operating room. It is important to discuss the patient's preferences regarding their DNR/DNI directive preoperatively; ideally this has been a discussion between the surgeon and the patient as well. It is important to provide "required reconsideration," explaining to the patient, for example, that under general anesthesia the patient is made apneic and so will require intubation. If a patient has significant co-morbidities a discussion between the patient and health care team may result in upholding the DNR/DNI order during the perioperative period. If a part or all of an advance directive is suspended for surgery, there should be a plan preoperatively for when and how the advance directive is reinstated.[14]

Fasting

Recent data suggest that preoperative fasting of clear liquids up to 2–3 hours prior to anesthesia does not pose an increased risk of aspiration compared to strict NPO for 8 hours. In a vulnerable patient population such as the elderly, providing nutrition for as long as possible during the perioperative period may confer additional benefit.

Surgical Prophylaxis

Elderly patients should be subject to the same risk stratification regarding surgical-site infection antibiotic prophylaxis and thromboprophylaxis as patients of any age.[14]

Conclusion

The geriatric population is a group of people above the age of 65 years with a wide range of physical capabilities and organ reserves. The effect of age-related illness on organ systems can be difficult to distinguish from the disease process itself, which poses a challenge in the perioperative setting. The preoperative visit is crucial in this population to establish the baseline health status of the individual, determine the level of optimization of the co-morbidities, provide a realistic risk assessment for the procedure and with this information formulate a plan of care that would provide optimum and efficient care to the elderly and minimize the risk of morbidity and mortality.

References

1. Polanczyk CA, Marcantonio E, Goldman L, et al. Impact of age on perioperative complications and length of stay in patients undergoing noncardiac surgery. *Ann Intern Med.* 2001; 134(8):637–643.

2. Weber DM. Laparoscopic surgery. *Arch Surg.* 2003; 138:1083–1088.

3. Liu LL, Leung JM. Predicting adverse postoperative outcomes in patients aged 80 years or older. *J Am Geriatr Soc.* 2000; 48:405–412.

4. Chow WB, Rosenthal RA, Merkow RP, et al. Optimal Preoperative Assessment of the Geriatric Surgical Patient: A Best Practices Guideline from the American College of Surgeons National Surgical Quality Improvement Program and the American Geriatrics Society. *J Am Coll Surg.* 2012; 215(4):453–466.

5. Bettelli G. Anaesthesia for the elderly outpatient: preoperative assessment and evaluation, anaesthetic technique and postoperative pain management. *Curr Opin Anesthesiol.* 2010; 23:726–731.

6. Cook DJ, Rooke GA. Priorities in perioperative geriatrics. *Anesth Analg.* 2003; 96:1823–1836.

7. Fleisher LA, Fleischmann KE, Auerbach AD, et al. 2014 ACC/AHA guideline on perioperative cardiovascular evaluation and management of patients undergoing noncardiac surgery: a report of the American College of Cardiology/American Heart Association Task Force on Practice Guidelines. *Circulation* 2014; 130:e278–e333.

8. White PF, White LM, Monk T, et al. Perioperative care for the older outpatient undergoing ambulatory surgery. *Anesth Analg.* 2012; 114(6):1190–1215.

9. Russell RM. Changes in gastrointestinal function attributed to aging. *Am J Clin Nutr.* 1992:55:1203S–1207S.

10. Grassi M, Petraccia L, Mennuni G, et al. Changes, functional disorders, and diseases in the gastrointestinal tract of eldery. *Nutr Hosp.* 2011; 26(4):659–668.

11. Dzankic S, Pastor D, Gonzalez C, Leung JM. The prevalence and predictive value of abnormal preoperative laboratory tests in eldery surgical patients. *Anesth Analg.* 2001; 93:301–308.

12. American Society of Anesthesiologists Task Force on Preanesthesia Evaluation. Practice Advisory for Preanesthesia Evaluation: An Updated Report by the American Society of Anesthesiologists Task Force on Preanesthesia Evaluation. *Anesthesiology* 2012; 116(3):1–17.

13. Chiang S, Gertan KA, Miller KL. Optimizing outcomes of surgery in advanced age–perioperative factors to consider. *Clin Obstet Gynecol.* 2007; 50(3):813–825.

14. Mohanty S, Rosenthal RA, Russell MM, et al. Optimal Perioperative Management of the Geriatric Patient: A Best Practices Guideline from the ACS NSQIP/American Geriatrics Society. *J Am Coll Surg.* 2016; 222(5):930–947.

Chapter 2

Ethical Issues in Perioperative Care of the Elderly: Informed Consent/Informed Refusal

Gail A. Van Norman

Key Points

- "Autonomy" is the ability of an individual to make decisions without undue influence by others or other impediments to meaningful choice.
- The informed consent process involves information and influence, both of which much meet certain ethical and legal standards.
- Legal and ethical standards require that the physician discuss the proposed treatment and its viable alternatives, the common risks (because they are likely to happen) and serious risks (because the consequences are severe).
- It is neither legal nor ethical to over-ride a competent patient's wishes in an emergency.
- "Competence" is a legal term that refers to adults who have not been judged to be incompetent. The competent patient: (i) is able to receive information relevant to the decision, (ii) can demonstrate some understanding of the consequences of the decision, including risks and benefits, (iii) can render a reasoned decision.
- An advance directive is a statement rendered by a competent patient outlining their wishes about specific aspects of medical care to guide treatment if they are unable to express themselves. A DNR (do not resuscitate) order is an example.

Introduction

Elderly patients present with a broad spectrum of physical disorders that may raise special ethical issues perioperatively, such as questions of autonomy and capacity to participate in medical decision-making, reliance on surrogate decision-makers, use of advance directives, and refusals and limitations of aspects of medical care. This chapter will address definitions and recommendations for improved decision-making in the elderly patient.

Autonomy

Respect for individual freedom is entrenched in Western political philosophy and informs contemporary commitments to patient autonomy. "Autonomy" is the ability of an individual to make decisions without undue influence by others or other impediments to meaningful choice.[1] In the US, the case of *Schloendorff v Society of New York Hospital* was one of the earliest tests of patient rights.[2] In *Schloendorff*, a woman had agreed to general anesthesia, for examination for pelvic pain. An unconsented surgery was performed while she was unconscious, and she sustained an injury to her arm that later necessitated amputation of the fingers of one hand. In his decision, Justice Cardozo stated, "Every human being of adult years and sound mind has the right to determine what shall be done to his own body." The legal concept of "informed" consent was cemented in *Salgo v Trustees of Leland Stanford Hospital* in 1957, when the court ruled that the patient's mere agreement to a procedure was insufficient, and that a meaningful discussion of risks and alternatives to the proposed treatment must be held.[3]

Patient "voluntarism" and "competence" are required elements of informed consent. Moreover, the informed consent process involves both *information* and *influence*, both of which must meet certain ethical and legal standards.

Competence

In the US, "competence" is a legal term that refers to adults older than 18 years of age who have not been judged to be incompetent. "Capacity" refers to the abilities of a person (adult or otherwise) to make decisions. In European literature these terms are often reversed.[4] For the purpose of this chapter, "capacity" and "competence" are used interchangeably, referring to a patient's ability to make decisions, regardless of age.

Competence may be compromised by many factors, e.g. overall burden of disease, underlying cerebrovascular disease and nonvascular causes of dementia, such as Alzheimer's disease and parkinsonism. Mild cognitive dysfunction affects 10–20% of people over age 65.[5] Medications and emotional disorders may raise concerns regarding a patient's competence. Further, a higher prevalence of noncognitive disorders in the elderly (impaired hearing, vision loss and poststroke communication challenges) can mimic incompetence, when the patient is perfectly capable of understanding and making decisions. Although capacity can be adversely impacted by conditions such as dementia, the presence of such factors is not sufficient evidence to establish that a patient lacks capacity. It has long been legally recognized that many patients suffering from dementia, for example, do have capacity for informed consent.[6]

Capacity is task-specific. A patient may not be able to carry out certain tasks (e.g. balancing a checkbook or driving a car), but nevertheless be capable of making health care decisions. Capacity may change with environmental factors: time of day, familiarity of surroundings, medication changes and the presence of distractions. When capacity is uncertain, expert consultation may be both advisable and necessary prior to proceeding with treatment.

Determining competence can be especially challenging in the immediate preoperative setting, which limits time and resources for making potentially complex determinations. Studies show that physicians understand patient decision-making poorly, and both paternalism and prejudice permeate physician behavior regarding informed consent. The elderly are particularly vulnerable to having their participation in medical decision-making inappropriately curtailed due to underestimation of their capacity to do so.

Functional capacity to make health care decisions must also be judged separately from bias about the quality of that decision. Competent patients have the right to make "bad" decisions – otherwise the term "informed consent" would be meaningless, and the physician would simply dictate the "good" decision. Refusal of treatment is not evidence of incompetence, but it is one of the most common reason physicians refer patients for competency evaluations.[7]

Physicians are poorly equipped to predict and understand patient choices. They often assign a lower quality of life than the patients themselves and are mistaken about patient preferences regarding life-extending therapies in around 30% of cases.[8] They frequently judge patient decisions to refuse therapy as "irrational."[9,10] Worse, physicians and other health care workers are likely to act on their own prejudices regarding the quality of life of handicapped patients.[11]

The competent patient shows three abilities. First, they are able to receive information relevant to the decision. This can be demonstrated by asking the patient to state back the proposed treatment and their understanding of it. Second, the patient demonstrates some understanding of the consequences of the decision, including risks and benefits. Finally, they render a reasoned decision. Patients demonstrating these abilities are usually competent, even if their decisions do not align with the opinion of their physician.[6,12,13]

Physicians are ethically obliged whenever possible to *promote* a patients' autonomy. When reversible conditions impede capacity, and capacity can be restored in time to have the medical therapy still meaningful, respect for patient autonomy requires that the physician take steps to restore the patient's autonomy, allowing them to participate in the decision. If a patient is too somnolent from medications to understand that they need a broken leg fixed, and surgery on the leg is nonemergent, then ethically surgery should wait until the patient has regained the capacity to consent. Proceeding to surgery to facilitate the surgery schedule is not ethically justifiable. Reversible impediments to decision-making can include language difficulties requiring an interpreter (including sign-language interpreters), and pain or anxiety.

It is neither legal nor ethical to over-ride a competent patient's wishes in an emergency. The decision of a Jehovah's Witness to not accept blood transfusions, for example, is binding, even if the cause of hemorrhage is a traumatic injury requiring emergency surgery. When a patient's wishes are unknown, and their capacity is *impeded* and will not be restored in time to allow the medical therapy to remain meaningful (e.g. an intoxicated patient presenting with a leaking aortic aneurism) then the physician is justified in proceeding, either with the consent of a surrogate decision-maker or under the ethical principle of treating to the patient's best interests.

The Problem of Premedication

Medication can interfere with patient autonomy if it causes the patient to be incapable of listening to or understanding the proposed treatments and alternatives. In one study, over half of surgeons believed that administration of pain medications to patients with acute pain would invalidate consent, and only 34% thought that consent could be obtained after making the patient comfortable. Informed consent was a consideration in withholding pain medications for 78% of the physicians.[14]

But in fact, some patients suffer from conditions that require treatment in order to *facilitate* competence. Pain can impede a patient's ability to listen to options and make an autonomous decision, and in certain cases must be treated before consent for other therapy can be obtained. Elderly patients can suffer from conditions such as cancer and degenerative arthritis that require chronic pain medications. Other patients can present with trauma or acute medical processes, such as bowel obstruction, that cause extreme pain, which will interfere with a patient's ability to understand their choices. Withholding pain medication to obtain a patient's consent in such cases can be construed as coercive, and may invalidate consent entirely.[14,15]

Administration of pain or anxiolytic medications does not automatically invalidate patient consent, provided the patient is still able to demonstrate the three steps in competence. If this were not true, then many patients on chronic pain medications would never be able to give consent. Furthermore, approximately one-quarter of patients self-prescribe pain or anxiolytic medications prior to surgery without their physician's knowledge.[16] Although some anxiolytic medications can interfere with memory, lack of recall of the informed consent process does not invalidate it. Many unpremedicated patients do not recall details of the informed consent process.[17,18]

When pain or anxiety poses an impediment to a reasoned discussion with a patient, these conditions should be treated judiciously to *promote* the patient's competence and to *facilitate* the informed consent process. Even if such premedication may diminish the patient's decision-making capacity, such medications should be administered as part of compassionate care – the presence of severe pain or anxiety compromises their capacity anyway. In no cases should *necessary* pain or anxiolytic medication be withheld in order to obtain consent.[19]

Voluntariness

Voluntariness is the embodiment of one of the most valued pursuits in Western culture – *freedom*. Indeed, some consider voluntariness to be *synonymous* with autonomy.[20] While absolute autonomy can be diminished by disease, psychiatric disorders, dependency disorders (drug and alcohol addiction) and other conditions, in this discussion we focus on voluntariness as it is constrained by other individuals or intentional agents.

Disclosure

Legal and ethical standards differ in determining what information is necessary to informed consent. US courts have relied on the reasonable person standard (whatever a reasonable person would want to know) and the subjective standard (information that applies to this particular patient only, e.g. the opera singer who wants to know the risks to her voice from intubation). In neither case is the physician required to present an exhaustive and potentially meaningless list of facts. Legal and ethical standards require that the physician discuss the proposed treatment and its viable alternatives, the common risks (because they are likely to happen) and serious risks (because the consequences are severe).

Risks should be discussed in terms that are meaningful to the patient. Stating that risk of death from an anesthetic is "1 in 25,000" may have little meaning to the patient, whereas stating that the risk of death from an anesthetic is "similar to risks the patient experiences while riding in a car," offers both the information that there is a risk of death, but that the risk is similar to common ones the patient assumes every day. This process is called "risk framing," and assists patients in contextualizing risk discussions.

Many anesthesiologists do not like to mention the risk of death for fear that the information will "harm" the patient by causing undue anxiety. Withholding information in this manner is exercising "therapeutic privilege" – a practice based in paternalism and the concept that the physician "knows what is best." While therapeutic privilege is allowed under some European laws, it is not supported under US law, and it violates the principle of respect for patient autonomy. Studies do not support the idea that patient anxiety is increased by detailed preoperative information compared to censored information.[21,22]

Some suggest such censoring causes patient and family mistrust,[23] and others show that patients prefer risk discussions, even if they might increase anxiety.[24]

Rarely, a patient may request to forgo risk discussion out of anxiety. In such cases, the physician can and should respect the patient's autonomous wish to curtail the discussion. This decision, however, rests with the patient rather than the physician, and should be documented in the patient's chart.

Influence

Influence and control are intertwined concepts constraining autonomy. The degree to which a form of influence is resistible in part tells us whether it is ethical, because it gives us an indication of how much the influence damages autonomy. Influence has many forms: threats, education, lies, emotional appeals, acts of love and others. Certain types of influence are unethical, while some forms of influence may be invited or even welcomed. Three broad categories of influence are coercions, manipulation and persuasion.

Coercion

Coercion is the most forceful form of influence. Coercion occurs when an intentional agent presents a credible threat of serious harm or force in order to control another's actions. For a threat to be credible, the recipient of the threat must believe that the coercer can effect it. What constitutes "serous harm" is generally in the judgment of the recipient.

An important aspect of coercion is that it must come from an intentional agent. Circumstances, while they can be compelling, do not have a goal or intention with regard to individuals, and therefore do not "coerce." Decisions and actions always involve circumstances that limit options. Pain, for example, cannot coerce, since it does not intend. Pain, however, can be used as a tool in a coercive threat.

Different degrees of coercion are surprisingly common in the perioperative setting. Denying a patient necessary analgesics or anxiolytics until they sign a consent form, for example, is coercive. Threatening a patient with refusal to do surgery unless they rescind their DNR directive invalidates the rescission by usurping the patient's autonomy, and may additionally invalidate the surgical consent itself. Coercion of a competent patient can only be justified to prevent imminent injury to themselves or others – as when a patient is behaving violently and requires containment. It is unethical in virtually all other medical circumstances.

Persuasion

Persuasion is on the opposite end of the spectrum of influential behaviors from coercion. Persuasion convinces an autonomous person to undertake an action through the merits of reason brought to bear by the convincer. The need to conform to the persuader's wishes is not compulsory, and therefore the receiver retains autonomy. Persuasion is not only ethical, but some argue that physicians are obliged to at least attempt to persuade patients to pursue a well-reasoned course of medical care.[25]

Manipulation

Manipulation refers to influence that is neither persuasive nor coercive. In health care decision-making, examples include presenting false, incomplete or exaggerated information. Lying, omitting key information or deliberately raising either false hopes or false alarms usurps patient autonomy by presenting a "false reality" in which the patient decides. Autonomous choice is impossible in such circumstances, because the choice itself is a false one, built out of assumptions that are deliberately forged to elicit a particular decision. Such manipulation of a competent person is always unethical.

Exaggerating the risks of a particular anesthetic technique in order to persuade a patient to accept one the physician wants them to choose is manipulative. Equally manipulative can be a chronic assault on an autonomous patient's decision by repeated entreaties or demands. In the Canadian case of *Beausoleil v Sisters of Charity*, an anesthesiologist subjected a patient to repeated discussions of spinal anesthesia until she finally assented. When the patient was paralyzed following anesthesia and sued, the judge determined that the consent was involuntary, because it rested on words that "denote defeat, exhaustion and abandonment of the will power."[26]

Other types of manipulation include use of rewards, offers and certain other types of encouragement. Socioeconomic deprivation, social isolation and other patient circumstances make elderly patients particularly vulnerable to inducements. Such influence is not coercive, but is often exploitative, and may be so compelling as to prevent a truly free choice.

Sadly, physicians and other health care providers frequently employ multiple forms of unethical influence. As Eliot Freidson stated:

> It is my impression that the clients are more often bullied than informed into consent, their resistance weakened in part by their desire for the general service if not the specific procedure, in part by the oppressive setting they find themselves in, and in part by the calculated intimidation, restriction of information and overt threats of rejection by the professional staff itself.[27]

Informed Refusal: DNR and Other Directives Limiting Medical Care in the Setting of Anesthesia and Surgery

Do Not Resuscitate (DNR) Orders

Informed consent is meaningless unless competent patients have the right to refuse treatments – otherwise there is no true choice. Legal rights of competent patients to refuse *any* medical therapy have long been codified in the US, in the Patient Self-Determination Act of 1990.[28] This federal law is based in constitutional protections of privacy and non-interference. Yet many physicians mistakenly feel that these rights are checked at the OR doors and that they can simply suspend do not resuscitate (DNR) orders during anesthesia and surgery.

Arguments that these rights can be suspended include: (1) resuscitation in the OR has a better prognosis than resuscitation in other hospital settings, (2) anesthesia is "nothing but ongoing resuscitation" and cannot be distinguished from other normal treatments in the OR and (3) patients who have DNR orders should seek invasive therapy.

Overall, in-hospital resuscitation has poor outcomes, with studies showing that about 40% of adult patients survive 1 hour, and only 6–20% survive to discharge.[29–32] From 30% to 74% of such survivors suffer significant neurologic impairments.[33] In the OR (for noncardiac surgery), statistics are still poor, but somewhat more favorable, with 46% of patients surviving for 1 hour, and approximately 34.5% surviving to discharge

(Figure 2.1).[34] These differences supply a legitimate argument for informing patients about the risk/benefit ratio of OR resuscitation and determining if they still wish to keep their DNR order in place. It is *not* a valid argument for unilaterally suspending a patient's rights to make a decision in light of new information.

The argument that "anesthesia is nothing but resuscitation" is particularly problematic, because it rests in a specious argument about the necessity of "resuscitation" in the OR, and in the manipulative misuse and misunderstanding of the term "resuscitation." For physicians, "resuscitation" is a generic term used to describe measures to restore or support normal function. Physicians term administration of fluids to dehydrated patients "fluid resuscitation," but no one mistakes it for being analogous to applying chest compressions to a patient whose has suffered a cardiac arrest. Patients, on the other hand, often refer to resuscitation as something that is done "when the heart stops." Cardiac arrest in noncardiac surgery is in fact rare, occurring in 1 to 3 cases out of 10,000 elective surgeries,[34,35] and is a complication that anesthesiologists and surgeons work diligently to avoid. Stating or implying that resuscitation from cardiac arrest is a routine part of anesthesia and noncardiac surgery is inaccurate and misleading.

The idea that invasive care should not be offered to patients who have DNR orders ignores the fact that invasive treatments may be necessary in the pursuit of comfort care. Bowel resection to prevent obstruction in a patient with advanced colon cancer,

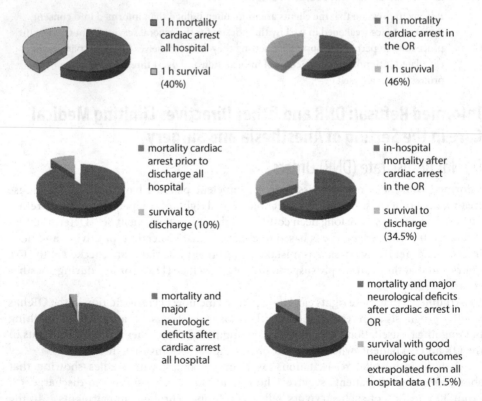

Figure 2.1 Outcomes of all in-hospital cardiac arrest compared to cardiac arrest in the operating room (OR). Note that survival with good neurologic outcomes (last chart) after cardiac arrest in the OR are unknown, and are extrapolated from in-hospital data.

placement of enteral tubes for hydration and nutrition and placement of invasive lines for administration of cancer treatments, fluids and medications are all examples of procedures that require procedural intervention to improve the quality of end of life.

In 1992 the American Society of Anesthesiologists published ethical guidelines for the care of patients with DNR and other orders limiting care,[36] concluding that in ethical management of DNR orders in the setting of anesthesia and surgery, the anesthesiologist should discuss the better prognosis of cardiopulmonary resuscitation in the OR, and should then respect patient decisions about their DNR orders. By 1995, the American College of Surgeons,[37] the Association of Operating Room Nurses[38] and the Joint Commission[39] had all published guidelines consistent with this opinion.

The requirement to respect DNR orders has been legally reinforced by civil cases that not only have awarded significant civil damages to patients who were resuscitated against their wills, but have also determined at times that the plaintiffs would have grounds for charges of *criminal battery*.[40,41]

Advance Directives (ADs)

DNR orders are one type of *advance directive* (AD) – a statement rendered by a competent patient outlining their wishes about specific aspects of medical care to guide treatment if they are unable to express themselves. ADs can authorize invasive treatments, or limit certain types of treatments (e.g. artificial nutrition and hydration). Other examples of ADs include blood transfusion refusals, living wills, wishes regarding organ donation and physician orders regarding life-sustaining treatment (POLST). The degree to which a physician must adhere to an advance directive is influenced by the nature of the directive, state law and, pragmatically, the degree to which survivors will support the life-sustaining order.

POLST orders deserve special mention, because they represent a type of DNR order that is meant to be applicable and legally enforceable outside of hospital settings (e.g. nursing facilities and the patient's own home) where the order guides out-of-hospital interventions by emergency medical responders. Currently 45 states recognize, endorse or are actively developing POLST orders.[42]

Surrogate Decision-Makers

Almost 60% of older adults do not have ADs to guide treatment decisions.[43] In such cases, physicians may have to rely on surrogate decision-makers (SDMs).

The concept that, once disease or disability has stolen a patient's ability to express themselves, others who are knowledgeable about the patient's wishes can express their wishes for them has long had strong legal support. In the US, the cases of Karen Ann Quinlan,[44] Nancy Cruzan[45] and Terri Schiavo[46] steadfastly protected the rights of patients to refuse even life-sustaining treatments through the SDMs.

SDMs include court-appointed guardians, persons holding durable powers of attorney for health care decision-making and family members.

However, relying on surrogate decision-makers is fraught with problems. The SDM is supposed to enact decisions that the patient would make, regardless of whether they personally agree with that decision. Like physicians, SDMs consistently rate quality of life poorer than seriously ill patients,[47,48] and in some studies SDMs were correct only a little over half of the time. Correlation between SDM and patient wishes was especially poor when it involved patients with dementia.[49]

Conclusion

Older patients with multisystem disease present greater challenges for anesthesiologists and surgeons. Making the right treatment decision with the patient goes beyond an understanding of the procedures and risks. It requires knowledge of the patient's capacity and wishes. Understanding the important differences in the various terms and definitions commonly used for consent and advance directive discussions is an important part of a complex issue.

References

1. Beauchamp TL, Childress JF. *Principles of Biomedical Ethics, 4th edn.* Oxford, Oxford University Press, 1994; 120.

2. Schloendorff v Society of New York Hospital, 311 NY 125, 127, 129;105 NE 92, 93, 1914.

3. Salgo v Leland Stanford, etc. Bd. Trustees, 154 Cal. App.2d 560.

4. Chalmers J. Capacity. In: Singer P, ed., *The Cambridge Textbook of Bioethics.* Cambridge, Cambridge University Press, 2008; 17–23.

5. Langa KM, Levine DA. The diagnosis and management of mild cognitive impairment: a clinical review. *JAMA.* 2014; 312:2551–2556.

6. Rizzolo P. Does a demented patient lose the right to refuse surgical intervention? *NC Med J.* 1992; 53:213–216.

7. Kornfeld DS, Muskin PR, Tahil FA. Psychiatric evaluation of mental capacity in the general hospital:a significant teaching opportunity. *Psychosomatics.* 2009; 50:468–473.

8. Wilson KA, Dowling AJ, Abdolell M, Tannock IF. Perception of the quality of life by patients, partners and treating physicians. *Qual Life Res.* 2000; 9:1041–52.

9. Covinsky KE, Fuller JD, Yaffe K, *et al.* Communication and decision-making in seriously ill patients: findings of the SUPPORT project. The Study to Understand Prognoses and Preferences for Outcomes and Risks of Treatments. *J Am Geriatr.* 2000; 48(Suppl):S187–S193.

10. van Kleffens T, van Leeuwen E. Physicians' evaluations of patients' decisions to refuse oncological treatment. *J Med Ethics.* 2005; 31:131–136.

11. Madorsky J. Is the slippery slope steeper for people with disabilities? *West J Med.* 1997; 166:410–411.

12. Culver C, Gert B. The inadequacy of incompetence. *Milbank Q.* 1990; 68:619–643.

13. Lo B. Assessing decision-making capacity. *Law Med Healthcare.* 1990; 18:193–201.

14. Graber MA, Ely JW, Clarke S, Kurtz S, Weir R. Informed consent and general surgeons' attitudes towards the use of pain medicines in the acute abdomen. *Am J Emer Med.* 1999; 17:113–116.

15. Etchells E, Sharpe G, Dykeman MJ, Meslin EM, Singer PA. Bioethics for clinicians: 4. Voluntariness. *CMAJ.* 1996; 155:1083–1086.

16. Amanor-Boadu D. Pattern of drug use in geriatric patients undergoing surgery under general anaesthesia. *Afr Med Med Sci.* 2002; 31:4–51.

17. Fusetti C, Lazzaro M, Trobia M, *et al.* Patients' point of view on informed consent: a prospective study in carpal tunnel surgery. *Am J Orthop (Belle Mead NJ).* 2013; 42:E111–E115.

18. Vallance JH, Ahmed M, Dhillon B. Cataract surgery and consent: recall, anxiety, and attitude toward trainee surgeons preoperatively and postoperatively. *J Cataract Refract Surg.* 2004; 30:1479–1485.

19. LaMance K. Informed consent for surgery lawyers. 2015. Available from: www .legalmatch.com/law-library/article/ informed-consent-for-surgery.html (Accessed May 31, 2015).

20. Beauchamp TL, Childress JF. *Principles of Biomedical Ethics, 4th edn.* Oxford, Oxford University Press, 1994; 163–164.

21. Wysocki WM, Mitus J, Komorowski AL, Karolewski K. Impact of preoperative information on anxiety and disease-related knowledge in women undergoing mastectomy for breast cancer:a randomized clinical trial. *Acta Chir Belg.* 2012; 112:111–115.

22. Inglis S, Farnill D. The effects of providing preoperative statistical anaesthetic-risk information. *Anaesth Intensive Care.* 1993; 21:799–805.

23. Kain ZN. Perioperative information and parental anxiety: the next generation. *Anes Analg.* 1999; 88:237–239.

24. Burkle CM, Pasternak JJ, Armstrong MH, Keegan MT. Patient perspectives on informed consent for anaesthesia and surgery: American attitudes. *Acta Anaesthesiol Scand.* 2013; 57:342–349.

25. Beauchamp TL, Childress JF. *Principles of Biomedical Ethics, 4th edn.* Oxford, Oxford University Press, 1994; 166.

26. Beausoleil v Sisters of Charity (1966), 56 DLR 65(QueCA), note 7 at 76.

27. Freidson E. *The Profession of Medicine.* New York, Dodd, Mead and Co, 1970; 376.

28. Omnibus Budget Reconciliation Act of 1990, P. L. 101-508, sec. 4206 and 4751, 104 Stat. 1388, 1388-115, and 1388-204 (classified respectively at 42 U.S.C. 1395cc(f) (Medicare) and 1396a(w) (Medicaid) (1994)).

29. Reisfield GM, Wallace SK, Munsell MF, et al. Survival in cancer patients undergoing in-hospital cardiopulmonary resuscitation: a meta-analysis. *Resuscitation.* 2006; 71:152–160.

30. Floom HL, Shukrullah I, Cuellar JR, et al. Long-term survival after successful inhospital cardiac arrest resuscitation. *Am Heart J.* 2007; 153:831–836.

31. Elshove-Bolk J, Guttormsen AB, Austlid I. In-hospital resuscitation of the elderly: characteristics and outcome. *Resuscitation.* 2007; 74:372–376.

32. Nadkarni VM, Larkin GL, Peberdy MA, et al. First documented rhythm and clinical outcome from in-hospital cardiac arrest among children and adults. *JAMA.* 2006; 295:50–57.

33. Kagawa E, Inoue I, Kawagoe T, et al. Assessment of outcomes and differences between in- and out-of-hospital cardiac arrest patients treated with cardiopulmonary resuscitation using extracorporeal life support. *Resuscitation.* 2010; 81:968–973.

34. Sprung J, Warner ME, Contreras MG, et al. Predictors of survival following cardiac arrest in patients undergoing noncardiac surgery: a study of 518,294 patients at a tertiary referral center. *Anesthesiology.* 2003; 99:259–269.

35. Biboulet P, Aubas P, Dubourdieu J, et al. Fatal and non fatal cardiac arrests related to anesthesia. *Can J Anaesth.* 2001; 48:326–332.

36. American Society of Anesthesiologists Committee on Ethics. *Ethical Guidelines for the Anesthesia Care of Patients with Do-Not-Resuscitate Orders or Other Directives that Limit Treatment.* Parkridge, IL, American Society of Anesthesiologists. Approved 2001, last amended Oct 16, 2013.

37. American College of Surgeons. Statement on advance directives by patients: do not resuscitate in the operating room. *ACS Bull.* 1994; 79:29.

38. AORN Position Statement: Perioperative care of patients with do-not-resuscitate orders. Denver, CO. 1995 Available at: www.AORN.org (Accessed May 31, 2015).

39. Joint Commission on Accreditation of Healthcare Organizations. Patient rights chapter. I: *Manual of the Joint Commission on Accreditation of Health Care Organizations.* Chicago, IL, Joint Commission on Accreditation of Health Care Organizations, 1994.

40. Snyder L. Refusing medical treatment: beyond the advance directive. *ABA Health Source.* 2007; 3(8). Available at: www.americanbar.org/content/newsletter/ publications/aba_health_esource_home/ snyder.html (Accessed May 30, 2015).

41. Martin RH. Liability for failing to follow advance directives. *Physicians News Digest.* 1999. Available at: physiciansnews .com/1999/09/14/liability-for-failing-to-follow-advance-directives/ (Accessed May 30, 2015).

42. www.polst.org (Accessed May 30, 2015).

43. Waite KR, Federman AD, McCarthy DM, *et al.* Literacy and race as risk factors for low rates of advance directives in older adults. *J Am Geriatr Soc.* 2013; 61:403–645.

44. In the Matter of Karen Quinlan, An Alleged Incompetent. 355 A2d 647 (NJ Super Ct Cir 1976).

45. Cruzan v Director, Missouri Department of Health, 497 U.S. 261 (1990).

46. Schiavo v Schiavo No. 05-11628 (11th Cir, March 25, 2005).

47. Scales DC, Tansey CM, Matte A, Herridge MS. Difference in reported pre-morbid health-related quality of life between ARDS survivors and their substitute decision-makers. *Intensive Care Med.* 2006; 32:1826–1831.

48. Pruchno RA, Lemay EP Jr., Feild L, Levinsky NG. Predictors of patient treatment preferences and spouse substituted judgments: the case of dialysis continuation. *Med Decis Making.* 2006; 26:112–121.

49. Shalowitz DI, Garrett-Mayer E, Wendler D. The accuracy of surrogate decision makers: a systematic review. *Arch Int Med.* 2006; 166:493–497.

Chapter

3

The Perioperative Management of Hypertension in the Elderly

Jeffrey B. Dobyns and Thomas R. Vetter

Key Points

- Isolated systolic hypertension, defined as a systolic blood pressure of greater than or equal to 140 mmHg with a diastolic blood pressure of less than 90 mmHg, is the most common type of hypertension in the elderly. Elevated systolic pressure results from reduced arterial compliance that occurs in the presence of rigid, atherosclerotic arteries, due to loss of elasticity in the aorta and large arteries.
- Substantial evidence demonstrates that chronic isolated systolic hypertension is associated with an increased longitudinal risk of stroke and heart failure, and that widened pulse pressure is an independent long-term predictor of cardiovascular complications and all-cause mortality.
- Benefits of treatment of isolated systolic hypertension in patients over 60 years of age include 36% reduction in incidence of hemorrhagic and ischemic stroke, 39% reduction in stroke deaths, 27% reduction in myocardial infarction, 23% reduction in cardiovascular morbid and fatal events, 64% reduction in the rate of heart failure and a 21% all-cause mortality reduction.
- Overly aggressive treatment of hypertension in elderly patients is associated with an increased incidence of stoke, depression, orthostasis, falls and cardiovascular morbidity, and decreased survival.
- Regardless of blood pressure, if the patient is experiencing a hypertensive crisis, nonemergent procedures should be postponed. Postponement of an elective procedure is justified if any evident end-organ dysfunction can be improved or if further evaluation could alter the anesthetic plan.
- The development, implementation and evolution of the Perioperative Surgical Home allows for medication review with elderly patients and the reduction of polypharmacy, as well as an opportunity to ensure appropriate stroke and cardiovascular risk reduction strategies are in place.

Introduction

Anesthesiologists have the opportunity to transform the perioperative care of surgical patients. By better integrating and coordinating perioperative care, anesthesiologists are in the unique position to enhance the patient care experience, mitigate perioperative risk and reduce costs for the patient, the health care institution and ultimately society. Perioperative management of hypertension in the elderly patient is one opportunity for the anesthesiologist to reduce surgical risk and improve outcomes.

Table 3.1 Stratification of hypertension according to current JNC8 guidelines

Hypertension class	Systolic blood pressure (mmHg)	Diastolic blood pressure (mmHg)
Normal	<120	<80
Prehypertension	120–139	80–89
Stage I	140–159	90–99
Stage II	≥160	≥100
Hypertensive urgency		>120 without evidence of end-organ dysfunction
Hypertensive emergency		>120 with evidence of end-organ dysfunction

From: James PA, Oparil S, Carter BL, *et al.* 2014 Evidence-based guideline for the management of high blood pressure in adults: report from the panel members appointed to the Eighth Joint National Committee (JNC 8). *JAMA*. 2014; 311(5):507–520.

In this chapter, we will discuss perioperative hypertension in the elderly patient and how it contributes to increased perioperative risk. Furthermore, we will detail how optimization of perioperative hypertension can mitigate risk and improve patient outcomes.

Epidemiology

Approximately 34 million Americans are currently over the age of 65, and this number is expected to reach 75 million by 2040, representing over 20% of the United States population.[1] The elderly are thus the largest growing segment of the United States population. The prevalence of hypertension among the elderly is as high as 60% to 80%.[1,2] A report from the Framingham Heart Study estimated that patients aged 55 to 65, who are not currently diagnosed as hypertensive, have a 90% lifetime risk of developing stage I hypertension and a 40% risk of developing stage II hypertension (Table 3.1).[3]

Pathophysiology of Hypertension in the Elderly

Isolated systolic hypertension, defined as a systolic blood pressure of greater than or equal to 140 mmHg with a diastolic blood pressure of less than 90 mmHg, is the most common type of hypertension in the elderly. Elevated systolic pressure results from reduced arterial compliance that occurs in the presence of rigid, atherosclerotic arteries, due to loss of elasticity in the aorta and large arteries. These vascular changes are reflected in an elevated systolic blood pressure, reduced diastolic pressure, and widened pulse pressure. Elderly patients with isolated systolic hypertension can experience large increases in systolic blood pressure, often to values of greater than 200 mmHg, during and after anesthesia, with only minor changes in diastolic blood pressure.[4]

Perioperative Risks of Hypertension

Substantial evidence demonstrates that chronic isolated systolic hypertension is associated with an increased longitudinal risk of stroke and heart failure, and that widened pulse pressure is an independent long-term predictor of cardiovascular complications and all-cause mortality. These patients therefore benefit greatly from therapies to reduce systolic pressure.[5-7] Isolated systolic hypertension is associated with a 40% increase in the probability of perioperative adverse cardiovascular events in patients undergoing coronary artery bypass surgery.[8] Patients presenting for carotid endarterectomy with systolic blood pressures of 200 mmHg or greater have a 10% incidence of postoperative hypertension and neurologic deficits, such as hyperperfusion syndrome, stroke or subarachnoid hemorrhage.[9] In patients with known or at high risk for coronary artery disease, perioperative hypertension is associated with a nearly fourfold increased risk of death. Perioperative hypertension is also associated with increased blood loss, cerebrovascular events and myocardial ischemia.[10] Patients with poorly controlled preoperative hypertension are more likely to experience intraoperative blood pressure lability and have an increased risk of adverse cardiovascular and cerebrovascular events, as well as other postoperative complications (e.g. acute renal failure).[11,12]

Benefits of Perioperative Hypertension Control

Meta-analyses of randomized trials have demonstrated that treatment of isolated systolic hypertension in patients over 60 years of age reduces the incidence of hemorrhagic and ischemic stroke by 36%.[13,14] Other longitudinal benefits include a 39% reduction in stroke deaths, 27% reduction in myocardial infarction, 23% reduction in cardiovascular morbid and fatal events, 64% reduction in the rate of heart failure and a 21% all-cause mortality reduction.[15] Treatment of hypertension improves diastolic function and reduces left ventricular mass.[16,17] An aldosterone receptor blocker (ARB), calcium channel blocker (CCB) and angiotensin converting enzyme inhibitor (ACEI) have the greatest effect on reduction of left ventricular hypertrophy, improvement of diastolic function and inhibition of ventricular remodeling (Figure 3.1).[16] Perioperative diastolic dysfunction is associated with an increased incidence of postoperative congestive heart failure, arrhythmias and prolonged mechanical ventilation. Two to eighteen months may be required for antihypertensive therapy to improve diastolic dysfunction.[12]

Patients with perioperative hypertension frequently demonstrate increased cardiovascular lability during the induction and maintenance of anesthesia. Given the pathophysiologic changes that occur with the aged vasculature, this lability in elderly patients can be dramatic and difficult to treat.[18] Furthermore, patients with poorly controlled or uncontrolled perioperative hypertension have a cardiovascular complication rate as high as 36%.[19] However, the cardiovascular complication rate was reduced to 16% in patients with controlled hypertension.

The primary goal of treating chronic hypertension in the elderly is not necessarily to reduce blood pressure, but to prevent the cardiovascular complications that result from such chronic hypertension.[20] However, hypertension treatment in the elderly is not without risk. Overly aggressive treatment of hypertension in elderly patients is associated with an increase incidence of stoke, depression, orthostasis, falls and cardiovascular morbidity, and decreased survival.[21,22] Advanced age is an independent risk factor for both perioperative stroke and major adverse cardiac events. When controlling hypertension in the elderly, one should consider their decreased cerebrovascular and cardiovascular reserve, as central vascular and cerebrovascular autoregulation remain abnormal for several weeks after hypertension has normalized.[23]

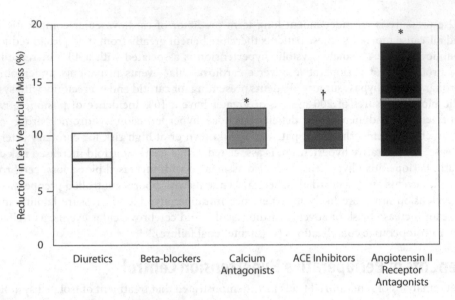

Figure 3.1 Change in left ventricular mass index by antihypertensive medication class.
From: Klingbeil AU, Schneider M, Martus P, Messerli FH, Schmieder RE. A meta-analysis of the effects of treatment on left ventricular mass in essential hypertension. *Am J Med*. 2003; 115(1):41–46. Reproduced with permission.

Predicting Perioperative Risk

The 2002 *ACC/AHA Guidelines on Perioperative Cardiovascular Evaluation and Management of Patients Undergoing Noncardiac Surgery* state that patients with severe hypertension undergoing elective surgery should have surgery postponed until the blood pressure is controlled.[24] The subsequent 2007 ACC/AHA version of these guidelines state that hypertension is a minor predictor of adverse cardiac outcome and that Stage I or II hypertension is not an *independent* risk factor for perioperative cardiac complications (Table 3.2).[25] The 2014 ACC/AHA guidelines make no mention of arterial hypertension.[26] Neither the Preoperative Cardiac Risk Index score nor the Revised Cardiac Risk Index (RCRI) considers hypertension in the calculation of perioperative risk.[27,28] Regardless, the clinical significance of co-morbid hypertension should not be underestimated. The American College of Surgeons' National Surgical Quality Improvement Program (NSQIP) risk model calculator considers age, hypertension and several other co-morbidities in a procedure-specific fashion and has a higher predictive accuracy rate than the RCRI.[29] Perioperative physicians should develop a familiarity with one risk calculation model and use it consistently for risk stratification.

Perioperative Blood Pressure Medication Management

Drug therapy for hypertension in elderly patients is indicated when the systolic blood pressure is greater than or equal to 160 mmHg.[20] While current evidence supports the use of diuretics or long-acting calcium channel blockers as first-line treatment, co-existing morbidities such as diastolic dysfunction should be considered.[7] Recent studies have also demonstrated that an ACEI is equally effective as a CCB and can alternatively be used as first-line therapy.[30] In the elderly patient, the choice of antihypertensive agent may be less

Table 3.2 Clinical predictors of increased perioperative risk of adverse cardiac events

- Major predictors
  - Unstable coronary syndromes
  - Recent myocardial infarction
  - Unstable or severe angina
  - Decompensated congestive heart failure
  - Significant arrhythmias
  - High-grade atrioventricular block
  - Symptomatic ventricular arrhythmias in the presence of underlying heart disease
  - Supraventricular arrhythmias with uncontrolled ventricular rate
  - Severe valvular disease
- Intermediate predictors
  - Mild angina pectoris
  - Prior myocardial infarction by history or pathological Q waves
  - Compensated or prior congestive heart failure
  - Diabetes mellitus
- Minor predictors
  - Advanced age (greater than 70 years)
  - Abnormal EKG (LVH, left bundle-branch block, ST-T abnormalities)
  - Rhythm other than sinus (atrial fibrillation)
  - Low functional capacity
  - History of stroke
  - Uncontrolled systemic hypertension

From: Priebe, HJ. The aged cardiovascular risk patient. *Br J Anaesth*. 2000; 85(5):763–768.
Jin F, Chung, F. Minimizing perioperative adverse events in the elderly. *Br J Anaesth*. 2001; 87(4):608–624.
Fleisher LA, Beckman JA, Brown KA, Calkins H, Chaikof E, Fleischmann KE, *et al.* ACC/AHA 2007 Guidelines
on Perioperative Cardiovascular Evaluation and Care for Noncardiac Surgery: Executive Summary: A Report
of the American College of Cardiology/American Heart Association Task Force on Practice Guidelines.
Anesth Analg. 2008; 106(3):685–712.

important than choosing a medication that achieves the target blood pressure and is well tolerated.

As a general rule, antihypertensive medications should be continued through the day of surgery, with a few exceptions.[31] For patients who take combination medications, such as a beta-blocker or CCB combined with a diuretic, the medication should be continued or withheld based upon the non-diuretic portion of the medication.

Angiotensin Converting Enzyme Inhibitors/Aldosterone Receptor Blockers

Studies of patients taking an ACEI or ARB and undergoing vascular surgery found that continuing the ACEI or ARB through the day of surgery resulted in significantly more hypotension and higher utilization of vasopressors.[32-34] Attenuation of the effects of phenylephrine and a decreased adrenergic vasoconstrictive response has also been demonstrated.[35]

An ACEI or ARB should be withheld on the morning of surgery and not reinstituted until the patient is euvolemic, unless the patient suffers from chronic heart failure. Neither an increase in in-hospital complications nor an increase in 30-day mortality has been shown in patients taking ACEI who withheld it on the morning of surgery.[36]

Calcium Channel Blockers

Two meta-analyses from 2003 observed that calcium channel blockers were associated with decreased ischemia and supraventricular tachycardia in patients undergoing both noncardiac and cardiac surgery; therefore, these medications should be continued perioperatively.[37,38] Calcium channel blockers, in particular nimodipine and nitrendipine, have also been shown in observational and laboratory studies to have a neuroprotective effect against the development of dementia.[39] While a meta-analysis did find evidence of a short-term benefit from nimodipine in measures of cognitive function and global impression, the review was not specific to the perioperative period, so no such recommendations could be made for its routine use.[40]

Diuretics

Hypovolemia resulting from diuretic use, coupled with the systemic vasodilation produced by intravenous and volatile anesthetic agents, may result in hypotension. While conventional practice is to withhold diuretics on the day of surgery, a 2010 randomized controlled trial noted that in elderly patients chronically treated with furosemide, continuing the dose on the day of surgery did not significantly increase the risk for intraoperative hypotension.[41] If the diuretic is withheld and signs and symptoms of hypervolemia develop, intravenous loop diuretics can be administered.

Beta-Blockers

Beta-blockers have several likely perioperative beneficial effects, including reduction of ischemia by decreasing myocardial oxygen demand, decreasing myocardial response to increased perioperative catecholamine release, prevention/control of cardiac arrhythmias, and reduction in 30-day and 1-year mortality.[42] Currently, however, the only evidence-based indication for perioperative beta-blockade is that they be continued in patients who have been taking them chronically.[26]

While beta-blockers may cause perioperative bradycardia and hypotension, abrupt withdrawal can result in significant morbidity and mortality.[42,43] Beta-blockers thus should be continued up to and including the day of surgery. If the beta-blocker was not taken on the day of surgery, it can be preoperatively orally administered or an intravenous formulation can be substituted.

Other Antihypertensives

Alpha-1 blockers are commonly used in elderly males to treat benign prostatic hypertrophy. Alpha-1 blockers should be continued through the day of surgery. However, tamsulosin (Flomax®) should be discontinued for several days prior to cataract surgery, due to its association with intraoperative floppy iris syndrome.[44]

Alpha-2 agonists, such as clonidine, may reduce cardiac ischemia, nonfatal myocardial infarction and cardiac death, and should be continued through the day of surgery. For those unable to take oral alpha-2 agonists in the perioperative period, transdermal formulations can be used. The transdermal formulation should be started 24–48 hours in advance of surgery. Alpha-2 agonists may decrease blood pressure lability, preoperative anxiety and anesthetic requirements.[45]

The prophylactic use of oral nitrates has not been associated with a reduction in perioperative coronary events.[46] They should be continued on the day of surgery, since the use of these medications typically implies co-existing ischemic heart disease.[47] As needed, topical or intravenous nitroglycerin can be substituted for oral nitrates.

Hydralazine is sometimes combined with oral nitrates in the treatment of New York Class 2, 3 and 4 heart failure, because of its associated decreased mortality and increase in left ventricular ejection fraction.[48] Abruptly stopping hydralazine may cause rebound hypertension, so hydralazine should be continued through the day of surgery.

Optimizing Perioperative Blood Pressure Management

While there is abundant evidence that the treatment of hypertension results in clinical benefits in the elderly and very elderly patient population, the treatment target remains obscure. The 2014 JNC8 recommends a blood pressure of less than 140/90 as a treatment goal for patients over age 60, while other data indicate that in patients over the age of 70, a blood pressure of 150/80 or higher should be accepted.[49-51] This latter target is supported by the HYVET trial, which concluded that blood pressure in the very elderly treated to a target of 150/80 was associated with reduced risk of death from stroke, heart failure or any-cause mortality.[15] There is no evidence to suggest that a lower blood pressure target in elderly patients with both hypertension and diabetes mellitus resulted in improved outcomes.[52] In the HYVET trial, cerebral blood flow decreased when blood pressure dropped below 140/65, and overshooting a target blood pressure was associated with worse outcomes.[53] In the SHEP trial, increased adverse cardiovascular events occurred in elderly patients with diastolic blood pressures below 65 mmHg (Figure 3.2).[54] If patients safely tolerate a blood pressure below this level, dose adjustment is not necessary.

Preoperative Management

Hypertension in the immediate preoperative period is multifactorial in origin, including pain, anxiety, hypertensive response to withholding of chronically administered antihypertensive medications, and a consequence of underlying medical conditions (primary or secondary hypertension). While the preoperative visit with the anesthesiologist may itself be anxiolytic, hypertension resulting from anxiety or pain can be treated, if indicated, with small doses of a benzodiazepine or short-acting opioid. The decision to treat such hypertension pharmacologically with antihypertensive medications is a clinical one, which should consider the immediate and delayed results of treatment. Elderly patients frequently have significant hypotension following the induction of anesthesia, and this hypotension may be very difficult to treat, particularly so if a long-acting antihypertensive medication like labetalol or hydralazine has been given immediately preoperatively.

Intraoperative Management

Hypertension is usually noted with laryngoscopy and intubation due to sympathetic stimulation. These brief episodes of hypertension can be treated with intravenous lidocaine, fentanyl or esmolol. While all three of these agents can be effective, only esmolol has been shown to reliably prevent laryngoscopy-associated hypertension and tachycardia.[55] Hypertension at the time of laryngoscopy and intubation should be treated with ultra-short-acting medications, as the institution of mechanical ventilation and the maintenance phase of anesthesia can result in significant hypotension, which again may be difficult to treat in the setting of longer-acting antihypertensive medications. Intravenous hydralazine should be used cautiously in elderly patients with ischemic heart disease, who may respond poorly to the reflex tachycardia that may result.

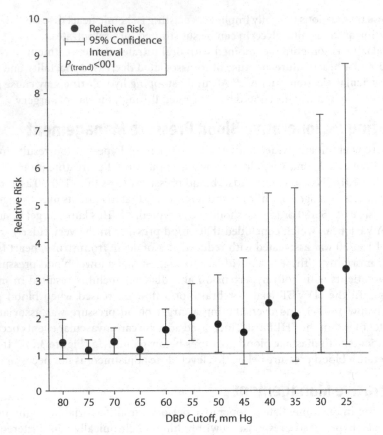

Figure 3.2 Relative risk of adverse cardiac events by diastolic blood pressure. DBP: diastolic blood pressure.
From: Somes GW, Pahor M, Shorr RI, *et al.* The role of diastolic blood pressure when treating isolated systolic hypertension. *Arch Intern Med.* 1999; 159(17):2004–2009. *Permission pending.*

Treatment of Hypertension in the Postanesthesia Care Unit

Hypertension is a common event in elderly patients while in the Postanesthesia Care Unit (PACU). It can be difficult to treat, and aggressive treatment may be necessary to prevent hypertensive end-organ damage, such as acute stroke, myocardial ischemia or arrhythmias. Hypertension in the PACU is also associated with increased admissions to the intensive care unit and mortality.[56] Hypertension may result from pain, anxiety, hypoxemia, hypercarbia, hypothermia, shivering, urinary retention, hypervolemia, bladder distention or discontinuation of chronic antihypertensive medications. While the underlying cause of the hypertension should be identified and treated, the ideal medication for treating hypertension in the PACU should be rapid-acting, predictable, safe and readily available.[57]

Preoperative Hypertension: Cancel or Proceed?

The decision to proceed with elective surgery or to delay for further blood pressure optimization should be individualized based upon consideration of a number of factors (Table 3.3).

Table 3.3 Considerations for delaying or proceeding with surgery

- Severity of hypertension
- Likelihood of co-existing myocardial ischemia
- Presence or absence of end-organ dysfunction
- Ventricular dysfunction
- Cerebrovascular effects of treatment
- Renal complications
- Emergent/urgent/elective status of the procedure
- Whether delay and additional medical management will alter the anesthetic plan or anticipated outcome

Guidelines and checklists are useful tools to aid and guide clinical decision-making, but the ultimate decision to proceed or cancel should be individualized to the patient and procedure. There is no reason to delay or cancel elective surgery in patients presenting preoperatively with prehypertension or stage I hypertension without evidence of existing metabolic or cardiovascular sequelae. However, patients presenting with stage II hypertension should have greater blood pressure control prior to undergoing elective surgery.[12] Regardless of blood pressure, if the patient is experiencing a hypertensive crisis, non-emergent procedures should be postponed.[12] Postponement of an elective procedure is justified if any evident end-organ dysfunction can be improved or if further evaluation could alter the anesthetic plan.

Role of the Preoperative Assessment Clinic and Perioperative Surgical Home

Elderly patients benefit greatly from a preoperative assessment clinic evaluation. The development, implementation, and evolution of the Perioperative Surgical Home allows for medication review with elderly patients and the reduction of polypharmacy, as well as an opportunity to ensure appropriate stroke and cardiovascular risk reduction strategies are in place. Review of the elderly patient's medications at the preoperative anesthesia visit potentially allows for elimination of duplicated medications, identification of medications that cross-react with one another (e.g. oral nitrates and sildenafil) and offers the potential to improve quality of life, decrease falls and possibly slow the decline in physical and cognitive function.

Summary

High-quality perioperative care for the elderly is not only a medical, but also a social and financial necessity. Hypertension is a very significant disorder in the elderly and is associated with a greater risk of cardiovascular morbidity and mortality. The goal of antihypertensive therapy should be the reduction and minimization of cardiovascular risks and maintenance of optimal postoperative quality of life and adequate functional capacity. Treatment of hypertension in the elderly is associated with a decreased incidence of dementia and improved intellectual functioning and thus sustained functional capacity and improved quality of life.

References

1. Aronow WS, Fleg JL, Pepine CJ, et al. ACCF/AHA 2011 expert consensus document on hypertension in the elderly: a report of the American College of Cardiology Foundation Task Force on Clinical Expert Consensus Documents developed in collaboration with the American Academy of Neurology, American Geriatrics Society, American Society for Preventive Cardiology, American Society of Hypertension, American Society of Nephrology, Association of Black Cardiologists, and European Society of Hypertension. *J Am Soc Hypertens*. 2011; 5(4): 259–352.

2. Egan BM, Zhao Y, Axon RN. US trends in prevalence, awareness, treatment, and control of hypertension, 1988-2008. *JAMA*. 2010; 303(20):2043–2050.

3. Vasan RS, Beiser A, Seshadri S, et al. Residual lifetime risk for developing hypertension in middle-aged women and men: The Framingham Heart Study. *JAMA*. 2002; 287(8):1003–1010.

4. Prys-Roberts C. Isolated systolic hypertension: pressure on the anaesthetist? *Anaesthesia*. 2001; 56(6):505–510.

5. Staessen JA, Fagard R, Thijs L, et al. Randomised double-blind comparison of placebo and active treatment for older patients with isolated systolic hypertension. The Systolic Hypertension in Europe (Syst-Eur) Trial Investigators. *Lancet*. 1997; 350(9080):757–764.

6. Gasowski J, Fagard RH, Staessen JA, et al. Pulsatile blood pressure component as predictor of mortality in hypertension: a meta-analysis of clinical trial control groups. *J Hypertens*. 2002; 20(1): 145–151.

7. SHEP Cooperative Research Group. Prevention of stroke by antihypertensive drug treatment in older persons with isolated systolic hypertension. Final results of the Systolic Hypertension in the Elderly Program (SHEP). *JAMA*. 1991; 265(24):3255–3264.

8. Aronson S, Boisvert D, Lapp W. Isolated systolic hypertension is associated with adverse outcomes from coronary artery bypass grafting surgery. *Anesth Analg*. 2002; 94(5):1079–1084, table of contents.

9. Karapanayiotides T, Meuli R, Devuyst G, et al. Postcarotid endarterectomy hyperperfusion or reperfusion syndrome. *Stroke*. 2005; 36(1):21–26.

10. Browner WS, Li J, Mangano DT; The Study of Perioperative Ischemia Research Group. In-hospital and long-term mortality in male veterans following noncardiac surgery. *JAMA*. 1992; 268(2):228–232.

11. Kheterpal S, Tremper KK, Englesbe MJ, et al. Predictors of postoperative acute renal failure after noncardiac surgery in patients with previously normal renal function. *Anesthesiology*. 2007; 107(6):892–902.

12. Sear JW. Perioperative control of hypertension: when will it adversely affect perioperative outcome? *Curr Hypertens Rep*. 2008; 10(6):480–487.

13. Staessen JA, Gasowski J, Wang JG, et al. Risks of untreated and treated isolated systolic hypertension in the elderly: meta-analysis of outcome trials. *Lancet*. 2000; 355(9207):865–872.

14. Perry HM Jr., Davis BR, Price TR, et al. Effect of treating isolated systolic hypertension on the risk of developing various types and subtypes of stroke: the Systolic Hypertension in the Elderly Program (SHEP). *JAMA*. 2000; 284(4):465–471.

15. Beckett NS, Peters R, Fletcher AE, et al. Treatment of hypertension in patients 80 years of age or older. *N Engl J Med*. 2008; 358(18):1887–1898.

16. Klingbeil AU, Schneider M, Martus P, Messerli FH, Schmieder RE. A meta-analysis of the effects of treatment on left ventricular mass in essential hypertension. *Am J Med*. 2003; 115(1):41–46.

17. Wachtell K, Bella JN, Rokkedal J, *et al.* Change in diastolic left ventricular filling after one year of antihypertensive treatment: The Losartan Intervention For Endpoint Reduction in Hypertension (LIFE) Study. *Circulation.* 2002; 105(9): 1071–1076.

18. Howell SJ, Sear JW, Foex P. Hypertension, hypertensive heart disease and perioperative cardiac risk. *Br J Anaesth.* 2004; 92(4):570–583.

19. Weksler N, Klein M, Szendro G, *et al.* The dilemma of immediate preoperative hypertension: to treat and operate, or to postpone surgery? *J Clin Anesth.* 2003; 15(3):179–183.

20. Wang JG, Staessen JA. Improved outcomes with antihypertensive medication in the elderly with isolated systolic hypertension. *Drugs Aging.* 2001; 18(5):345–353.

21. Kim BS, Bae JN, Cho MJ. Depressive symptoms in elderly adults with hypotension: different associations with positive and negative affect. *J Affect Disord.* 2010; 127(1–3):359–364.

22. Devereaux PJ, Yang H, Yusuf S, *et al.* Effects of extended-release metoprolol succinate in patients undergoing non-cardiac surgery (POISE trial): a randomised controlled trial. *Lancet.* 2008; 371(9627):1839–1847.

23. Foex P, Sear JW. The surgical hypertensive patient. *Cont Edu in Anaesth, Crit Care Pain.* 2004; 4:139–143.

24. Eagle KA, Berger PB, Calkins H, *et al.* ACC/AHA guideline update for perioperative cardiovascular evaluation for noncardiac surgery: executive summary a report of the American College of Cardiology/American Heart Association Task Force on Practice Guidelines (Committee to Update the 1996 Guidelines on Perioperative Cardiovascular Evaluation for Noncardiac Surgery). *Circulation.* 2002; 105(10):1257–1267.

25. Fleisher LA, Beckman JA, Brown KA, *et al.* ACC/AHA 2007 guidelines on perioperative cardiovascular evaluation and care for noncardiac surgery: executive summary: a report of the American College of Cardiology/American Heart Association Task Force on Practice Guidelines (Writing Committee to Revise the 2002 Guidelines on Perioperative Cardiovascular Evaluation for Noncardiac Surgery). *Anes Analg.* 2008; 106(3):685–712.

26. Fleisher LA, Fleischmann KE, Auerbach AD, *et al.* 2014 ACC/AHA guideline on perioperative cardiovascular evaluation and management of patients undergoing noncardiac surgery: a report of the American College of Cardiology/American Heart Association Task Force on Practice Guidelines. *J Am Coll Cardiol.* 2014; 64(22):e77–e137.

27. Goldman L, Caldera DL, Nussbaum SR, *et al.* Multifactorial index of cardiac risk in noncardiac surgical procedures. *N Engl J Med.* 1977; 297(16):845–850.

28. Lee TH, Marcantonio ER, Mangione CM, *et al.* Derivation and prospective validation of a simple index for prediction of cardiac risk of major noncardiac surgery. *Circulation.* 1999; 100(10):1043–1049.

29. Gupta PK, Gupta H, Sundaram A, *et al.* Development and validation of a risk calculator for prediction of cardiac risk after surgery. *Circulation.* 2011; 124(4):381–387.

30. Collaboration BPLTT. Effects of angiotensin converting enzyme inhibitors, calcium antagonists and other blood pressure lowering drugs on mortality and major cardiovascular morbidity: first cycle of analyses from a program of prospectively designed collaborative overviews of major randomised trials. *Lancet.* 2000; 355(9246):1955–1964.

31. Fleisher LA. Preoperative evaluation of the patient with hypertension. *JAMA.* 2002; 287(16):2043–2046.

32. Coriat P, Richer C, Douraki T, *et al.* Influence of chronic angiotensin-converting enzyme inhibition on anesthetic induction. *Anesthesiology.* 1994; 81(2):299–307.

33. Bertrand M, Godet G, Meersschaert K, *et al.* Should the angiotensin II antagonists be discontinued before surgery? *Anesth Analg.* 2001; 92(1):26–30.

34. Ryckwaert F, Colson P. Hemodynamic effects of anesthesia in patients with ischemic heart failure chronically treated with angiotensin-converting enzyme inhibitors. *Anesth Analg.* 1997; 84(5):945–949.

35. Licker M, Schweizer A, Hohn L, Farinelli C, Morel DR. Cardiovascular responses to anesthetic induction in patients chronically treated with angiotensin-converting enzyme inhibitors. *Can J Anaesth.* 2000; 47(5):433–440.

36. Turan A, You J, Shiba A, *et al.* Angiotensin converting enzyme inhibitors are not associated with respiratory complications or mortality after noncardiac surgery. *Anesth Analg.* 2012; 114(3):552–560.

37. Wijeysundera DN, Beattie WS. Calcium channel blockers for reducing cardiac morbidity after noncardiac surgery: a meta-analysis. *Anesth Analg.* 2003; 97(3):634–641.

38. Wijeysundera DN, Beattie WS, Rao V, Karski J. Calcium antagonists reduce cardiovascular complications after cardiac surgery: a meta-analysis. *J Am Coll Cardiol.* 2003; 41(9):1496–1505.

39. Wildburger NC, Lin-Ye A, Baird MA, Lei D, Bao J. Neuroprotective effects of blockers for T-type calcium channels. *Mol Neurodegener.* 2009; 4:44.

40. Lopez-Arrieta JM, Birks J. Nimodipine for primary degenerative, mixed and vascular dementia. *Cochrane Database Syst Rev.* 2002(3):CD000147.

41. Khan NA, Campbell NR, Frost SD, *et al.* Risk of intraoperative hypotension with loop diuretics: a randomized controlled trial. *Am J Med.* 2010; 123(11):1059. e1–8.

42. Wallace AW, Au S, Cason BA. Association of the pattern of use of perioperative beta-blockade and postoperative mortality. *Anesthesiology.* 2010; 113(4):794–805.

43. Shammash JB, Trost JC, Gold JM, *et al.* Perioperative beta-blocker withdrawal and mortality in vascular surgical patients. *Am Heart J.* 2001; 141(1):148–153.

44. Bell CM, Hatch WV, Fischer HD, *et al.* Association between tamsulosin and serious ophthalmic adverse events in older men following cataract surgery. *JAMA.* 2009; 301(19):1991–1996.

45. Milne B. Alpha-2 agonists and anaesthesia. *Can J Anaesth.* 1991; 38(7):809–813.

46. Cohn S. *Perioperative Medication Management.* London, Springer-Verlag, 2011.

47. Hollevoet I, Herregods S, Vereecke H, Vandermeulen E, Herregods L. Medication in the perioperative period: stop or continue? A review. *Acta Anaesthesiol Belg.* 2011; 62(4):193–201.

48. Taylor AL, Ziesche S, Yancy C, *et al.* Combination of isosorbide dinitrate and hydralazine in blacks with heart failure. *N Engl J Med.* 2004; 351(20):2049–2057.

49. Xhignesse P, Saint-Remy A, Krzesinski JM. [Management of arterial hypertension in the elderly]. *Rev Med Liege.* 2014; 69(5-6):294–300.

50. Ogihara T, Saruta T, Rakugi H, *et al.* Target blood pressure for treatment of isolated systolic hypertension in the elderly: valsartan in elderly isolated systolic hypertension study. *Hypertension.* 2010; 56(2):196–202.

51. James PA, Oparil S, Carter BL, *et al.* 2014 evidence-based guideline for the management of high blood pressure in adults: report from the panel members appointed to the Eighth Joint National Committee (JNC 8). *JAMA.* 2014; 311(5):507–520.

52. Arguedas JA, Leiva V, Wright JM. Blood pressure targets for hypertension in people with diabetes mellitus. *Cochrane Database Syst Rev.* 2013(10):CD008277.

53. Rhoney D, Peacock WF. Intravenous therapy for hypertensive emergencies, Part 1. *Am J Health Syst Pharm.* 2009; 66(15):1343–1352.

54. Young JH, Klag MJ, Muntner P, *et al.* Blood pressure and decline in kidney function: findings from the Systolic Hypertension in the Elderly Program (SHEP). *J Am Soc Nephrol.* 2002; 13(11):2776–2782.

55. Helfman SM, Gold MI, DeLisser EA, Herrington CA. Which drug prevents tachycardia and hypertension associated with tracheal intubation: lidocaine, fentanyl, or esmolol? *Anesth Analg*. 1991; 72(4):482–486.

56. Rose DK, Cohen MM, DeBoer DP. Cardiovascular events in the postanesthesia care unit: contribution of risk factors. *Anesthesiology*. 1996; 84(4):772–781.

57. Varon J, Marik PE. Perioperative hypertension management. *Vasc Health Risk Manag*. 2008; 4(3):615–627.

Chapter

4

Heart Failure

Rabya S. Saraf, Mario E. Montealegre and
Robina Matyal

Key Points

- Heart failure (HF) prevalence in older patients is approximately 22%, and heart failure mortality is estimated at 50% within 5 years of diagnosis.
- Heart failure is commonly categorized as *systolic or diastolic*. In systolic HF, there is an impaired contraction of the left ventricle (LV), whereas in diastolic HF the LV muscle suffers from impaired relaxation, which increases LV end diastolic pressures. In both cases, activation of compensatory mechanisms results in LV remodeling, increased dysfunction and changes in LV geometry (e.g. dilation, increased sphericity, mitral valve regurgitation).
- The most common risk factors for HF include hypertension, arrhythmias, congenital heart disease, diabetes mellitus, myocardial infarction and cardiomyopathy. Other associated factors include dyslipidemia, endothelial inflammation, alcohol abuse, cigarette smoking, micronutrient deficiency and a family history of cardiovascular disease.
- Takotsubo cardiomyopathy is a transient condition characterized by apical ballooning and ventricular systolic dysfunction that is accelerated by physical and/or emotional stress. Associated acute HF is common and it may manifest as pulmonary edema or cardiogenic shock.
- HF patients undergoing major surgical procedures have a higher risk of death and hospital readmission. Elderly patients are more likely to present with diastolic HF.
- Implantable cardioverter defibrillators (ICD) or cardiac resynchronization therapy (CRT) may be recommended in patients with chronic HF. These devices have been shown to increase survival and improve morbidity when used in conjunction with pharmacological therapy.

Introduction

According to the American Heart Association,[1] heart failure (HF) is "a complex clinical syndrome that can result from any structural or functional cardiac disorder that impairs the ability of the ventricle to fill or eject blood."[1] HF is a progressive, chronic disease that affects virtually every organ system. Providing care for HF patients results in high economic costs.[1] The worldwide prevalence of HF is over 23 million cases. In the United States, the prevalence is 6 million with an incidence of 500,000 cases each year.[1] Unlike cardiovascular diseases such as coronary artery disease and stroke, HF prevalence and mortality are increasing, and its prognosis remains poor.[2] About 5% of medical admissions to hospitals are due to chronic HF, and of those about 40% die within 1 year of hospitalization.[3] HF increases exponentially with age, with the prevalence in patients ≥80 years old approximately 22.4%.[4] Despite recent advances in HF treatment, it is still associated with a high mortality rate, with almost 50% of patients dying within 5 years of diagnosis.[5]

As the geriatric population increases, a larger number of noncardiac surgical procedures are being performed in the elderly.[6] The anesthetic implications of HF are important, as it increases the risk of major perioperative adverse cardiac events and death, particularly in the elderly.[6] Furthermore, geriatric patients that present with HF usually have multiple associated co-morbidities, such as hypertension, diabetes mellitus, chronic lung disease, atrial fibrillation, renal dysfunction and degenerative neurologic disease that significantly impact treatment plans and mandate a multidisciplinary approach.[7] In this chapter we will discuss HF in the geriatric patient and its perioperative implications for noncardiac surgery.

Pathophysiology of Heart Failure

HF pathophysiology involves cardiac and renal dysfunction, as well as skeletal muscle abnormalities and impairment of neurohormonal patterns necessary for adequate ventricular function.[2]

Heart failure can be left-sided, right-sided or global. Left-sided HF (also called left ventricular (LV) HF) can be systolic failure or diastolic failure. Right-sided heart failure is usually secondary to LV failure, but may be precipitated by diseases of the pulmonary vasculature and/or lung parenchyma.[1] Global heart failure occurs when both right and left ventricles fail. Originally, LV HF was synonymous with a depressed ejection fraction (i.e. systolic HF). Elderly patients are particularly prone to developing diastolic HF. In an HF patient, the presence of an enlarged left atrium without mitral valve disease suggests diastolic HF.[8]

In systolic HF, there is an impaired contraction of the LV, whereas in diastolic HF the LV muscle suffers from impaired relaxation, which increases LV end diastolic pressures.[8] In both cases, activation of compensatory mechanisms results in LV remodeling, increased dysfunction and changes in LV geometry (e.g. dilation, increased sphericity, mitral valve regurgitation).[8] Compensatory mechanisms affect multiple organ systems, and can be evidenced by changes such as increased renin secretion, increased sympathetic nervous system tone, salt and water retention, etc.[8]

Risk Factors

Multiple risk factors have been associated with HF. Chronic arterial hypertension, arrhythmias, congenital heart disease, diabetes mellitus, myocardial infarction and cardiomyopathy are among the most frequent.[2] Other associated factors include dyslipidemia, endothelial inflammation, alcohol abuse, cigarette smoking, micronutrient deficiency and a family history of cardiovascular disease or HF.[2]

Gender Differences

In the United States, the prevalence of HF is about 1.98% in Caucasian women, 3% in African-American women and 1.8% in Mexican-American women. Asian women have a lower prevalence, although this could be because of incomplete statistics for this group.[9]

The Health, Aging and Body Composition Study tracked heart failure incidence for 60 months and suggested that both Caucasian and African-American women displayed a lower incidence of HF than men.[10] In a community-based study, HF was estimated to have an annual mortality of about 21% for men and 17% for women.[11] Women usually have smaller and stiffer hearts, smaller stroke volume and higher resting heart rates when compared to men.[12] Female patients also have smaller coronary arteries with less collateral circulation.[12] These differences can affect heart physiology and may partly account for the differences in HF progression between both sexes.[9]

Specific co-morbidities are also more common in one gender than the other. Women with HF tend to present with more hypertension, diabetes and a preserved LV ejection fraction, whereas men are more likely to have ischemic heart disease and myocardial infarction.[13] Diastolic heart failure is seen more often in elderly postmenopausal women, since it is associated with hypertension, obesity and diabetes mellitus, whereas systolic heart failure is seen more commonly in men because of its association with coronary artery disease.[13]

Takotsubo Cardiomyopathy

Takotsubo cardiomyopathy is becoming increasingly recognized as a mechanism of acute HF. Most commonly presenting in postmenopausal women, Takotsubo cardiomyopathy is a transient condition characterized by apical ballooning and ventricular systolic dysfunction that is accelerated by physical and/or emotional stress.[14] The most common patient symptom is chest pain followed by dyspnea. Acute HF is common in Takotsubo cardiomyopathy, and it may manifest as pulmonary edema or cardiogenic shock.[15]

Diagnosis of Heart Failure

Heart failure can result from any cardiomyopathy that injures the heart.[4] Diagnosing HF requires a thorough physical examination, a detailed patient history and multiple investigative tests to identify and contribute to a clinical diagnosis.[16] These include a 12-lead resting ECG, plasma BNP/NT-proBNP concentration, transthoracic echocardiography, exercise testing, ECG monitoring and coronary arteriography.[17] Progressively increasing fatigue and shortness of breath, orthopnea, paroxysmal nocturnal dyspnea and nocturia are some of the frequent symptoms associated with HF.[9] Neurologic symptoms, such as disorientation, confusion and altered mood may be observed as well if there is reduced cerebral perfusion. Abdominal pain (due to liver capsule distension) and other gastrointestinal symptoms (due to bowel edema) can also be observed.[18] Signs of HF include peripheral edema, jugular venous distension and a displaced point of maximal impulse. Peripheral edema may be manifested as hepatomegaly, ascites, scrotal edema, pitting edema of the legs, S3 gallop, pulmonary congestion and pleural effusion (usually right-sided).[9] The presence of resting sinus tachycardia, peripheral vasoconstriction and reduced pulse pressure are associated with severe HF.[9]

Identifying biomarkers for HF is important for diagnostic and therapeutic purposes. An ideal biomarker should be specific and sensitive enough to monitor changes in the disease's progression, as well as noninvasive, and have low cost.[19] Biomarkers for HF can be broadly categorized into myocardial stress (BNP, NT-proBNP), damage (troponins and heart-type fatty-acid binding protein (H-FABP)), extracellular matrix (matrix metalloproteinase (MMP) and galectin-3), oxidative stress (8-hydroxy-2'-deoxyguanosine

(8-OHdG)), inflammation (C-reactive protein and pentraxin-3), and renal function markers (creatinine and cystitis C).[19] Taken altogether, these biomarkers have shown to provide accurate assessments for prognosis and risk stratification.[19]

Management of Heart Failure

Primary prevention of HF consists of early diagnosis and treatment of the underlying causes and risk factors (cardiovascular, noncardiovascular or patient-related).[20] Secondary prevention consists of preventing chronic HF decompensation that may be a cause of mortality or hospitalization. Recurrence of acute HF episodes causes further impairment in cardiac and kidney function, which in turn deteriorates the patient's clinical outcome.[20] Current AHA guidelines have outlined management goals for each stage of HF. Recommendations for stage A include management of hypertension, metabolic syndrome and dyslipidemia, smoking cessation and regular exercise, discouragement of alcohol intake and illicit drug use, and treatment with ACE inhibitors for vascular disease or diabetes, with statins if appropriate.[18] Stage B entails all measures from stage A along with the use of beta-blockers as appropriate and implantable defibrillators, valve surgery or revascularization in selected patients.[18] Stage C entails all measures from stages A and B along with diuretics, ACE inhibitors/beta-blockers and digitalis in selected patients.[18] Guideline-based indications should be followed for resynchronization therapy, implantable defibrillators or surgery. Finally, stage D includes advanced care measures, including heart transplant and permanent mechanical circulatory support, among others.[18,21,22]

Interventional Management

Some patients with HF are suitable candidates for implantable cardioverter defibrillators (ICD) or cardiac resynchronization therapy (CRT). These devices have been shown to increase survival and improve morbidity in some patient populations with chronic HF when used in conjunction with pharmacological therapy.[7]

Currently, the only curative treatment for end-stage HF is heart transplantation, with a survival rate of roughly 50% after 10 years.[23] However, despite the vast number of heart transplants performed each year, the risk of complications and challenges in terms of long-term stabilization are still significant. Immunosuppressive drugs are effective only to a certain extent and have their own adverse side effects.[23]

Ventricular assist device (VAD) therapy is a type of mechanical circulatory support system.[23,24] The main advantage of VADs over transplant is their availability (i.e. there is no waiting list); a patient in need will receive one immediately, provided all the criteria are met. However, as with most developing therapies, there is a risk of complications, including bleeding, infection and thromboembolic events.[25]

Gender Differences in Management

Men and women respond differently to the same HF therapy. For example, a study showed that digitalis therapy is associated with a worse survival rate in women.[26] This can be explained by the fact that digitalis therapy can have a negative impact in the upper ranges of blood concentration levels, which are more often found in women than in men.[26] The Bisoprolol Study showed that if the quality of treatment given to women was raised to the same standard as the one afforded to men, they had a more positive outcome for systolic HF.[27] It also showed that men in the placebo group did significantly worse than women in the placebo group, whereas women in the placebo group had a similar outcome to the men in the bisoprolol treatment group. This suggests that being a woman has a risk-lowering effect similar to treatment with beta-blockers.[27] Hormone replacement therapy has shown some benefits in the clinical course of HF patients; however, the side effects are significant. Therefore, its use as a form of treatment is not frequent.[28,29]

Perioperative Care

Implications of High-Risk Noncardiac Surgery

According to the 2013 ACC/AHA guidelines, HF patients undergoing major surgical procedures have a higher risk of death and hospital readmission.[1] Recently, it has been suggested that HF poses a higher risk than coronary artery disease in patients undergoing major noncardiac surgery.[1] Poor exercise tolerance is one of the three largest adverse perioperative outcome predictors according to the AHA guidelines, with the others being active cardiac conditions and high-risk procedures.[1]

The geriatric population with HF is different in terms of risk assessment, disease presentation and progression, and patient profile. Elderly patients are more likely to present with diastolic HF. Perioperative management of these patients is summarized in Table 4.1. HF is a significant risk factor when it comes to perioperative complications and calls for specific strategies and recommendations to be implemented.[30] Elderly patients are four times as likely to require surgery compared to the rest of the population. Elderly patients undergoing general surgery are also more likely to present with co-morbidities such as cardiovascular disease and have higher rates of perioperative mortality and morbidity.[22] Preoperative screening tests used to determine risk of complications include ejection fraction and natriuretic peptides, stress tests and exercise capacity tests. Patients with significantly decreased LV ejection fraction (<30%) have been shown to have a larger number of perioperative events as compared to patients with moderate or mild LV dysfunction.[31]

Preoperative Evaluation

Generally, there are three aims of preoperative care: (i) identifying and treating potentially life-threatening cardiac disease, (ii) conducting only necessary tests, (iii) implementing appropriate medical therapy and/or interventional strategies. Preoperative evaluation of patients presenting with a history of HF should include a clinical assessment of symptoms and their effect on daily activities, as well as LV function and volume status assessments. Identifying and treating active cardiac conditions (e.g. atrial fibrillation with rapid ventricular response) is also important. Elective surgical procedures should be postponed if HF is a new diagnosis, so that LV function can be properly evaluated and, if possible, stabilized and improved.

In HF patients, optimization of pharmacological therapy should be attempted before elective surgery. Newly prescribed treatment for HF in the perioperative period should ideally be nonaggressive, in order to avoid complications such as bradycardia and hypotension.[6] Patients should be near euvolemic with stable blood pressure and stable end-organ function prior to surgery. Chronic HF is controlled by adjusting therapy

Table 4.1 Heart failure with preserved ejection fraction in the elderly patient[8]

Factors associated with HFpEF in the elderly

- Left ventricular hypertrophy
- Fibrosis and amyloid deposition causing increased stiffness
- Ischemia causing decreased ATP and impaired calcium homeostasis resulting in reduced relaxation
- Increased myocardial collagen content
- Increased arterial stiffness causing higher afterload

Diagnosis of HFpEF

- Symptoms of HF
- Evidence of LV diastolic dysfunction by echocardiography or cardiac catheterization

Perioperative management of HFpEF

Preoperative
- Perform a thorough preoperative assessment with a focus on HF symptoms and their effect on activities of daily living
- Perform cardiac testing if it will change perioperative management
- Echocardiographic evidence of increased left atrial size in the absence of mitral valve disease is a sign of diastolic dysfunction
- Assess current treatments and their associated side effects (e.g. electrolyte abnormalities, volume depletion)
- Discontinue ACEIs and ARBs
- Continue beta-blockers and digoxin

Intraoperative
- Preload decrease can cause profound hypotension due to frequent diuretic use, pre-existing renal function impairment and decreased thirst response to hypovolemia
- Vasodilator and negative cronotropic effects of anesthetic drugs should be managed aggressively
- Careful monitoring of volume status and prevention of fluid overload
- Direct arterial pressure monitoring may be useful
- For major surgery consider central venous pressure, pulmonary artery catheterization or transesophageal echocardiography monitoring
- Avoid hypoxemia and hypercapnia because patients frequently have co-existing pulmonary hypertension
- Avoid arrythmias
- Maintain blood pressure within 10% of baseline levels
- Avoid decreases in diastolic blood pressure due to its association with myocardial ischemia
- Opioid drugs during induction may be beneficial due to their minimal hemodynamic effects
- Regional anesthesia can be used safely, but the associated decrease in vascular resistance should be assessed and managed

Postoperative
- Postoperative ICU care and monitoring in selected cases
- Aggressive treatment of pain
- Prevent hypoxemia and hypercapnia
- Restoration of vascular tone on emergence of general anesthesia or resolution of neuraxial block can precipitate pulmonary edema
- Restart HF treatment when possible

with beta-blockers, ACE inhibitors and loop diuretics. Consistent use of beta-blockers in patients with HF has been shown to reduce mortality in patients with HF and thus should be continued perioperatively.[6] It has also been reported that patients with HF tend to have anemia. Some studies have shown benefits of intravenous iron therapy in terms of surgical outcome; however, randomized trials studying the mortality of these patients are not available. Although an observational study has shown a decreased incidence of major adverse cardiac events after the administration of erythropoietin to anemic patients weekly for 5 weeks before surgery, it cannot confirm a causal relationship between therapy for anemia and improved postoperative results.[6]

Intraoperative and Postoperative Management

In general, perioperative management of HF should be focused on preventing an acute exacerbation of HF.[8] Prevention of myocardial ischemia, arrhythmias and infection is essential. Careful fluid therapy and management of blood loss to avoid anemia is also important. Drugs that depress LV contractility or cause nephrotoxicity should be avoided.[8] General anesthetic agents are often used for patients with HF, although a high proportion of them produce at least some degree of impairment of LV contractility and changes in vascular tone.[8] Opioids tend to be beneficial since they cause an inhibition of adrenergic activation.[8] Arterial oxygenation should be optimized and pulmonary congestion reduced by positive pressure ventilation and positive end-expiratory pressure. For major surgical procedures performed on patients with HF, invasive pressure monitoring is recommended.[8]

Regional anesthesia is another option for HF patients undergoing surgery. There is a slight decrease in systemic vascular resistance under regional anesthesia, which has the benefit of increasing cardiac output.[8] However, this decrease in systemic vascular resistance has a tendency to fluctuate and can be hard to treat if significant. Patients who have transplanted hearts need special consideration since they have increased susceptibility to infection.[23]

Patients with HF are at an increased risk of acute valvular dysfunction, myocardial ischemia, pulmonary edema, ischemia or arrhythmias.[22] These should be treated as they would be in a nonsurgical setting.[22] Fluid management is of utmost importance, since an overload can worsen HF. Fluid administration can be guided by using a pulmonary artery catheter.[31] However, in patients with diastolic HF and poor ventricular compliance, making an accurate assessment of LV end diastolic volume is challenging.[31] An alternative method to monitor ventricular filling, wall motion and valve function is using transesophageal echocardiography.[30]

Postoperative Management

Close monitoring in the intensive care unit is recommended for most elderly patients with acute HF who have undergone surgery. Adequate pain management is necessary in the HF patient; because uncontrolled pain may precipitate hypoxemia (especially in abdominal and thoracic surgery) or myocardial ischemia (due to tachycardia and hypertension).[32] Furthermore, restarting of HF treatments should be done promptly, to prevent an acute exacerbation of HF due to discontinuation of treatment.[32]

Conclusion

HF is an increasingly prevalent, multifaceted disease that results in significant challenges during the perioperative management of elderly patients. Despite great advances in HF treatment that have allowed for improved prognoses and better quality of life, there is still much to be accomplished in terms of preventive strategies and curative methods.

References

1. Yancy CW, Jessup M, Bozkurt B, *et al.* 2013 ACCF/AHA guideline for the management of heart failure: a report of the American College of Cardiology Foundation/American Heart Association Task Force on practice guidelines. *Circulation.* 2013; 128(16):e240–e327.

2. Liu L, Eisen HJ. Epidemiology of heart failure and scope of the problem. *Cardiol Clin.* 2014; 32(1):1–8, vii.

3. Holdright DR, Dayer M, Cowie MR. Heart failure: diagnosis and healthcare burden. *Clin Med.* 2004; 4(1):13–18.

4. Wong CY, Chaudhry SI, Desai MM, Krumholz HM. Trends in comorbidity, disability, and polypharmacy in heart failure. *Am J Med.* 2011; 124(2):136–143.

5. Levy D, Kenchaiah S, Larson MG, *et al.* Long-term trends in the incidence of and survival with heart failure. *N Engl J Med.* 2002; 347(18):1397–1402.

6. Upshaw J, Kiernan MS. Preoperative cardiac risk assessment for noncardiac surgery in patients with heart failure. *Curr Heart Fail Rep.* 2013; 10(2):147–156.

7. Swedberg K, Cleland J, Cowie MR, *et al.* Successful treatment of heart failure with devices requires collaboration. *Eur J Heart Fail.* 2008; 10(12):1229–1235.

8. Bardia A, Montealegre-Gallegos M, Mahmood F, *et al.* Left atrial size: an underappreciated perioperative cardiac risk factor. *J Cardiothor Vasc Anesth.* 2014; 28(6):1624–1632.

9. Taylor AL. Heart failure in women. *Curr Heart Fail Rep.* 2015; 12(2):187–195.

10. Taylor T. *Emergency Ultrasound Guidelines.* 2010:1–38.

11. Roger VL, Weston SA, Redfield MM, *et al.* Trends in heart failure incidence and survival in a community-based population. *JAMA.* 2004; 292(3): 344–350.

12. Matyal R. Newly appreciated pathophysiology of ischemic heart disease in women mandates changes in perioperative management: a core review. *Anesth Analg.* 2008; 107(1):37–50.

13. Meyer S, van der Meer P, Massie BM, *et al.* Sex-specific acute heart failure phenotypes and outcomes from PROTECT. *Eur J Heart Fail.* 2013; 15(12):1374–1381.

14. Sharkey SW, Lesser JR, Zenovich AG, *et al.* Acute and reversible cardiomyopathy provoked by stress in women from the United States. *Circulation.* 2005; 111(4):472–479.

15. Akashi YJ, Goldstein DS, Barbaro G, Ueyama T. Takotsubo cardiomyopathy: a new form of acute, reversible heart failure. *Circulation.* 2008; 118(25):2754–2762.

16. Cowie MR, Wood DA, Coats AJ, *et al.* Incidence and aetiology of heart failure: a population-based study. *Eur Heart J.* 1999; 20(6):421–428.

17. Dolgin M. *Nomenclature and Criteria for Diagnosis of Diseases of the Heart and Great Vessels.* New York, Little, Brown Medical Division; 1994.

18. Hunt SA, Abraham WT, Chin MH, *et al.* 2009 focused update incorporated into the ACC/AHA 2005 Guidelines for the Diagnosis and Management of Heart Failure in Adults: A Report of the American College of Cardiology Foundation/American Heart Association Task Force on Practice Guidelines developed in collaboration with the International Society for Heart and Lung Transplantation. *J Am Coll Cardiol.* 2009; 53(15):e1–e90.

19. Takeishi Y. Biomarkers in heart failure. *Int Heart J.* 2014; 55(6):474–481.

20. Farmakis D, Parissis J, Lekakis J, Filippatos G. Acute heart failure: epidemiology, risk factors, and prevention. *Rev Esp Cardiol (Engl Ed).* 2015; 68(3):245–248.

21. Schocken DD, Benjamin EJ, Fonarow GC, *et al.* Prevention of heart failure: a scientific statement from the American Heart Association Councils on Epidemiology and Prevention, Clinical Cardiology, Cardiovascular Nursing, and High Blood Pressure Research; Quality of Care and Outcomes Research Interdisciplinary Working Group; and Functional Genomics and Translational Biology Interdisciplinary Working Group. *Circulation.* 2008; 117(19):2544–2565.

22. Poldermans D, Bax JJ, Boersma E, *et al.* Guidelines for pre-operative cardiac risk assessment and perioperative cardiac management in non-cardiac surgery. *Eur Heart J.* 2009; 30(22):2769–2812.

23. Garbade J, Barten MJ, Bittner HB, Mohr FW. Heart transplantation and left ventricular assist device therapy: two comparable options in end-stage heart failure? *Clin Cardiol.* 2013; 36(7):378–382.

24. Rose EA, Gelijns AC, Moskowitz AJ, *et al.* Long-term use of a left ventricular assist device for end-stage heart failure. *N Engl J Med.* 2001; 345(20):1435–1443.

25. Slaughter MS, Rogers JG, Milano CA, *et al.* Advanced heart failure treated with continuous-flow left ventricular assist device. *N Engl J Med.* 2009; 361(23):2241–2251.

26. Rathore SS, Curtis JP, Wang Y, Bristow MR, Krumholz HM. Association of serum digoxin concentration and outcomes in patients with heart failure. *JAMA.* 2003; 289(7):871–878.

27. Simon T, Mary-Krause M, Funck-Brentano C, Jaillon P. Sex differences in the prognosis of congestive heart failure: results from the Cardiac Insufficiency Bisoprolol Study (CIBIS II). *Circulation.* 2001; 103(3):375–380.

28. Modena MG, Muia N, Aveta P, Molinari R, Rossi R. Effects of transdermal 17beta-estradiol on left ventricular anatomy and performance in hypertensive women. *Hypertension.* 1999; 34(5):1041–1046.

29. Rossouw JE, Prentice RL, Manson JE, *et al.* Postmenopausal hormone therapy and risk of cardiovascular disease by age and years since menopause. *JAMA.* 2007; 297(13):1465–1477.

30. Hernandez AF, Whellan DJ, Stroud S, *et al.* Outcomes in heart failure patients after major noncardiac surgery. *J Am Coll Cardiol.* 2004; 44(7):1446–1453.

31. Healy KO, Waksmonski CA, Altman RK, *et al.* Perioperative outcome and long-term mortality for heart failure patients undergoing intermediate- and high-risk noncardiac surgery: impact of left ventricular ejection fraction. *Congest Heart Fail.* 2010; 16(2):45–49.

32. Stoelting RK, Dierdorf SF, McCammon RL. *Anesthesia and Co-Existing Disease.* London, Churchill Livingston, 2002.

Dementia

5

Angela Georgia Catic

Key Points

- Dementia is a general term used to describe cognitive decline from a prior level of function that is severe enough to interfere with daily activities. Most common causes are Alzheimer's disease, vascular dementia, Lewy body disease, Parkinson disease with dementia and frontotemporal dementia.
- Alzheimer's disease (AD) is the most common type of dementia and accounts for 60% to 80% of cases. AD affects 15% of individuals ≥65 and 45% of those ≥85 years of age.
- Characteristic histopathologic features of AD include neuritic plaques, extracellular deposits containing Aβ and other proteins, neurofibrillary tangles and intracellular deposits containing tau and ubiquitin.
- Cholinesterase inhibitors (ChEIs) function by increasing cholinergic transmission by inhibiting cholinesterase at the synaptic cleft. Three ChEIs, donepezil, glanatamine and rivastigmine, are approved by the Food and Drug Administration (FDA) for use in early to moderate AD.
- 70% to 90% of patients with Lewy body dementia (DLB) suffer from parkinsonian symptoms, including bradykinesia, akinesia, facial masking, limb rigidity and gait disorders. Patients with DLB can experience severe neuroleptic sensitivity reactions with confusion, autonomic dysfunction and exacerbation of parkinsonism with the use of antipsychotics. Conventional antipsychotics (like haloperidol) should be avoided in patients with DLB.
- Older patients with dementia have an increased risk (41%) of developing delirium during the postoperative period.

Introduction

Dementia, a decline in cognition from a prior level of function that leads to impairment in daily activities, currently impacts 35.6 million individuals worldwide. Understanding the basics of diagnosis and how to differentiate dementia from other common conditions impacting mental status, including delirium and depression, is key to optimizing postoperative care in the elderly. Although all etiologies of dementia share certain features in common, familiarity with the unique characteristics of the most common types of dementia, including Alzheimer's disease, vascular dementia, Lewy body dementia and frontotemporal dementia, will allow increased diagnostic accuracy and appropriate treatment. During the postoperative period, special attention should be given to accurate pain assessment and delirium prevention in patients carrying a dementia diagnosis.

Dementia

Dementia is a general term that encompasses a broad spectrum of cognitive dysfunction. Areas of cognition in which deficits can be present include learning and memory, language, executive function, complex attention, perceptual-motor and social cognition. There are currently 35.6 million people with dementia worldwide and, with the aging of the population, this number is anticipated to increase by 7.7 million new cases each year.[1] To provide optimal care to elders during the perioperative period, it is necessary to possess a basic, working knowledge regarding the diagnosis of dementia, most common etiologies and treatment options.

Diagnosis of Dementia

Although the diagnosis of dementia is best made by primary care physicians or appropriate specialists (i.e. geriatrician or neurologist), it is important for all providers to have a basic understanding of how to diagnose dementia and differentiate it from other common conditions that impact cognition in the elderly. A careful clinical assessment during which information is obtained from the patient and other reliable informants regarding any changes in memory or cognition from baseline, the time course of deterioration, associated symptoms, including gait disturbance, urinary incontinence and headache, co-morbid medical conditions, behavioral issues, substance abuse, medication history and family history of dementia is the first step in diagnosis. If concerns arise during this evaluation, the patient should undergo a thorough physical examination, including a careful neurologic exam, depression screen and mental status testing. A variety of mental status tests are available, but the Montreal Cognitive Assessment (MoCA) is commonly used as it is available free of charge on the internet (www.mocatest.org), is offered in several different languages and is less dependent on culture and education than the Mini-Mental State Examination (MMSE).[2] Routine laboratory testing, comprising a complete blood count, electrolytes, renal function tests, thyroid stimulating hormone, liver function tests and vitamin B12 level should be obtained to evaluate for possibly treatable causes of cognitive impairment including thyroid abnormalities and renal dysfunction. Additional tests such as HIV testing, rapid plasma regain (RPR), heavy metals screen and toxicology can be obtained on an as-needed, individual basis. Genetic testing and cerebrospinal fluid assays are available, but seldom indicated in geriatric patients. The utility of neuroimaging is controversial, but in practice is often performed during diagnostic workup for cognitive decline. The American Academy of Neurology recommends structural imaging with a noncontrast head CT or MRI during routine evaluation of patients with dementia.[3] In contrast, the American Geriatrics Society does not recommend routine imaging. However, they note that imaging may be especially useful in the following cases: onset of symptoms at <65 years of age, sudden onset or rapid progression of symptoms, focal or asymmetrical findings on neurologic exam, concern for normal pressure hydrocephalus or history of recent head trauma.[4]

To optimize perioperative care, it is important to differentiate dementia from other conditions that cause cognitive changes among elders. It can be difficult to distinguish delirium from dementia, especially in the inpatient setting. However, understanding the

Table 5.1 Differentiating dementia versus delirium

	Dementia	Delirium
Attention	Normal until end-stage	Impaired
Consciousness	Clear	Fluctuating
Speech	Ordered to aphasic	Disorganized to incoherent
Onset	Insidious	Abrupt
Duration	Months to years	Hours to days

characteristic features of delirium and obtaining an accurate history of the patient's cognitive baseline is very useful in differentiating the two conditions (Table 5.1). Typically dementia is characterized by an insidious progressive decline; in contrast the hallmarks of delirium include an abrupt onset and a fluctuating course, which is a notable change from the patient's baseline. Depression and pseudodementia can also be confused with dementia as both can present with significant cognitive impairment, with or without alterations of mood in the elderly. Furthermore, even if a patient is determined to suffer depression, it is important to realize that late-life depression is associated with a significantly increased risk of developing dementia in the future and patients should be screened regularly for the development of cognitive deficits.[5,6]

Etiologies of Dementia

There are multiple causes of dementia. However, among patients ≥65 years, the most common causes are Alzheimer's disease, vascular dementia, Lewy body disease, Parkinson disease with dementia and frontotemporal dementia (Table 5.2). Reversible causes of dementia, while rare, are important to consider as patients may improve following treatment. The most common etiologies of potentially reversible dementia include thyroid abnormalities, vitamin B12 deficiency, neurosyphilis and normal pressure hydrocephalus.

Alzheimer's Disease

Epidemiology

Alzheimer's disease (AD), the most common type of dementia, accounts for 60% to 80% of cases.[7] Although there are rare cases of inherited AD that occur in younger individuals, the majority of cases occur after 60 years of age, with incidence and prevalence increasing exponentially with age. AD affects 15% of individuals ≥65 and 45% of those ≥85 years of age. Due to superior longevity, 75% of elderly AD patients are female.[7]

Pathogenesis

While the exact pathogenesis of AD remains unclear, it appears to be related to abnormal metabolism, deposition, and clearance of amyloid-β (Aβ) and tau. The presence of neuritic plaques, extracellular deposits containing Aβ and other proteins, and neurofibrillary tangles, intracellular deposits containing tau and ubiquitin, are characteristic histopathologic features. While rare cases are caused by a genetic defect, the majority of instances occurring in elders are sporadic and of unknown cause.

Table 5.2 Types of dementia and characteristics

Type of dementia	Cognitive symptoms	Motor symptoms	Progression	Brain changes
Alzheimer's disease	Memory, language, visuospatial	Late apraxia	Gradual decline over ~10 years	Plaques and tangles. Global atrophy. Small hippocampal volumes
Vascular dementia	Early impairment in executive function is common. Exact symptoms dependent on location of ischemia	Symptoms dependent on location of ischemia	Stepwise decline with subsequent ischemic episodes	Cerebral white matter lesions
Lewy body dementias	Fluctuating symptoms with characteristic hallucinations and visuospatial deficits	Parkinsonism	Gradual decline. If dementia develops ≥1 year after motor symptoms, it is classified as Parkinson disease with dementia. If dementia develops prior to or within 1 year of motor symptoms, it is classified as dementia with Lewy bodies	Lewy bodies and neurites. Global atrophy
Frontotemporal dementia	Prominent changes in social behavior or personality. Language deficits	None	Gradual but faster than Alzheimer's disease	Degeneration of the frontotemporal lobes. Abnormal protein inclusions in the cytoplasm and nuclei of neuronal and glial cells

Clinical Features

Memory impairment is the hallmark feature of AD and is almost always present at the time of initial presentation. Among patients with AD, declarative memory for events and facts is most significantly impaired, while procedural memory and motor learning can be spared until late in the disease. Early in the disease course, language dysfunction and impaired visuospatial skills are also quite common. Language dysfunction often presents as word-finding difficulties, reduced vocabulary and anomia, and can progress to para-phasic errors, impoverished speech content and impaired comprehension later in the disease course. Deficits in executive function are often subtle in early AD. However, later in the course, patients may suffer from poor insight, reduced reasoning skills, poor judg-ment and an inability to complete tasks. Concurrent psychiatric symptoms are common, with 50% of patients suffering from depression and up to 90% experiencing behavioral and psychiatric symptoms of dementia (BPSD) at some point in their disease.[8,9]

Treatment

Pharmacologic treatment options, which may improve symptoms or delay decline in AD, include acetylcholinesterase inhibitors and memantine, an antagonist at the N-methyl-D-aspartate (NMDA) receptor. Cholinesterase inhibitors (ChEIs) function by increasing cholinergic transmission by inhibiting cholinesterase at the synaptic cleft. Three ChEIs, donepezil, glanatamine and rivastigmine, are approved by the Food and Drug Administration (FDA) for use in early to moderate AD. Donepezil and the rivastigmine transdermal patch are also approved for severe AD.[7] Improvement in cognitive function, global clinical status and performance of activities of daily living (ADL) has been demonstrated with all of the ChEIs.[10-12] Possible side effects include nausea, vomiting, diarrhea and bradycardia due to AV block.[13] If treatment is stopped, the medication should be tapered and cognition reassessed within 3 months so therapy can be resumed if a significant decline is detected.[14] Memantine, approved for moderate to severe AD, has demonstrated improved cognition, global function and ADL performance compared to placebo.[15,16] However, there is debate if memantine results in clinically significant improvements.[17] It is commonly used in conjunction with a ChEI. Possible side effects include nausea, vomiting, diarrhea, dizziness, confusion, and increased anxiety or agitation.[18] The dose should be adjusted for patients with impaired renal function (creatinine clearance <29 ml/min). Importantly, there is no currently available treatment that can reverse or permanently halt the underlying neurodegenerative process. In AD and other dementias, nonpharmacologic management should be included in all treatment plans.

Vascular Dementia

Epidemiology

Although vascular disease is considered the second most common cause of dementia, accounting for 10% to 20% of cases, the relationship between cerebral vascular disease and dementia is poorly characterized.[19] It is estimated that the prevalence of vascular dementia (VaD) among individuals over age 65 years ranges between 1.2% and 4.2%.[20] The incidence of VaD is higher among men than women.[21]

Pathogenesis

There are a large number of possible etiologic mechanisms for VaD, with the most common being small vessel disease or lacunes, chronic subcortical ischemia and large artery infarcts. Small vessel disease or lacunes occur exclusively in the subcortical region and affect the basal ganglia, caudate, thalamus, internal capsule, cerebellum and brainstem.[22] Chronic subcortical ischemia occurs in the periventricular white matter and leads to loss of tissue elements including neurons, oligodendrocytes and myelinated axons.[23] Small artery disease, both due to subcortical ischemia and lacunar infarctions, is most commonly due to lipohyalinosis or microatheroma affecting small penetrating arteries. Risk factors for these etiologies of VaD include aging, hypertension and diabetes. Large artery infarctions are usually cortical, although they can also occur in the subcortical area. Cerebrovascular disease resulting in clinically significant VaD is dependent on the following: (i) volume of lesions, (ii) number of cerebral injuries, (iii) location of cerebral injury, (iv) white matter ischemia secondary to small vessel disease and (v) co-occurrence of AD or another dementing illness.

Clinical Features

Depending on the etiology of VaD, the clinical pattern can be predominantly subcortical or cortical. Subcortical pathology often impacts the frontal lobe and other cortico-cortical circuits leading to focal motor signs, gait disturbances with unsteadiness and falls, urologic symptoms, pseudobulbar palsy, personality and mood changes, including emotional lability and apathy, and cognitive issues, including memory deficits and abnormal executive function. The progression of subcortical VaD may occur in a gradual or stepwise pattern. The clinical characteristics of cortical VaD are dependent on the area of the brain affected. For example, involvement of the medial frontal lobe often results in executive dysfunction and apathy, while involvement of the right parietal lobe can cause hemineglect, confusion, agitation and visuospatial impairments.

Treatment

While ChEIs and memantine are approved for treatment of AD, they are frequently used in patients with VaD and have been studied in this population as well. Cholinergic dysfunction has been well documented in VaD.[24] However, results of studies to evaluate the effect of ChEIs on VaD have been mixed and evidence supporting clinically significant improvement is unclear.[25] Studies of memantine in VaD have been limited in size and number. They have demonstrated improvement on cognitive scales, but not on clinical global impression or activities of daily living.[25]

Management of cardiovascular risk factors, while prudent in all types of dementia, is especially important in VaD. Focus should be placed on optimizing blood pressure and diabetes management. While studies of lipid-lowering medications have not shown a reduction in cognitive decline, the studies were underpowered to show this effect and cholesterol management in accordance with current guidelines is most likely reasonable in elders with VaD.[26,27]

Lewy Body Dementias

Epidemiology

In approximately 50% of patients with Parkinson disease, the characteristic symptoms of tremor, rigidity, bradykinesia and postural instability are accompanied by dementia within 10 years following diagnosis.[28] If the dementia develops at least 1 year after the onset of motor symptoms, it is classified as Parkinson disease with dementia (PDD). If patients develop dementia prior to or within 1 year of the onset of motor symptoms, they are classified as having dementia with Lewy bodies (DLB). These two etiologies account for up to 30% of all dementias.[29,30] While the age of onset is generally earlier than in AD, with a mean age of 75 years, many patients suffer from mixed pathology on postmortem examination.[31,32] Men are affected more frequently than women.[32]

Pathogenesis

Lewy bodies are eosinophilic, intracytoplasmic neuronal inclusions.[33] In Lewy body dementias, these are seen in deep cortical layers throughout the brain, including the anterior frontal and temporal lobes, the cingulate gyrus, the insula, the substantia nigra and the locus ceruleus.[28] Lewy neurites, degenerating neuronal processes that stain positively for ubiquitin and alpha-synuclein, are present in many areas of the brain, including the hippocampus, the transentorhinal cortex, the amygdala and brainstem nuclei.[28] Concurrent deposition of Aβ and tau, as is seen in AD, is also often noted on postmortem exam.[28] Additional structural and neurochemical abnormalities that have been noted include increased density of postsynaptic muscarinic acetylcholine receptors, loss of dopamine levels in the caudate nucleus, loss of neurons in the substantia nigra and decreased binding of 5-HT2 receptors.[34,35,36]

Clinical Features

Consensus criteria for diagnosing DLB were developed by the Consortium on Dementia with Lewy Bodies.[37] According to the parameters, a diagnosis of DLB requires: (i) progressive cognitive decline and (ii) two of the following core features: fluctuating cognition, recurrent, well-formed, detailed visual hallucinations or spontaneous features of parkinsonism or (iii) one of the following suggestive features in conjunction with one core feature: REM sleep disorder, severe neuroleptic sensitivity or low dopamine transporter uptake in the basal ganglia on SPECT or PET. Fluctuations in cognition and levels of alertness affect up to 80% of patients with DLB and can occur early in the disease course.[38] These episodes may be very mild or more significant and can manifest as drowsiness, increased confusion and episodes of staring into space.[39] The periods of fluctuation can last from seconds to days. Visual hallucinations are an early sign in DLB, compared to the other dementias, and affect approximately 75% of patients.[39,40] These are often recurrent, well-formed images of people or animals. However, they can also be more abstract in character. Approximately 70% to 90% of patients with DLB suffer from parkinsonian symptoms, including bradykinesia, akinesia, facial masking, limb rigidity and gait disorders.[41] Tremors are usually less common and severe than in Parkinson disease. Supportive features of DLB that are commonly noted but not specific include repeated falls, syncope, severe autonomic dysfunction, non-visual hallucinations, systematized delusions and depression.[37]

Treatment

Cholinesterase inhibitors are a first-line treatment in DLB and studies have shown positive effects on cognition, as well as fluctuations, psychotic symptoms and parkinsonian symptoms.[42] Memantine, in contrast, has not been found to have significant effects on motor function, cognition or activities of daily living.[43] Importantly, patients can experience severe neuroleptic sensitivity reactions with confusion, autonomic dysfunction and exacerbation of parkinsonism with the use of antipsychotics. Conventional antipsychotics should be avoided in patients with DLB. If it is absolutely necessary to use a neuroleptic, the lowest dose possible of an atypical antipsychotic, such as olanzapine, would be recommended. A geriatric medicine, geriatric psychiatry, or neurology consult should be considered in this situation.

Frontotemporal Dementia

Epidemiology

Frontotemporal dementia (FTD), previously known as Pick disease, includes several variants, including behavioral variant FTD (bvFTD) and primary progressive aphasia (PPA). It is a relatively common etiology of early-onset dementia and is responsible for 20% to

50% of dementia in individuals younger than 65 years.[44] It is the fourth leading cause of dementia, following AD, VaD and LBD, among individuals over age 65 years of age.[45] Although FTD has occurred in patients ranging from age 20 to 80 years of age, the mean age of onset is 58 years.[46] The occurrence in men and women is fairly equal.

Pathogenesis

In general, FTD is defined by degeneration of the frontotemporal lobes and abnormal protein inclusions in the cytoplasm and nuclei of neuronal and glial cells.[47] The specific subtypes of FTD can be classified based on the pattern of protein deposition. The inclusions are comprised of hyperphosphorylated tau protein in approximately half of cases of FTD. Microscopically, microvacuolation and neuronal loss, swollen neurons, loss of myelin and astrocytic gliosis are present. In 40% of cases of FTD, there is a family history of the disease, with 10% to 25% of cases exhibiting an autosomal dominant pattern of behavior. bvFTD is the most prominent subtype, with a strong family history. Genes most commonly exhibiting mutations associated with FTD include C9ORF72, MPAT and GRN.[48]

Clinical Features

While individual features of the FTD variants differ, they are uniformly characterized by prominent changes in social behavior or personality or aphasia. bvFTD, which accounts for approximately 70% of FTD cases, is the most common subtype of FTD.[49] Marked changes in personality and behavior are the diagnostic hallmark of this variant. These changes are a significant shift from the premorbid baseline and can include disinhibition, apathy, lack of empathy, hyperorality, dietary changes, including food fetishes, and compulsive behaviors, including stereotyped speech or repetitive behaviors. Cognitive functions, including memory and praxis, are usually relatively preserved.[50] Cognitive testing is usually significant for intact memory, but impaired executive functions. PPA is a language disorder characterized by changes in the ability to speak, read, write and understand what others are saying. It can be divided into three clinical subtypes: nonfluent/agrammatic variant PPA (PNFA), semantic variant PPA (svPPA) and logopenic variant PPA (lvPPA).[51] To diagnose one of these FTD subtypes, patients must first meet the basic criteria for PPA, including significant damage to language, with limited impairment in other cognitive domains. Second, assessment is performed to clarify in which of the main language domains deficits are present: verbal generation, understanding of words and syntax, naming, semantic knowledge and reading/ spelling. PNFA accounts for 25% of FTD and is characterized by grammatical errors and/or laborious speech in the setting of preserved comprehension.[52] svPPA accounts for 20–25% of FTD and is characterized by impaired naming ability and word comprehension.[52] The production of speech is preserved. In lvPPA, there is impaired ability in repeating sentences, spontaneous speech and single word extracting. Unlike other subtypes of FTD, behavior and personality changes do not usually occur until later in the disease process.[47]

Treatment

At this time, there is no FDA approved therapy for FTD. In contrast to many of the other dementias, medications targeting the cholinergic system are largely ineffective.[53] Memantine has also failed to show improvements in cognition or function.[53] Some studies have suggested the utility of using selective serotonin reuptake inhibitors or serotonin norepinephrine reuptake in treating behavioral disturbances.

Postoperative Care

Special considerations regarding postoperative care in elders with dementia include opti-mization of pain management and delirium prevention. Pain assessment can be challeng-ing in elders with moderate or advanced dementia. It may be necessary to present multiple pain assessment tools before finding one the patient is able to understand. If surgery is nec-essary in nonverbal elders with advanced dementia, an observational pain assessment tool, such as the Pain Assessment in Advanced Dementia (PAINAD) scale, should be utilized.[54] While no particular analgesic administration route is superior in elders with dementia, patient-controlled analgesia should be avoided if the patient is unable to independently understand how to use the pump and decide when to self-administer the medication.

Compared to their cognitively intact peers, elders with dementia have an increased risk (41%) of developing delirium during the postoperative period.[55] Nonpharmacologic delir-ium prevention measures should be employed to optimize cognition, both prior to surgery and during the postoperative period. These include frequent reorientation, allowing family to be present whenever possible, normalization of the sleep/wake cycle, early mobilization as tolerated and ensuring the patient has all necessary assistive devices, including their eyeglasses, hearing aids and dentures. Tethers, including intravenous lines, Foley catheters and telemetry leads, should be minimized as soon as clinically reasonable. Patients should have their bowel and bladder habits assessed on a daily basis to ensure they do not develop urinary retention, constipation or fecal impaction. Optimizing pain management is criti-cal in reducing the risk of postoperative delirium, as undertreated pain is a well-known risk factor for the development of delirium in elders.[56]

Conclusion

With the aging of America, the number of elders suffering from dementia is anticipated to grow dramatically over the next several decades. As many of these individuals will be undergoing surgical procedures, it is important to have a basic understanding of the most common types of dementia, including their diagnosis and treatment. In the postoperative period, close attention should be paid to accurate pain assessment and delirium prevention.

References

1. World Health Organization. Dementia fact sheet No. 362. April 2012. Available from: www.who.int/mediacentre/factsheets/fs362/en/ (Accessed June 30, 2017).

2. Dong Y, Lee WY, Basri NA, et al. The Montreal Cognitive Assessment is superior to the Mini-Mental State Examination in detecting patients at higher risk of dementia. Int Psychogeriatr. 2012; 24(11):1749–1755.

3. Knopman DS, DeKosky ST, Cummings JL, et al. Practice parameter: diagnosis of dementia (an evidence-based review). Report of the Quality Standards Subcommittee of the American Academy of Neurology. Neurology. 2001; 56:1143.

4. American Geriatrics Society. A guide to dementia diagnosis and treatment. Available from: unmfm.pbworks.com/f/American+Geriatric+Society+Dementia+Diagnosis+03-09-11.pdf (Accessed July 19, 2017).

5. Diniz BS, Butters MA, Albert SM, et al. Late-life depression and risk of vascular dementia and Alzheimer's disease: systematic review and meta-analysis of community-based cohort studies. Br J Psychiatry. 2013; 202:329.

6. Barnes De Yaffe K, Byers AL, et al. Midlife vs late-life depressive symptoms and risk of dementia: differential effects of Alzheimer disease and vascular dementia. Arch Gen Psychiatry. 2012; 69:493.

7. Cummings JL, Isaacson RS, Schmitt FA, Velting DM. A practical algorithm for managing Alzheimer's disease: what, when, and why? *Ann Clin Transl Neurol.* 2015; 2(3):307–323.

8. Chi S, Yu JT, Tan MS, Tan L. Depression in Alzheimer's disease: epidemiology, mechanisms, and management. *J Alzheimer's Dis.* 2014; 42(3):739–755.

9. Staedtler AV, Nunez D. Nonpharmacologic therapy for the management of neuropsychiatric symptoms of Alzheimer's disease: linking evidence to practice. *Worldviews Evid Based Nurs.* 2015; 12(2):108–115.

10. Cummings J, Froelich L, Black SE, *et al.* Randomized, double-blind, parallel-group, 48-week study for efficacy and safety of a higher-dose rivastigmine patch (15 vs. 10 cm²) in Alzheimer's disease. *Dement Geriatr Cogn Disord.* 2012; 33:341–353.

11. Birks J. Cholinesterase inhibitors for Alzheimer's disease. *Cochrane Database Syst Rev.* 2006(1):CD005593.

12. Raina P, Santaguida P, Ismaila A, *et al.* Effectiveness of cholinesterase inhibitors and memantine for treating dementia: evidence review for a clinical practice guideline. *Ann Intern Med.* 2008; 148:379–397.

13. Hogan DB. Long-term efficacy and toxicity of cholinesterase inhibitors in the treatment of Alzheimer disease. *Can J Psychiatry.* 2014; 59(12):618–623.

14. Herrmann N, Lanctot KL, Hogan DB. Pharmacological recommendations for the symptomatic treatment of dementia: the Canadian Consensus Conference on the Diagnosis and Treatment of Dementia 2012. *Alzheimer Res Ther.* 2013; 5(Suppl 1):S5.

15. Reisberg B, Doody R, Stoffler A, *et al.* Memantine in moderate-to-severe Alzheimer's disease. *N Engl J Med.* 2003; 348:1333–1341.

16. Grossberg GT, Manes F, Allegri RF *et al.* The safety, tolerability, and efficacy of once-daily memantine (28 mg): a multinational, randomized, double-blind,

placebo-controlled trial in patients with moderate-to-severe Alzheimer's disease taking cholinesterase inhibitors. *CNS Drugs.* 2013; 27:469–478.

17. Schwarz S, Froelich L, Burns A. Pharmacologic treatment of dementia. *Curr Opin Psychiatry.* 2012; 25(6):542–550.

18. Lo D, Grossberg GT. Use of memantine for the treatment of dementia. *Expert Rev Neurother.* 2011; 11(1):1359–1370.

19. Lobo A, Launer LJ, Fratiglioni L, *et al.* Prevalence of dementia and major subtypes in Europe: a collaborative study of population-based cohorts. Neurologic Diseases in the Elderly Research Group. *Neurology.* 2000; 54:S4.

20. Hebert R, Brayne C. Epidemiology of vascular dementia. *Neuroepidemiology* 1995; 14:240.

21. Ruitenberg A, Ott A, van Swieten JC, *et al.* Incidence of dementia: does gender make a difference? *Neurobiol Aging.* 2001; 22(4):575–580.

22. Smith EE, Schneider JA, Wardlaw JM, Greenberg SM. Cerebral microinfarcts: the invisible lesions. *Lancet Neurol.* 2012; 11(3):272–282.

23. Chui H. Vascular dementia, a new beginning: shifting focus from clinical phenotype to ischemic brain injury. *Neurol Clin.* 2000; 18(4):951–978.

24. Jellinger KA. Pathology and pathogenesis of vascular cognitive impairment: a critical update. *Front Aging Neurosci.* 2013; 5:17.

25. Kavirajan H, Schneider LS. Efficacy and adverse effects of cholinesterase inhibitors and memantine in vascular dementia: a meta-analysis of randomized controlled trails. *Lancet Neurol.* 2007; 6(9):782–792.

26. Shepherd J, Blauw GJ, Murphy MB, *et al.* Pravastatin in elderly individuals at risk of vascular disease (PROSPER): a randomized controlled trial. *Lancet.* 2002; 360(9346):1623–1630.

27. Stone NJ, Robinson JG, Lichtenstein AH, *et al.* 2013 ACC/AHA guideline on the treatment of blood cholesterol to reduce atherosclerotic cardiovascular risk in

adults: a report of the American College of Cardiology/American Heart Association Task Force on Practice Guidelines. *Circulation.* 2014; 129(25 Suppl 2): S1–S45.

28. Cosgrove J, Alty JE, Jamieson S. Cognitive impairment in Parkinson's disease. *PGMJ.* 2015; 91(1074):212–220.

29. Vann Jones SA, O'Brien JT. The prevalence and incidence of dementia with Lewy bodies: a systematic review of population and clinical studies. *Psychol Med.* 2014; 44(4):673–683.

30. Fujimi K, Sasaki K, Noda K, *et al.* Clinicopathological outline of dementia with Lewy bodies applying the revised criteria: the Hisayama study. *Brain Pathol.* 2008; 18(3):317–325.

31. McKeith IG. Dementia with Lewy bodies. *Br J Psychiatry.* 2002; 180:144–147.

32. Savica R, Grossardt BR, Bower JH, *et al.* Incidence of dementia with Lewy bodies and Parkinson disease dementia. *JAMA Neurol.* 2013; 70(11):1396–1402.

33. Lewy FH. Paralysis agitans. In: Lawandowsky M, ed., *Handbuch der Neurologie.* Berlin, Springer-Verlag, 1912; 920.

34. Perry EK, Marshall E, Perry RH, *et al.* Cholinergic and dopaminergic activities in senile dementia of Lewy body type. *Alzheimer Dis Assoc Disord.* 1990; 4(2):87–95.

35. Ballard C, Piggott M, Johnson M, *et al.* Delusions associated with elevated muscarinic binding in dementia with Lewy bodies. *Ann Neurol.* 2000; 48(6):868–876.

36. Piggott MA, Marshall EF, Thomas N, *et al.* Striatal dopaminergic markers in dementia with Lewy bodies. Alzheimer's and Parkinson's diseases: rostrocaudal distribution. *Brain.* 1999; 122(Pt 8):1449–1468.

37. McKeith IG, Dickson DW, Lowe J, *et al.* Diagnosis and management of dementia with Lewy bodies: third report of the DLB Consortium. *Neurology.* 2005; 65(12):1863–1872.

38. McKeith IG, Galasko D, Kosaka K, *et al.* Consensus guidelines for the clinical and pathological diagnosis of dementia with Lewy bodies (DLB): report of the Consortium on DLB International Workshop. *Neurology.* 1996; 47(5):1113–1124.

39. Weisman D and McKeith I. Dementia with Lewy Bodies. *Semin Neurol.* 2007; 27(1):042–047.

40. Galvin JE, Pollack J, Morris JC. Clinical phenotype of Parkinson disease dementia. *Neurology.* 2006; 67(9):1605–1611.

41. Aarsland D, Ballard C, McKeith I, *et al.* Comparison of extrapyramidal signs in dementia with Lewy bodies and Parkinson's disease. *J Neuropsychiatry Clin Neurosci.* 2001; 13(3):374–379.

42. Ikeda M, Mori E, Kosaka K, *et al.* Long-term safety and efficacy of donepezil in patients with dementia with Lewy bodies: results from a 52-week, open-label, multicenter extension study. *Dement Geriatr Cogn Disord.* 2013; 36(3–4):229–241.

43. Matsunaga S, Kishi T, Iwata N. Memantine for Lewy body disorders: systematic review and meta-analysis. *Am J Geriatr Psychiatry.* 2015; 23(4):373–383.

44. Cardarelli R, Kertesz A, Knebl JA. Frontotemporal dementia: a review for primary care physicians. *Am Fam Physician.* 2010; 82(11):1372–1377.

45. Arvanitakis Z. Update on frontotemporal dementia. *Neurologist.* 2010; 16(1):16–22.

46. Johnson JK, Diehl J, Mendez MF, *et al.* Frontotemporal lobar degeneration: demographic characteristics of 353 patients. *Arch Neurol.* 2005; 62(2):925–930.

47. Xiao-dong P, Xiao-chun C. Clinic, neuropathology and molecular genetics of frontotemporal dementia: a mini-review. *Transl Neurodegener.* 2013; 2(1):8.

48. Sieben A, Van Langenhove T, Engelborghs S, *et al.* The genetics and neuropathology of frontotemporal lobar degeneration. *Acta Neuropathol.* 2012; 124(3):353–372.

49. Ratnavialli E, Brayne C, Dawson K, Hodges JR. The prevalence of frontotemporal dementia. *Neurology.* 2002; 58(11):1615–1621.

50. Piguet O, Hornberger M, Mioishi E, Hodges JR. Behavioral-variant frontotemporal dementia: diagnosis, clinical staging, and management. *Lancet Neurol.* 2011; 10(2):162–172.

51. Gorno-Tempini ML, HIllis AE, Weintraub S, *et al.* Classification of primary progressive aphasia and its variants. *Neurology.* 2011; 76(11):1006–1014.

52. Johnson JK, Diehl J, Mendez MF, *et al.* Frontotemporal lobar degeneration: demographic characteristics of 353 patients. *Arch Neurol.* 2005; 62(6):925–930.

53. Nardell M and Tampi RR. Pharmacological treatments for frontotemporal dementias: a systematic review of randomized controlled trials. *Am J Alzheimers Dis Other Demen.* 2014; 29(2):123–132.

54. Warden V, Hurley AC, Volicer L. Development and psychometric evaluation of the Pain Assessment in Advanced Dementia (PAINAD) scale. *J Am Med Dir Assoc.* 2003; 4(1):9–15.

55. Hamrick I, Meyer F. Perioperative management of delirium and dementia in the geriatric surgical patient. *Langenbecks Arch Surg.* 2013; 398(7):947–955.

56. Morrison RS, Magaziner J, Gilbert M, *et al.* Relationship between pain and opioid analgesics on the development of delirium following hip fracture. *J Gerontol A Biol Sci Med Sci.* 2003; 58(1):76–81.

Postoperative Cognitive Issues

Christopher G. Hughes and Charles H. Brown IV

Key Points

- Diagnostic features of delirium include: disturbance in attention and awareness, acute onset and fluctuating course, and disordered cognition, not better explained by another neurocognitive disorder or severely reduced arousal. Delirium is associated with important long-term consequences, including mortality, morbidity and need for extended care.
- Three subtypes of delirium have been described based on psychomotor features: hypoactive, hyperactive and mixed delirium. Outcomes have been demonstrated to be poor after both hypoactive and hyperactive delirium.
- Incidence of delirium is highest after cardiac surgery (12–52%) and following traumatic hip fracture (13–40%). Hypoactive delirium comprises between 57–78% of delirious episodes and may often be overlooked.
- Etiology of delirium is multifactorial and hypotheses include changes in neurotransmitters (particularly cholinergic deficiency and/or dopamine excess), increased neuroinflammation, changes in cerebral perfusion and direct effects of anesthetic agents.
- Perioperative strategies to reduce the risk of delirium include nonpharmacologic delirium prevention protocols, optimization of pain control with multimodal analgesia, ensuring adequate volume status, avoiding deliriogenic medications and consideration of reduction in depth of anesthesia.
- Postoperative cognitive dysfunction (POCD) is a reduction in memory, concentration and information processing compared to the preoperative period. Accurate data on the true incidence have been hampered by heterogeneous definitions of POCD.
- Baseline patient vulnerabilities are key risk factors for both delirium and POCD. Important common risk factors include: age, lower level of education, baseline cognitive impairment and cerebrovascular disease.

Introduction

There is increasing evidence that postoperative delirium and cognitive decline are common among older adults after surgery. As would be expected, preservation of cognitive status is an important goal for patients, with evidence that older adults with limited life expectancy often place greater weight on preservation of cognitive and functional status than on survival.[1] Nevertheless, neither baseline nor postoperative cognitive status is routinely measured in a rigorous manner,[2] and effective strategies to preserve brain function after surgery are limited. This chapter outlines the epidemiology, causes and consequences of delirium and cognitive decline after surgery, as well as potential perioperative strategies to reduce these complications.

Postoperative Delirium

Definition and Diagnosis

The gold standard for delirium diagnosis is a comprehensive psychiatric evaluation using criteria based on the 5th edition of the *Diagnostic and Statistical Manual of Mental Disorders* (DSM) from the American Psychiatric Association.[3] Key diagnostic features of DSM-5-based delirium include: disturbance in attention and awareness, acute onset and fluctuating course, and disordered cognition, not better explained by another neurocognitive disorder or severely reduced arousal. In the clinical and research settings, several methods have been validated for delirium diagnosis, including the Confusion Assessment Method (CAM)[4] and the Memorial Delirium Assessment Scale.[5] The CAM (Table 6.1) was derived from key DSM criteria and can be administered by nonphysicians, with a sensitivity of 94–100% and specificity of 91–94%.[4] The CAM instrument is widely used[6] and has been adapted for several specific patient populations, including intubated intensive care unit patients (CAM-ICU).[7] In the absence of a formal delirium assessment, the sensitivity of delirium diagnosis in routine clinical practice is low (15–31%).[8]

Beyond diagnostic criteria, there are several ways to further classify patients with symptoms of delirium. First, three subtypes of delirium have been described based on psychomotor features – hypoactive, hyperactive and mixed delirium[9] – and, importantly, outcomes have been demonstrated to be poor after both hypoactive and hyperactive delirium.[10] Second, delirium severity may be rated using the Delirium Rating Scale-Revised-98[11] or the CAM-S,[12] and the severity of delirium has been associated with increased hospital length of stay and mortality,[12] among other outcomes. Finally, subsyndromal delirium has been described as occurring when a patient exhibits symptoms of delirium without fulfilling DSM-5 criteria and may presage the imminent development of delirum.[13]

Table 6.1 Summary of Confusion Assessment Method[6] (CAM) diagnostic criteria

Criteria	Explanation
Acute onset and fluctuating course	Is there evidence of change in mental status from baseline, and does mental status change during the course of the day?
Inattention	Does the patient have difficulty focusing attention, such as distractibility?
Disorganized thinking	Is the patient's thinking disorganized, as evidenced by rambling thoughts or illogical flow of ideas?
Altered level of consciousness	Is the patient's consciousness anything other than "alert?"

Epidemiology

The incidence of delirium is likely underestimated in routine clinical practice, and hypoactive delirium is the least well recognized without formal delirium assessment.[8,14] Generally, the reported incidence of delirium using rigorous and validated assessments has been highest after cardiac surgery[10,15,16] (12–52%) and surgery for traumatic hip fracture[17-19] (13–40%), although a high incidence of delirium after other types of surgeries (13–33%) has also been reported.[20,21] Factors that contribute to the wide range in estimates include methodology of delirium assessment, types of surgeries and underlying co-morbidities in patients undergoing distinct types of surgeries.[22] Hypoactive delirium is quite common, reported to comprise between 57% and 78% of delirious episodes.[10,23]

Risk Factors and Pathophysiology

The development of delirium is often multifactorial, involving the interaction of a vulnerable patient with a perioperative insult.[24] Several prediction models for delirium have been developed in both cardiac and noncardiac surgery. In cardiac surgery, the most well-known model[16] incorporates measures of cognitive status, depression, cerebrovascular disease and albumin levels, while in noncardiac surgery, risk factors include age >70, alcohol abuse, poor cognitive or functional status, electrolyte abnormalities, and thoracic or aortic surgery.[25] The importance of baseline vulnerability is further substantiated by reports that frailty, a geriatric syndrome identifying vulnerable patients, is highly associated with postoperative delirium.[26,27]

Nevertheless, the pathophysiology of delirium has not been well defined, and each individual episode of delirium likely results from complex and multifactorial causes. Leading hypotheses for the etiology of delirium include changes in neurotransmitters[28] (particularly cholinergic deficiency and/or dopamine excess), increased neuroinflammation,[29,30] changes in cerebral perfusion[31,32] and direct effects of anesthetic agents.[33] Each of these potential etiologies has been the basis for trials to prevent postoperative delirium, as will be further described below.

Consequences

Although delirium was once thought to be a transient and self-limiting complication, it has become increasingly clear that delirium is associated with important long-term consequences, including mortality,[34-36] morbidity[37] and the need for extended care.[38] Importantly, delirium has also been associated with cognitive decline.[39,40] However, a limitation of the vast majority of current studies is their observational design, so that it is not fully clear whether delirium simply identifies patients with poor postoperative prognosis, or whether delirium contributes to causing poor outcomes. Indeed, the long-term independent effects of delirium have been questioned, with recent evidence suggesting that the association of delirium and mortality may be explained by unmeasured confounding variables.[41] This distinction is critical to determine whether efforts to prevent delirium can prevent long-term consequences. There is some evidence that particular characteristics of delirium (such as severity or reversibility) may be associated with different outcomes, so future work is needed to further examine the importance of delirium characteristics.

Principles of Anesthetic and Perioperative Management to Reduce the Risk of Delirium

General Considerations

Strategies to prevent and manage delirium should encompass the entire perioperative period. Preoperatively, it is important to assess risk for delirium in older adults in order to optimize both intra- and postoperative prevention strategies. General anesthetic principles include optimization of volume status, avoidance of electrolyte abnormalities, pain control and limiting potential triggering agents.[42] Guidelines for prevention and management of delirium have been developed by the American Geriatrics Society[43] (recommendations summarized in Table 6.2), the Society of Critical Medicine[44] and the National Institute for Health and Care Excellence.[45]

Nonpharmacologic Approaches

The strongest evidence for delirium prevention in hospitalized patients is structured clinical protocols such as the Hospital Elder Life Program,[46] which focuses on reducing cognitive impairment, sleep deprivation, immobility, visual impairment, hearing impairment and dehydration. The evidence is less strong after surgery, but several trials in surgical patients have been effective.[47,48] Proactive geriatric consultation has been shown to reduce the incidence of delirium after hip fracture surgery.[49]

Pain Management and Sedation

It is important to control postoperative pain in older adults, with higher baseline and postoperative pain scores independently associated with delirium.[50,51] Opioids are a

Table 6.2 Summary of pertinent recommendations from the American Geriatrics Society guidelines on postoperative delirium[43]

Recommendation	Strength	Quality
Implement multicomponent nonpharmacologic intervention programs delivered by an interdisciplinary team for the entire hospitalization for at-risk older adults	Strong	Moderate
Optimize postoperative pain control, preferably with nonopioid pain medications	Strong	Low
Avoid medications that induce postoperative delirium	Strong	Low
Avoid newly prescribing cholinesterase inhibitors	Strong	Low
Do not prescribe antipsychotic or benzodiazepine medications for treatment of postoperative delirium in patients who are not agitated or a potential harm to self or others	Strong	Low
Consider a regional anesthetic technique to improve pain control and prevent postoperative delirium	Weak	Low
For treatment of agitated delirium, antipsychotic agents may be used at the lowest effective dose for the shortest possible duration. Avoid benzodiazepines as first-line treatment for agitated delirium	Weak	Low
Depth of anesthesia monitors may be used	Insufficient	Low
There is insufficient evidence to recommend for or against (a) prophylactic antipsychotic medications or (b) specialized hospital units	N/A	Low

mainstay, but are potentially deliriogenic, so multimodal analgesia should be considered, as some trials have shown benefit for both nonopioid medications[52,53] and regional anesthesia.[54,55] Among opioids, meperidine has been associated with the development of postoperative delirium and should be avoided,[56] while differences in other opioids appear small.[57] Benzodiazepines have been consistently associated with the development of postoperative delirium in both medical and surgical populations,[56,58,59] and thus should be given sparingly, especially if long-acting. However, older patients are at high risk for alcohol abuse and withdrawal, and pertinent history should be obtained, which may warrant benzodiazepines to prevent withdrawal. For postoperative sedation, several studies have demonstrated a potential benefit to dexmedetomidine, but further studies are needed.[58,60]

Other Important Drugs Affecting the Risk of Delirium

Generally, polypharmacy is to be avoided in older adults given multiple drug interactions that can have deleterious central nervous system effects.[61] The Beers Criteria list drugs that are potentially inappropriate for older adults,[62] and in the perioperative period, the most pertinent drugs to avoid are those with anticholinergic effects (including diphenhydramine)[56], benzodiazepines and meperidine.

The results of trials examining prophylactic antipsychotic agents to reduce the incidence of delirium have been inconsistent,[63,64] and for the ICU population, recent guidelines from the Society of Critical Care Medicine[44] and American Geriatrics Society[43] provide no recommendation for using either haloperidol or atypical antipsychotics to prevent delirium. The anti-inflammatory effects of steroids were recently investigated in a large trial in cardiac surgery patients. Randomization to dexamethasone 1 mg/kg did not result in reduced delirium incidence compared to placebo.[65] Although cholinergic deficiency has been hypothesized to lead to delirium, the prophylactic administration of acetylcholinesterase inhibitors has no benefit in reducing delirium,[66] and when given as a delirium treatment, has been shown to increase mortality.[67] Antidepressants should be continued during the postoperative period, so abrupt withdrawal does not cause an increase in symptoms of depression or confusion.[68]

Depth of Anesthesia and Regional Versus General Anesthesia

Depth of anesthesia may represent a modifiable target to reduce the incidence of postoperative delirium in older adults. Indeed, there is some evidence in laboratory cell models and in animal studies that anesthetic agents may be directly neurotoxic due to multiple mechanisms, including neuronal apoptosis[69] and increased oligomerization and production of Alzheimer's-associated amyloid-β protein,[70,71] and breakdown of the blood–brain barrier.[33]

In elective surgery, studies of regional versus general anesthesia have shown little consistent benefit to regional anesthetic techniques in reducing postoperative delirium.[72,73] On the other hand, in urgent hip fracture repair surgery, a Cochrane review did find that spinal anesthesia may reduce postoperative confusional state compared with general anesthesia.[74] However, a significant limitation of these studies has been failure to measure depth of anesthesia as well as exclusion of the most vulnerable patients. Thus, it is unclear whether the potential anesthetic-sparing effects of regional anesthesia were fully utilized, leading to further studies in which the depth of anesthesia was measured.

Four randomized controlled trials have demonstrated that using a processed electroencephalogram to optimize depth of anesthesia can reduce postoperative delirium.

However, the results may not be generalizable. In one trial, all patients received spinal anesthesia (not feasible for all surgeries) and were extremely vulnerable (dementia prevalence of 35% and 1-year mortality of 25%).[19] In three other studies,[75–77] all patients were exposed to general anesthesia, thereby reducing the ability to create a large difference between groups. Thus, studies in populations that are more generalizable to the vast majority of older adults undergoing surgery are needed, as are studies with greater ability to examine large differences in depth of anesthesia.

Blood Pressure

There is no clear agreement on the effect of hemodynamic management on postoperative delirium, with evidence both supporting[78,79] and refuting[80,81] the importance of hypotension on postoperative cognitive outcomes. Given the common occurrence of intraoperative hypotension in older adults,[73] optimization of blood pressure, and hence cerebral perfusion, may represent a strategy to reduce the risk of postoperative delirium. However, defining hypotension is problematic, with more than 50 definitions in the literature.[82] A wide range of blood pressure at the lower limit of cerebral autoregulation in patients undergoing cardiac surgery has been demonstrated using innovative methods to measure real-time cerebral autoregulation, thus demonstrating the potential for cerebral hypoperfusion in the intraoperative period.[83] On the other hand, elevated blood pressure may also be a risk factor for postoperative delirium, based on studies in both cardiac surgery and hip fracture surgery.[32,84] Further research is necessary to develop strategies to optimize blood pressure management for older adults.

Transfusion

Both anemia and transfusion have generally been associated with poor outcomes after surgery, and delirium is no exception. However, demonstrating a causal relationship is difficult. A recent randomized trial[85] (ancillary to the FOCUS study[86]) demonstrated no impact of transfusion targets of 10 g/dl versus 8 g/dl on the severity or incidence of delirium after hip fracture surgery. Of the largest randomized studies of transfusion triggers in postoperative patients, this trial is important because of the high age of participants (mean age 82 years) with results generalizable to older adults.

Postoperative Cognitive Dysfunction

Definition and Diagnosis

Postoperative cognitive dysfunction (POCD) is a reduction in memory, concentration and information processing compared to the preoperative period.[87] There are no current standardized diagnostic criteria for POCD; however, it is generally considered a mild neurocognitive disorder, which the DSM-5 defines as new deficits in ≥1 neurocognitive domains that do not interfere with capacity for independence in everyday activities (which would be considered a major neurocognitive disorder) and do not meet criteria for delirium, other mental disorders or dementia.[3] Diagnosing POCD, therefore, requires a battery of neuropsychological testing (scores 1–2 standard deviations below the norm are typical for mild impairment) and comparison between preoperative and postoperative testing, but there is no consensus regarding which specific tests should be used. The International Study of Postoperative Cognitive Dysfunction (ISPOCD) group has recommended that POCD batteries focus on memory, attention, sensorimotor speed and cognitive flexibility, and the battery utilized in their studies consists of the Visual Verbal Learning Test, Concept Shifting Task, Stroop Colour–Word Test and Letter Digit Coding Test.[88,89] The reported characteristics and the magnitude of these postoperative impairments are varied due to the lack of standardized diagnostic criteria, inconsistent assessment intervals and utilization of diverse neuropsychological tests. Furthermore, studies examining POCD are often limited by lack of longitudinal assessments, lack of adjustment for potential confounders in the postoperative period and the absence of appropriate control groups, and comparative cognitive outcomes data from postsurgical patients versus other models of cognitive decline are generally lacking in the medical literature. Despite these limitations, POCD is an important concern to patients, families and perioperative clinicians.

Epidemiology

The reported incidence of POCD varies primarily with the type of surgery and age of the cohort examined. One of the earliest prospective studies examined patients >60 years old undergoing major noncardiac surgery, performing a psychometric battery at 1 week and 3 months after surgery.[81] POCD occurred in approximately 25% of patients at 1 week and in 10% of patients at 3 months. Even higher rates of POCD were seen in a more recent study of patients >55 years old requiring major elective noncardiac surgery, with a 54% incidence at 6 weeks and 46% incidence at 1 year.[90] A study of patients undergoing cardiac bypass surgery found cognitive decline in 53% at hospital discharge, 24% at 6 months and 42% at 5 years after surgery.[91] A subsequent study of on-pump and off-pump coronary artery bypass surgery patients found that 50% of patients had cognitive decline 5 years after surgery.[92] A large study that included patients >18 years of age undergoing major noncardiac surgery found POCD to be present in 37% of young (18–39 years old), 30% of middle-aged (40–59 years old) and 41% of elderly (>59 years old) patients at hospital discharge.[93] At 3 months after surgery, these rates decreased to 6%, 6% and 13%, respectively. Additional studies examining lower-risk surgical patients have found rates of POCD ranging from 5% to 20%.[75,80,94–96] Thus, the incidence of POCD in high-risk patients (elderly and cardiac surgery patients in particular) may be as high as 50% up to 5 years after surgery, whereas younger, lower-risk patients have a much lower, but variable, reported incidence. The evolution of POCD symptoms over time has also been examined. Some studies have shown consistent rates of cognitive deficits over months and years,[90,91] while others have shown drastic decreases in rates of POCD from the early postoperative time period to later assessments.[81,93] One cohort study of elderly patients undergoing major noncardiac surgery requiring general anesthesia found a 25% incidence of POCD 1 week after surgery, which subsequently decreased to 10% at 3 months and 1–2 years after surgery.[97] A smaller study found that POCD was common 1 week after cardiac (44%) and thoracic (33%) surgery and that nearly all patients recovered to preoperative levels within 8 weeks of surgery, with up to 25% improving beyond preoperative level.[98] A meta-analysis examining POCD after cardiac surgery found the presence of early POCD, but showed improvement relative to baseline in cognitive measures at 3 months and further improvement at 6–12 month follow-up.[99] These data suggest that POCD is reversible in most patients. Although biases in study design, such as measurement error, practice effect or drop-out, need to be accounted for, these data also raise the intriguing possibility that postoperative cognitive *improvement* may be feasible, potentially due to improvement in health after correction of a surgical condition.

Risk Factors and Pathophysiology

The cause of POCD is unknown and likely multifactorial, with pain and inflammatory pathways being proposed mechanisms, similar to postoperative delirium and potentially paralleling the acute brain dysfunction and long-term cognitive impairment witnessed in patients with critical illness. To date, the majority of published studies have focused on POCD incidence and risk factors. When examining risks for POCD, factors can be separated into baseline patient characteristics, operative surgical and anesthetic techniques, and the postoperative course (Table 6.3). The baseline patient characteristics most associated with POCD, according to large prospective studies, include advancing age, lower education level, cerebrovascular disease and preoperative cognitive impairment.[81,93,100] For example, a recent study of hip joint replacement patients performed a neuropsychological battery before surgery and at three time points postoperatively and demonstrated that patients with pre-existing cognitive impairment have an increased incidence of POCD and cognitive decline up to 1 year after surgery.[95]

The contribution of operative factors to POCD is less clear. Some studies have shown that general anesthesia, duration of anesthesia, and surgical factors may play a role in POCD.[72,81,101] Additionally, a prospective cohort study nested within a randomized controlled trial of optimization of anesthesia depth and cerebral oxygen saturation found that POCD was significantly reduced at 1, 12 and 52 weeks postoperatively in patients who received the optimization protocol.[102] The majority of data, however, indicate surgery and anesthesia are not implicated in the development of POCD.[103,104] For instance, cognitive outcomes are similar after invasive surgery requiring general anesthesia versus percutaneous procedures requiring moderate sedation,[105-107] and cognitive outcomes after cardiac surgery requiring cardiopulmonary bypass are similar to those of off-pump cardiac surgery and to those of patients with coronary artery disease without intervention.[108-111] Choice of regional versus general anesthesia for surgery does not alter rates of cognitive deficits.[80,112,113] The results from studies examining depth of anesthesia have been inconsistent, with increased depth of anesthesia resulting in worse,[76] equivalent[75] or improved[114] cognitive outcomes after surgery. Finally, a retrospective study of non-demented and mild dementia patients found no difference in cognitive trajectories in patients with noncardiac surgery, hospitalization for major medical illness or control, and found no correlation with surgery or major illness and progression of clinical dementia ratings.[115] Thus, surgical and anesthetic factors may not be strongly associated with the development of POCD.

Table 6.3 Potential risk factors for postoperative cognitive dysfunction

Baseline Characteristics	Operative Factors	Postoperative Course
Advanced age	General anesthesia	Delirium
Lower education	Anesthesia depth	Infection
Cerebrovascular disease	Cardiac surgery	Critical illness
Cognitive impairment		Additional operations

The patient's postoperative course likely does contribute to the development of POCD. Delirium in the recovery room after general anesthesia portends subsequent delirium in the hospital and impaired cognition at discharge.[116] In elderly (≥60 years old) patients undergoing noncardiac surgery, postoperative delirium was associated with functional decline at 3 months.[96] In cardiac surgery patients, those with postoperative delirium had cognitive decline up to a year after surgery versus patients without delirium (who return to preoperative cognition within days of surgery).[39] Postoperative delirium in the surgical intensive care unit has been associated with a decline in physical and social functioning, and increased dependence in activities of daily living,[117] and survivors of critical illness without pre-existing dementia have a high incidence of global cognition and executive function deficits up to 1 year after discharge, which is most strongly associated with delirium during the hospitalization.[118] Thus, acute brain dysfunction in the postoperative period is a major risk factor for long-term brain dysfunction in surgical patients.

Consequences

A few studies have examined the long-term outcomes from POCD. In a large prospective observational study of noncardiac surgery patients followed for a median of 8.5 years, POCD at 3 months was associated with an increased risk of mortality (hazard ratio 1.63, $p = 0.01$).[119] In addition, POCD at 1 week was associated with a much higher risk of leaving the labor market due to disability or early retirement (hazard ratio 2.26, $p = 0.01$).[119] The same cohort of patients was then studied approximately 3 years later to examine whether POCD was associated with the development of dementia, including Alzheimer's disease, vascular dementia and frontotemporal dementia.[120] No significant association was found between POCD at 1 week or 3 months and subsequent diagnosis of dementia.

Principles of Anesthetic and Perioperative Management to Reduce the Risk of POCD

When confronted with a patient at high risk for POCD, there is currently little direct evidence to guide clinicians in techniques to decrease the incidence or magnitude of POCD. Improvement in physical conditioning and nutritional status preoperatively when able may improve the patient's cognitive resilience to the stress of the perioperative period.[121] Maintaining adequate cerebral perfusion and avoiding overly deep anesthesia in the operating room may prove to be beneficial.[102] Strategies to prevent surgical site infection, promote wound healing and decrease the risk for subsequent surgeries[122] may also reduce the risk of POCD. Techniques to decrease postoperative delirium outlined previously in this chapter may lead to improved long-term brain outcomes as well. Finally, in patients with surgical processes that require intensive care unit admission, adherence to clinical practice guidelines[44] for analgesia and sedative regimens (e.g. adequate treatment of pain and targeted light sedation techniques avoiding benzodiazepines) and use of prevention and treatment strategies for delirium will likely decrease the risk of POCD.

Summary

In summary, delirium occurs frequently after surgery in older adults and is associated with long-term consequences, including cognitive decline. Delirium after surgery results from the interaction of a vulnerable patient and a perioperative insult. Similarly,

POCD occurs frequently, with the highest reported incidence in elderly and cardiac surgery patients. Although POCD may be reversible in the majority of patients, it also may have significant impact on survival and quality of life. Current data suggest that baseline patient characteristics and postoperative delirium are most strongly associated with POCD. Future research into the standardization of diagnoses, characterization of common deficits, mechanisms of delirium and POCD, and strategies to reduce the incidence and magnitude of these complications are required to reduce the public health burden of neurocognitive changes after surgery in older adults.

References

1. Fried TR, Bradley EH, Towle VR, Allore H. Understanding the treatment preferences of seriously ill patients. *N Engl J Med*. 2002; 346(14):1061–1066.

2. Crosby G, Culley D. Preoperative cognitive assessment of the elderly surgical patient: a call for action. *Anesthesiology*. 2011; 114:1265–1268.

3. American Psychiatric Association. *Diagnostic and Statistical Manual of Mental Disorders, Fifth Edition, 5th edn.* Washington, DC, American Psychiatric Association, 2013.

4. Inouye S, van Dyck C, Alessi C, *et al.* Clarifying confusion: the confusion assessment method. A new method for detection of delirium. *Ann Intern Med*. 1990; 113(12):941–948.

5. Breitbart W, Rosenfeld B, Roth A, *et al.* The Memorial Delirium Assessment Scale. *J Pain Symptom Manage*. 1997; 13(3):128–137.

6. Wei L, Fearing M, Sternberg E, Inouye SK. The Confusion Assessment Method: a systematic review of current usage. *J Am Geriatr Soc*. 2008; 56:823–830.

7. Ely EW, Margolin R, Francis J, *et al.* Evaluation of delirium in critically ill patients: validation of the Confusion Assessment Method for the Intensive Care Unit (CAM-ICU). *Crit Care Med*. 2001; 29(7):1370–1379.

8. Inouye SK, Foreman MD, Mion LC, *et al.* Nurses' recognition of delirium and its symptoms: comparison of nurse and researcher ratings. *Arch Int Med*. 2001; 161(20):2467–2473.

9. Yang FM, Marcantonio ER, Inouye SK, *et al.* Phenomenological subtypes of delirium in older persons: patterns, prevalence, and prognosis. *Psychosomatics*. 2009; 50(3):248–254.

10. Stransky M, Schmidt C, Ganslmeier P, *et al.* Hypoactive delirium after cardiac surgery as an independent risk factor for prolonged mechanical ventilation. *J Cardiothor Vasc Anesth*. 2011; 25:968–974.

11. Trzepacz P, Mittal D, Torres R. Validation of the Delirium Rating Scale-Revised-98: comparison with the Delirium Rating Scale and the Cognitive Test for Delirium. *J Neuropsychiatry Clin Neurosci*. 2001; 13(2):229–242.

12. Inouye SK, Kosar CM, Tommet D, *et al.* The CAM-S: development and validation of a new scoring system for delirium severity in 2 cohorts. *Ann Intern Med*. 2014; 160(8):526–533.

13. Cole MM, McCusker JJ, Dendukuri NN, Han LL. The prognostic significance of subsyndromal delirium in elderly medical inpatients. *J Am Geriatr Soc*. 2003; 51(6):754–760.

14. Inouye SK, Leo-Summers L, Zhang Y, *et al.* A chart-based method for identification of delirium: validation compared with interviewer ratings using the Confusion Assessment Method. *J Am Geriatr Soc*. 2005; 53(2):312–318.

15. Koster S, Hensens AG, Schuurmans MJ, van der Palen J. Consequences of delirium after cardiac operations. *Ann Thorac Surg*. 2012; 93(3):705–711.

16. Rudolph JL, Jones RN, Levkoff SE, *et al.* Derivation and validation of a preoperative prediction rule for delirium after cardiac surgery. *Circulation*. 2009; 119(2):229–236.

17. Kalisvaart K, Vreeswijk R. Risk factors and prediction of postoperative delirium in elderly hip-surgery patients: implementation and validation of a medical risk factor model. *J Am Geriatr Soc.* 2006; 54:817–822.

18. Bickel H, Gradinger R, Kochs E, Forstl H. High risk of cognitive and functional decline after postoperative delirium. *Dement Geriatr Cogn Disord.* 2008; 26:26–31.

19. Sieber F, Zakriya K, Gottschalk A, *et al.* Sedation depth during spinal anesthesia and the development of postoperative delirium in elderly patients undergoing hip fracture repair. *Mayo Clin Proc.* 2010; 85:18–26.

20. Benoit AG, Campbell BI, Tanner JR, *et al.* Risk factors and prevalence of perioperative cognitive dysfunction in abdominal aneurysm patients. *J Vasc Surg.* 2005; 42(5):884–890.

21. Ansaloni L, Catena F, Chattat R, *et al.* Risk factors and incidence of postoperative delirium in elderly patients after elective and emergency surgery. *Br J Surg.* 2010; 97:273–280.

22. Brown CH IV, Dowdy D. Risk factors for delirium: are systematic reviews enough? *Crit Care Med.* 2015; 43(1):232–233.

23. Albrecht JS, Marcantonio ER, Roffey DM, *et al.* Stability of postoperative delirium psychomotor subtypes in individuals with hip fracture. *J Am Geriatr Soc.* 2015; 63:970–976.

24. Inouye S, Westendorp R, Sazynski J. Delirium in elderly people. *Lancet.* 2014; 383:911–922.

25. Marcantonio ER, Goldman L, Mangione CM, *et al.* A clinical prediction rule for delirium after elective noncardiac surgery. *JAMA.* 1994; 271(2):134–139.

26. Leung JM, Tsai TL, Sands LP. Preoperative frailty in older surgical patients is associated with early postoperative delirium. *Anesth Analg.* 2011; 112(5):1199–1201.

27. Jung P, Pereira M, Hiebert B, *et al.* The impact of frailty on postoperative delirium in cardiac surgery patients.

J Thorac Cardiovasc Surg. 2015; 149:869–875.

28. Hshieh TT, Fong TG, Marcantonio ER, Inouye SK. Cholinergic deficiency hypothesis in delirium: a synthesis of current evidence. *J Gerontol A Biol Sci Med Sci.* 2008; 63(7):764–772.

29. Dantzer R, O'Connor JC, Freund GG, Johnson RW, Kelley KW. From inflammation to sickness and depression: when the immune system subjugates the brain. *Nat Rev Neurosci.* 2008; 9(1):46–56.

30. van Munster BC, Aronica E, Zwinderman AH, *et al.* Neuroinflammation in delirium: a postmortem case-control study. *Rejuv Res.* 2011; 14(6):615–622.

31. Fong TG, Bogardus ST, Daftary A, *et al.* Cerebral perfusion changes in older delirious patients using 99mTc HMPAO SPECT. *J Gerontol A Biol Sci Med Sci.* 2006; 61(12):1294–1299.

32. Hori D, Brown C, Ono M, *et al.* Arterial pressure above the upper cerebral autoregulation limit during cardiopulmonary bypass is associated with postoperative delirium. *Br J Anaesth.* 2014; 113(6):1009–1017.

33. Acharya NK, Goldwaser EL, Forsberg MM, *et al.* Sevoflurane and isoflurane induce structural changes in brain vascular endothelial cells and increase blood–brain barrier permeability: possible link to postoperative delirium and cognitive decline. *Brain Res.* 2015; 1620:29–41.

34. Gottesman R, Grega M, Bailey M, *et al.* Delirium after coronary artery bypass graft surgery and late mortality. *Ann Neurol.* 2010; 67:338–344.

35. Ely EW, Shintani A, Truman B, *et al.* Delirium as a predictor of mortality in mechanically ventilated patients in the intensive care unit. *JAMA.* 2004; 291(14):1753–1762.

36. Pisani MA, Kong SY, Kasl SV, *et al.* Days of delirium are associated with 1-year mortality in an older intensive care unit population. *Am J Respir Crit Care Med.* 2009; 180:1092–1097.

37. Martin B, Buth K, Arora R, Baskett R. Delirium as a predictor of sepsis in postcoronary artery bypass grafting patients: a retrospective cohort study. *Crit Care*. 2010; 14:R171.

38. House A, Holmes J. Occurrence and outcome of delirium in medical in-patients: a systematic literature review. *Age Ageing*. 2006; 35:350–364.

39. Saczynski JS, Marcantonio ER, Quach L, *et al.* Cognitive trajectories after postoperative delirium. *N Engl J Med*. 2012; 367(1):30–39.

40. MacLullich AM, Beaglehole A, Hall RJ, Meagher DJ. Delirium and long-term cognitive impairment. *Int Rev Psychiatry*. 2009; 21(1):30–42.

41. Gottschalk A, Hubbs J, Vikani AR, Gottschalk LB, Sieber FE. The impact of incident postoperative delirium on survival of elderly patients after surgery for hip fracture repair. *Anesth Analg*. 2015; 121(5):1336–1343.

42. Sieber F, Barnett S. Preventing postoperative complications in the elderly. *Anesthesiol Clin*. 2011; 29:83–97.

43. American Geriatrics Society Expert Panel on Postoperative Delirium in Older Adults. American Geriatrics Society abstracted clinical practice guideline for postoperative delirium in older adults. *J Am Geriatr Soc*. 2015; 63:142–150.

44. Barr J, Fraser GL, Puntillo K, *et al.* Clinical practice guidelines for the management of pain, agitation, and delirium in adult patients in the intensive care unit. *Crit Care Med*. 2013; 41(1):263–306.

45. Young J, Murthy L, Westby M, *et al.* Diagnosis, prevention, and management of delirium: summary of NICE guidance. *BMJ*. 2010; 341:c3704.

46. Inouye S, Bogardus S, Charpentier P, *et al.* A multicomponent intervention to prevent delirium in hospitalized older patients. *NEJM*. 1999; 340:669–676.

47. Lundström M, Olofsson B, Stenvall M, *et al.* Postoperative delirium in old patients with femoral neck fracture: a randomized intervention study. *Aging Clin Exp Res*. 2007; 19(3):178–186.

48. Chen C, Lin MT, Tien YW, *et al.* Modified Hospital Elder Life Program: effects on abdominal surgery patients. *J Am Coll Surg*. 2011; 213(2):245–252.

49. Marcantonio E, Flacker J, Wright R, Resnick N. Reducing delirium after hip fracture: a randomized trial. *J Am Geriatr Soc*. 2001; 49:516–522.

50. Lynch E, Lazor M, Gellis J, *et al.* The impact of postoperative pain on the development of postoperative delirium. *Anesth Analg*. 1998; 86:781–785.

51. Vaurio LE, Sands LP, Wang Y, Mullen EA, Leung JM. Postoperative delirium: the importance of pain and pain management. *Anesth Analg*. 2006; 102(4):1267–1273.

52. Krenk L, Rasmussen LS, Hansen TB, *et al.* Delirium after fast-track hip and knee arthroplasty. *Br J Anaesth*. 2012; 108:607–611.

53. Leung JM, Sands LP, Rico M, *et al.* Pilot clinical trial of gabapentin to decrease postoperative delirium in older patients. *Neurology*. 2006; 67(7):1251–1253.

54. Kinjo S, Lim E, Sands LP, Bozic KJ, Leung JM. Does using a femoral nerve block for total knee replacement decrease postoperative delirium? *BMC Anesthesiol*. 2012; 12(1):4.

55. Mouzopoulos G, Vasiliadis G, Lasanianos N, *et al.* Fascia iliaca block prophylaxis for hip fracture patients at risk for delirium: a randomized placebo-controlled study. *J Orthopaed Traumatol*. 2009; 10(3):127–133.

56. Marcantonio ER, Juarez G, Goldman L, *et al.* The relationship of postoperative delirium with psychoactive medications. *JAMA*. 1994; 272(19):1518–1522.

57. Fong HK, Sands LP, Leung JM. The role of postoperative analgesia in delirium and cognitive decline in elderly patients: a systematic review. *Anesth Analg*. 2006; 102(4):1255–1266.

58. Riker R, Shehabi Y, Bokesch P, *et al.* Dexmedetomidine vs midazolam for sedation of critically ill patients. *JAMA*. 2009; 301:489–499.

59. Pandharipande P, Pun B, Herr D, *et al.* Effect of sedation with dexmedetomidine vs lorazepam on acute brain dysfunction in mechanically ventilated patients: the MENDS randomized controlled trial. *JAMA.* 2007; 298(22):2644–2653.

60. Maldonado JR, Wysong A, van der Starre P, *et al.* Dexmedetomidine and the reduction of postoperative delirium after cardiac surgery. *Psychosomatics.* 2009; 50(3):206–217.

61. Hogan D. Revisiting the O complex: urinary incontinence, delirium and polypharmacy in elderly patients. *Can Med Assoc J.* 1997; 157:1071–1077.

62. The American Geriatrics Society 2012 Beers Criteria Update Expert Panel. American Geriatrics Society Updated Beers Criteria for Potentially Inappropriate Medication Use in Older Adults. *J Am Geriatr Soc.* 2012; 60(4):616–631.

63. Hakim S, Othman A, Naoum D. Early treatment with risperidone for subsyndromal delirium after on-pump cardiac surgery in the elderly. *Anesthesiology.* 2012; 116:987–997.

64. Kalisvaart K, De Jonghe J, Bogaards M. Haloperidol prophylaxis for elderly hip-surgery patients at risk for delirium: a randomized placebo-controlled study. *J Am Geriatr Soc.* 2005; 53:1658–1666.

65. Sauër A-MC, Slooter A, Veldhuijzen D, *et al.* Intraoperative dexamethasone and delirium after cardiac surgery. *Anesth Analg.* 2014; 119(5):1046–1052.

66. Gamberini M, Bolliger D, Lurati Buse GA, *et al.* Rivastigmine for the prevention of postoperative delirium in elderly patients undergoing elective cardiac surgery: a randomized controlled trial. *Crit Care Med.* 2009; 37(5):1762–1768.

67. van Eijk MD, Roes K, Honing M, *et al.* Effect of rivastigmine as an adjunct to usual care with haloperidol on duration of delirium and mortality in critically ill patients: a multicentre, double-blind, placebo-controlled randomised trial. *Lancet.* 2010; 376(9755):1829–1837.

68. Fava M. Prospective studies of adverse events related to antidepressant discontinuation. *J Clin Psychiatry.* 2006; 67(Suppl 4):14–21.

69. Xie Z, Dong Y, Maeda U, Alfille P, Culley DJ. The common inhalation anesthetic isoflurane induces apoptosis and increases amyloid β protein levels. *Anesthesiology.* 2006; 104:988–994.

70. Zhang B, Dong Y, Zhang G, *et al.* The inhalation anesthetic desflurane induces caspase activation and increases amyloid β-protein levels under hypoxic conditions. *J Biol Chem.* 2008; 283(18):11866–11875.

71. Zhang Y, Dong Y, Wu X, *et al.* The mitochondrial pathway of anesthetic isoflurane-induced apoptosis. *J Biol Chem.* 2010; 285:4025–4037.

72. Mason SE, Noel-Storr A, Ritchie CW. The impact of general and regional anesthesia on the incidence of postoperative cognitive dysfunction and postoperative delirium: a systematic review with meta-analysis. *J Alz Dis.* 2010; 22(Suppl 3):67–79.

73. Marcantonio ER, Goldman L, Orav EJ, Cook EF, Lee TH. The association of intraoperative factors with the development of postoperative delirium. *Am J Med.* 1998; 105(5):380–384.

74. Parker MJ, Handoll HH, Griffiths R. Anaesthesia for hip fracture surgery in adults. *Cochrane Database Syst Rev.* 2004(4):CD000521.

75. Radtke FM, Franck M, Lendner J, *et al.* Monitoring depth of anaesthesia in a randomized trial decreases the rate of postoperative delirium but not postoperative cognitive dysfunction. *Br J Anaesth.* 2013; 110(Suppl 1):i98–i105.

76. Chan MT, Cheng BC, Lee TM, Gin T; Coda Trial Group. BIS-guided anesthesia decreases postoperative delirium and cognitive decline. *J Neurosurg Anesthesiol.* 2013; 25:33–42.

77. Whitlock EL, Torres BA, Lin N, *et al.* Postoperative delirium in a substudy of cardiothoracic surgical patients in the BAG-RECALL clinical trial. *Anesth Analg.* 2014; 118:809–817.

78. Yocum GT, Gaudet JG, Teverbaugh LA, *et al.* Neurocognitive performance in hypertensive patients after spine surgery. *Anesthesiology*. 2009; 110(2):254–261.

79. Patti R, Saitta M, Cusumano G, Termine G, Di Vita G. Risk factors for postoperative delirium after colorectal surgery for carcinoma. *Eur J Oncol Nurs*. 2011; 15(5):519–523.

80. Williams-Russo P, Sharrock NE, Mattis S, Szatrowski TP, Charlson ME. Cognitive effects after epidural vs general anesthesia in older adults. A randomized trial. *JAMA*. 1995; 274(1):44–50.

81. Moller J, Cluitmans P, Rasmussen L, *et al.* Long-term postoperative cognitive dysfunction in the elderly: ISPOCD1 study. *Lancet*. 1998; 351:857–861.

82. Bijker JB, van Klei WA, Kappen TH, *et al.* Incidence of intraoperative hypotension as a function of the chosen definition: literature definitions applied to a retrospective cohort using automated data collection. *Anesthesiology*. 2007; 107(2):213–220.

83. Joshi B, Ono M, Brown C, *et al.* Predicting the limits of cerebral autoregulation during cardiopulmonary bypass. *Anesth Analg*. 2012; 114(3):503–510.

84. Wang NY, Hirao A, Sieber F. Association between intraoperative blood pressure and postoperative delirium in elderly hip fracture patients. *PLoS One*. 2015; 10(4):e0123892.

85. Gruber-Baldini AL, Marcantonio E, Orwig D, *et al.* Delirium outcomes in a randomized trial of blood transfusion thresholds in hospitalized older adults with hip fracture. *J Am Geriatr Soc*. 2013; 61(8):1286–1295.

86. Carson JL, Terrin ML, Noveck H. Liberal or restrictive transfusion in high-risk patients after hip surgery. *N Engl J Med*. 2011; 365:2453–2462.

87. Monk TG, Price CC. Postoperative cognitive disorders. *Curr Opin Crit Care*. 2011; 17(4):376–381.

88. Rasmussen LS, Larsen K, Houx P, *et al.* The assessment of postoperative cognitive function. *Acta Anaesthesiol Scand*. 2001; 45(3):275–289.

89. Krenk L, Rasmussen LS. Postoperative delirium and postoperative cognitive dysfunction in the elderly: what are the differences? *Minerva Anestesiol*. 2011; 77(7):742–749.

90. McDonagh DL, Mathew JP, White WD, *et al.* Cognitive function after major noncardiac surgery, apolipoprotein E4 genotype, and biomarkers of brain injury. *Anesthesiology*. 2010; 112(4): 852–859.

91. Newman MF, Kirchner JL, Phillips-Bute B, *et al.* Longitudinal assessment of neurocognitive function after coronary-artery bypass surgery. *NEJM*. 2001; 344(6):395–402.

92. van Dijk D, Spoor M, Hijman R, *et al.* Cognitive and cardiac outcomes 5 years after off-pump vs on-pump coronary artery bypass graft surgery. *JAMA*. 2007; 297(7):701–708.

93. Monk TG, Weldon BC, Garvan CW, *et al.* Predictors of cognitive dysfunction after major noncardiac surgery. *Anesthesiology*. 2008; 108(1):18–30.

94. Ottens TH, Dieleman JM, Sauer AM, *et al.* Effects of dexamethasone on cognitive decline after cardiac surgery: a randomized clinical trial. *Anesthesiology*. 2014; 121(3):492–500.

95. Silbert B, Evered L, Scott DA, *et al.* Preexisting cognitive impairment is associated with postoperative cognitive dysfunction after hip joint replacement surgery. *Anesthesiology*. 2015; 122(6):1224–1234.

96. Quinlan N, Rudolph JL. Postoperative delirium and functional decline after noncardiac surgery. *J Am Geriatr Soc*. 2011; 59(Suppl 2):S301–S304.

97. Abildstrom H, Rasmussen LS, Rentowl P, *et al.* Cognitive dysfunction 1-2 years after non-cardiac surgery in the elderly. ISPOCD group. International Study of PostOperative Cognitive Dysfunction. *Acta Anaesthesiol Scand*. 2000; 44(10):1246–1251.

98. Bruce KM, Yelland GW, Smith JA, Robinson SR. Recovery of cognitive function after coronary artery bypass graft operations. *Ann Thorac Surg*. 2013; 95(4):1306–1313.

99. Cormack F, Shipolini A, Awad WI, et al. A meta-analysis of cognitive outcome following coronary artery bypass graft surgery. Neurosci Biobehav Rev. 2012; 36(9):2118–2129.

100. Selnes OA, Gottesman RF, Grega MA, et al. Cognitive and neurologic outcomes after coronary-artery bypass surgery. N Engl J Med. 2012; 366(3):250–257.

101. Papaioannou A, Fraidakis O, Michaloudis D, Balalis C, Askitopoulou H. The impact of the type of anaesthesia on cognitive status and delirium during the first postoperative days in elderly patients. Eur J Anesthesiol. 2005; 22(7):492–499.

102. Ballard C, Jones E, Gauge N, et al. Optimised anaesthesia to reduce post operative cognitive decline (POCD) in older patients undergoing elective surgery, a randomised controlled trial. PLoS One. 2012; 7(6):e37410.

103. Nadelson MR, Sanders RD, Avidan MS. Perioperative cognitive trajectory in adults. Br J Anesth. 2014; 112(3):440–451.

104. Silbert B, Evered L, Scott DA. Cognitive decline in the elderly: is anaesthesia implicated? Best Pract Res Clin Anaesthesiol. 2011; 25(3):379–393.

105. Evered L, Scott DA, Silbert B, Maruff P. Postoperative cognitive dysfunction is independent of type of surgery and anesthetic. Anesth Analg. 2011; 112(5):1179–1185.

106. Hlatky MA, Bacon C, Boothroyd D, et al. Cognitive function 5 years after randomization to coronary angioplasty or coronary artery bypass graft surgery. Circulation. 1997; 96(9 Suppl):II-11–14; discussion II-15.

107. Lal BK, Younes M, Cruz G, et al. Cognitive changes after surgery vs stenting for carotid artery stenosis. J Vascul Surg. 2011; 54(3):691–698.

108. Selnes OA, Grega MA, Bailey MM, et al. Neurocognitive outcomes 3 years after coronary artery bypass graft surgery: a controlled study. Ann Thorac Surg. 2007; 84(6):1885–1896.

109. Selnes OA, Grega MA, Bailey MM, et al. Cognition 6 years after surgical or medical therapy for coronary artery disease. Ann Neurol. 2008; 63(5):581–590.

110. Selnes OA, Grega MA, Bailey MM, et al. Do management strategies for coronary artery disease influence 6-year cognitive outcomes? Ann Thor Surg. 2009; 88(2):445–454.

111. Shroyer AL, Grover FL, Hattler B, et al. On-pump versus off-pump coronary-artery bypass surgery. N Engl J Med. 2009; 361(19):1827–1837.

112. Silbert BS, Evered LA, Scott DA. Incidence of postoperative cognitive dysfunction after general or spinal anaesthesia for extracorporeal shock wave lithotripsy. Br J Anaesth. 2014; 113:784–791.

113. Rasmussen LS, Johnson T, Kuipers HM, et al. Does anaesthesia cause postoperative cognitive dysfunction? A randomised study of regional versus general anaesthesia in 438 elderly patients. Acta Anaesthesiol Scand. 2003; 47(3):260–266.

114. Farag E, Chelune GJ, Schubert A, Mascha EJ. Is depth of anesthesia, as assessed by the Bispectral Index, related to postoperative cognitive dysfunction and recovery? Anesth Analg. 2006; 103(3):633–640.

115. Avidan MS, Searleman AC, Storandt M, et al. Long-term cognitive decline in older subjects was not attributable to noncardiac surgery or major illness. Anesthesiology. 2009; 111(5):964–970.

116. Neufeld KJ, Leoutsakos JM, Sieber FE, et al. Outcomes of early delirium diagnosis after general anesthesia in the elderly. Anesth Analg. 2013; 117(2):471–478.

117. Abelha FJ, Luis C, Veiga D, et al. Outcome and quality of life in patients with postoperative delirium during an ICU stay following major surgery. Crit Care. 2013; 17(5):R257.

118. Pandharipande PP, Girard TD, Jackson JC, et al. Long-term cognitive impairment after critical illness. N Engl J Med. 2013; 369(14):1306–1316.

119. Steinmetz J, Christensen KB, Lund T, et al. Long-term consequences of postoperative cognitive dysfunction. Anesthesiology. 2009; 110(3):548–555.

120. Steinmetz J, Siersma V, Kessing LV, *et al.*
Is postoperative cognitive dysfunction
a risk factor for dementia? A cohort
follow-up study. *Br J Anaesth.* 2013;
110(Suppl 1):i92–i97.

121. AGS/NIA Delirium Conference Writing
Group, Planning Committee and Faculty.
The American Geriatrics Society/National
Institute on Aging Bedside-to-Bench

Conference: research agenda on delirium
in older adults. *J Am Geriatr Soc.* 2015;
63(5):843–852.

122. Anderson DJ, Podgorny K, Berrios-Torres
SI, *et al.* Strategies to prevent surgical site
infections in acute care hospitals: 2014
update. *Infect Control Hosp Epidemiol.*
2014; 35(Suppl 2):S66–S88.

Renal and Metabolic Aging

Rita S. Patel and Michael C. Lewis

Key Points

- Age-related metabolic changes have a direct effect on the pharmacokinetics and pharmacodynamics of anesthetic drugs; alterations are due to both specific anatomical changes of organs as well as a decrease in physiological function.
- The volume of distribution in the elderly patient is reduced for hydrophilic drugs due to a decrease in total body water, and increased for lipophilic drugs due to an increase in body fat. Increase in total body fat favors deposition of drugs that are lipophilic, increasing the amount of drug found in adipose tissue and increasing the plasma concentration.
- Age-related decreases in hepatic blood flow affect metabolism by decreasing the first-pass metabolism of drugs with high hepatic extraction ratios and reducing the clearance of hepatically metabolized drugs. The greatest effect is seen on those drugs with high extraction ratios.
- The glomerular filtration rate (GFR) as well as creatinine clearance decreases with aging. Creatinine clearance, often used as a measure of GFR, declines even in the face of normal creatinine concentrations.
- In stressful states, for instance with surgery, age-related changes within the tubule lead to a decreased ability to retain sodium, preventing concentration of urine or even excretion of free water. This can lead to an inability to maintain sodium homeostasis, often resulting in dehydration in the elderly patient.
- Older patients are also more susceptible to dehydration due to an attenuation in the thirst response after periods of fasting.

Introduction

Aging is not a pathologic condition. Rather it represents senescence of biologic processes. It has long been noted that there is a tendency towards a decrease in performance of regulatory biologic processes with progressive aging and an inability to maintain homeostasis during stressful conditions.[1] This phenomenon is especially prevalent in those individuals with decreased functional reserve.[2] Functional reserve is the body's ability to compensate for changes represented as physiological or pathological stress.[3] Adequate functional reserve is demonstrated when one can maintain homeostasis during increased physiologic demand. In contrast, decreased functional reserve is said to be present when there is a decline in the ability to maintain a steady state during stress. Often this is due to the presence of co-morbid disease. Functional reserve can vary; not all elderly individuals are alike and interindividual variability is an important factor for consideration when taking care of elderly patients.[2]

The US aging population continues to expand. There is an increasing life expectancy due to improvement in living conditions and advances in medicine.[4] It is predicted that by the year 2030, the populations of those 65 and 85 years of age and older will surpass 74 million and 9 million, respectively.[5] As a consequence of the expanding aging population with increased morbidity it is reasonable to expect a parallel increase in the elderly surgical population. Indeed, it has been estimated that almost half of those aged 65 will undergo surgery at least once in their lifetime.[6]

As the surge in the elderly surgical population[7] becomes a reality there is an increased necessity for anesthesiologists taking care of these patients to understand their changing physiological processes. Clearly grasping the principles underlying the metabolic physiology of the aging patient, and how it is altered from their younger counterparts, will aid in anesthesia decision-making.

The elderly surgical population represents a unique group as compared with their younger counterparts, as age-associated co-morbid conditions can potentially affect perioperative outcomes. Consequently, it is important that an anesthesiologist caring for such a patient is aware of not only co-morbid conditions, but the pharmacology of the medications necessary for treating these ailments. An understanding of how basic age-related changes in physiology affect changes in the pharmacokinetics and pharmacodynamics of older patients is necessary.[2] This chapter aims to focus on the changes in the hepatic and renal systems and their specific effect on the pharmacokinetics and pharmacodynamics of drugs in the elderly.

Pharmacokinetics and Pharmacodynamics

Senescent-related metabolic changes have a direct effect on the pharmacokinetics and pharmacodynamics of anesthetic drugs in the elderly. Such alterations are due to both specific anatomical changes of organs, as well as a decrease in function.

Pharmacokinetics is the process by which a drug is absorbed, distributed, metabolized and excreted. Absorption of a drug depends on the route of administration, and changes in organ system can alter absorption. For example, orally administered medications may be affected by decreases in gastric acid content, decreased motility and emptying, and even reduced blood flow to gastric tissue due to decreased cardiac output.[1,8,9] Although these alterations are seen in the elderly, their impact on altering oral drug dosage are minimal.[1,10]

The distribution of drug within various compartments is also altered due to age-related changes in body composition.[1,9] The volume of distribution in the aging patient is reduced for hydrophilic drugs due to a decrease in total body water, and increased for lipophilic drugs due to an increase in body fat.[1,2,9] Increase in total body fat favors deposition of drugs that are lipophilic, increasing the amount of drug found in adipose tissue and increasing the plasma concentration.[2,9] A reduction in dose is recommended for these types of medication.[2,9] An example of this phenomenon is seen with fentanyl, a highly lipophilic opioid that has a large volume of distribution, which will have an increased plasma concentration, as well as a longer half-life in this population.[7]

Along with the changes described above, there is a decrease in total body protein, a reduction in lean body mass,[7] termed sarcopenia and a reduction in proteins such as albumin that are an essential part of the transport mechanism of certain medications. Albumin is the primary transport carrier protein for most acidic drugs in plasma.[2] With aging, there is a 10–20% reduction in albumin production.[11] Decreased levels of albumin theoretically reduce the amount of bound drug, increasing the unbound and active form of the drug, and therefore enhance the risk of toxicity.[9] α_1-Acid glycoprotein, responsible for transporting basic drugs in the plasma, may be unchanged or slightly elevated in the elderly.[11] This rise may be associated with an increase in inflammatory disease seen with aging.[12] Despite the overall alterations in transport protein binding, the degree of binding is unchanged or only slightly reduced compared to a younger adult, and seems to have little clinical relevance in the absence of severe malnutrition or hypoalbuminemia.[1,11] It has been noted that there is a decrease in plasma cholinesterase production, especially in elderly men, that may result in prolonged actions of drugs such as succinylcholine.[4]

Pharmacokinetics are also affected by decreases in hepatic metabolism and renal clearance. These are discussed in the following sections.

Pharmacodynamics refers to the pharmacological effects of the drug at the receptors of the target organs.[13] The extent of the age-related pharmacodynamic effects can be measured in terms of potency, efficacy, slope of the graph of efficacy range and variability in concentration.[14] Aging affects pharmacodynamics, independent of any co-morbid pathology,[10] and these effects can be at the receptor level or from diminishing functional reserve.[13] A good illustration of this phenomenon can be seen with an attenuated response to β-receptor antagonists as the receptors downregulate with age.[13] Another example is of a heightened response to propofol due to more dramatic fluctuations in blood concentrations than those seen in younger adults.[10,14,15] A general recommendation is to reduce the doses of anesthetic drugs given to the elderly due to changes in the pharmacodynamics at the receptors.[2,14]

It has been estimated that 20–50% of elderly patients are taking many medications, referred to as polypharmacy, due to the co-existence of several co-morbid conditions.[1] Moreover, multiple co-morbid conditions can account for the changes seen in pharmacokinetic and pharmacodynamic properties of medications.[1]

Hepatic Function

Aging affects hepatic structure and consequently function. Cardiac output decreases by approximately 1% per year after the age of 30, leading to a parallel decline in hepatic blood flow of about 60% by the age of 90.[11] Reduction in both splanchnic and hepatic blood flow will occur, regardless of disease, accounting for the decrease in hepatic size from liver involution.[1] Decreased liver blood flow results in a decreased size of the liver. Aging leads to a reduction of 30% of liver weight by the age of 90 years, with liver totaling 2.5% of bodyweight at 50 years and only 1.6% of bodyweight at 90 years.[1,11] Although the overall mass of the liver diminishes with age, the volume within the individual hepato cytes appears to be unaffected between 20 to 90 years of age.[11] There is some controversy as to whether the age-related effects on liver size affect drug metabolism and clearance, the degree of this effect and whether it has any clinical relevance in the elderly patient.[11] Some studies have shown a correlation of decreased liver size with diminished drug clearance, while others have shown no correlation, suggesting there are other factors involved with drug clearance in the elderly.[11] There are no significant changes noted in relation to aging on liver function tests or other routine clinical tests of the liver, suggesting that overall drug metabolism in the elderly is relatively well preserved until at least 80 years of age, in the absence of known liver disease.[1,13]

Metabolism of drugs by the liver occurs in two phases. Phase 1 reactions typically inactivate functionally active drugs to inactive metabolites by processes of oxidation, reduction and hydrolysis. This phase of metabolism is responsible for creating polar metabolites within enzymes such as the cytochrome P450 systems.[1,9] These processes may also lead to functionally active metabolites, termed prodrugs.[9] It is unclear how aging affects phase 1 metabolism by the cytochrome P450 system. It is thought by some that the efficiency of phase 1 metabolism may be lessened in the elderly, leading to prolongation of the half-life of drugs dependent on this phase of metabolism.[9,11] There is variability in the degree of reduction of drug clearance on those that are reliant on phase 1 metabolism, and can result in up to a 30–50% reduction in their clearance.[10] Drugs such as lidocaine and midazolam will have less hepatic clearance as a result of this effect. The quantity of cytochrome P450 enzymes reduced by approximately 30–50% in the elderly compared to younger counterparts.[16] Although there are fewer enzymes available, changes within the hepatic endothelium are thought to contribute to reduced metabolic clearance in the elderly, rather than the functional capability per se of these enzymes.[16]

Phase 2 metabolism by the liver is responsible for converting the products of phase 1 metabolism to a more water-soluble compound, there by facilitating excretion. Phase 2 involves conjugation through addition of polar groups by processes of glucuronidation, methylation, sulfation and acylation.[1,11] Phase 2 metabolism appears to be relatively unaffected by aging, unlike phase 1 metabolism in fit elderly patients,[1,11] although in frail elderly patients reduced conjugation has been observed.[7,10]

In summary, the changes on hepatic drug clearance due to aging have been studied extensively, with questions still remaining as to whether liver function is compromised. The alterations in drug clearance observed appear to be due to changes in hepatic blood flow, liver size and changes in the endothelium, and not due to age-related changes in the enzymes responsible for drug metabolism.[10] The effect of decreased hepatic blood flow affects metabolism by decreasing the first-pass metabolism of drugs with high hepatic extraction ratios and reducing the clearance of hepatically metabolized drugs.[10,16] The greatest effect is seen on those drugs with high extraction ratios, as their plasma concentration will be increased with the decrease in clearance for elimination.[1] The reduction in first-pass metabolism may also affect activation of prodrugs by having a reduced plasma concentration of drug available, leading to a decreased or delayed effect.[10,12]

Renal Function

Age-related structural and functional changes can be seen in the kidneys leading to a consequent compromise in homeostasis.[17] Decreased cardiac output leads to a reduction in renal blood flow and therefore renal size, as seen with the liver.[17] The alterations in renal structure are related to decreases in weight, renal and cortical area, and the number of glomeruli.[18] Kidney size actually increases until 40–50 years, then begins to decline with age.[17] This fluctuation in size is related not just to decreases in glomeruli, but also to tubule-interstitial changes from infarction, scarring and fibrosis.[17–19] Scarring and fibrosis of glomeruli are most notably seen in the cortical zone, with a loss of functioning glomeruli of up to 50% by the age of 80.[4,19] Along with these changes in the number of tubules, there is a decrease in volume and length of tubule, as well as an increase in diverticula and atrophy.[17,18]

Reduced cardiac output and other concomitant diseases in the elderly lead to a decrease in renal flow. There are also decreases in glomerular filtration rate (GFR), as well as creatinine clearance due to increasing age.[10,17,18] A decline in GFR from approximately 130 to 80 ml/min can be seen between the ages of 30 and 80, with an acceleration of the decline after the age of 65.[18] Creatinine clearance, often used as a measure of GFR, also declines in a similar fashion, even in the face of normal creatinine concentrations.[10,12,20] The decrease in GFR is not as great as the decrease in renal plasma flow, creating an increase in filtration fraction and a state of hyperfiltration.[18,19] This can be seen more prominently in the deeper glomeruli and may be an adaptive compensation to help preserve function due to the reduced number of functional glomeruli.[18]

Hypertension and diabetes are co-morbid conditions that are often associated with worsening glomerulosclerosis and arteriolar sclerosis of the afferent, efferent and cortical systems, accelerating the effects that are already in place due to aging.[17-19] The consequences of these co-morbid conditions often seen in the elderly are thought to increase mean arterial pressure, further causing a decline in GFR; however, this may not be clinically relevant until there is a decrease in functional reserve.[17,19]

Typically under nonstressed conditions, aging has little effect on the kidney's ability to maintain fluid balance. Functional reserve of the kidney may be preserved in the healthy older adult, and electrolyte balance is maintained in a similar way to a younger counterpart. However, in stressful states, for instance with surgery, the changes within the tubule lead to a decreased ability to retain sodium, preventing concentration of urine, or even excretion of free water.[17,18,21-23] Because the adaptive responses are lessened, there is an inability to maintain sodium homeostasis, often resulting in dehydration in the elderly patient.[17] These patients are more susceptible to dehydration, not only as a result of a decreased ability to perform these functions, but also due to an attenuation in the thirst response.[21,22,24]

In the aging kidney the remaining functional renal tubules become less responsive to autoregulation from a reduced sensitivity to the hormonal influence of aldosterone, vasopressin and atrial natriuretic peptide (ANP).[17] Increased ANP secretion is responsible for reduction in renin, and therefore aldosterone concentrations, contributing to dehydration and electrolyte imbalances.[21] Suppression of renin compounded with downregulation of the renin angiotensin system contribute to hyponatremia and hyperkalemia often seen in the elderly.[17] Reduction in antidiuretic hormone (ADH) can reduce the ability to respond to decreases in extracellular fluid by concentrating urine.[21,24] Consequences of electrolyte disturbances could impact cardiac function and possibly cause arrhythmias.[23]

In general, healthy older individuals maintain acid–base homeostasis and have normal electrolytes under baseline conditions. However, due to an impaired ability to excrete hydrogen ion load, the elderly are more prone to metabolic acidosis, especially when stressed or when function is further compromised by acute or chronic diseases.[24]

The acute stress response to surgery includes secretion of ADH leading to increased water retention, as well as increased renin and aldosterone secretion, also promoting additional water and sodium absorption, making the elderly patient susceptible to retention of salt and water.[21,22] Caution should be taken with fluid management in the perioperative setting, with close monitoring of fluid balance using blood pressure, pulse rate and urine output as guides.[21,23]

Table 7.1 Physiologic changes of aging and their pharmacokinetic consequences

Pharmacokinetic mechanism	Changes in the elderly	Consequence
Absorption	↑ gastric pH	
	↓ gastric motility and emptying	↓ absorption
	↓ gastric blood flow	
Distribution	↓ total body water	↓ V_D of hydrophilic drugs
	↑ body fat	↑ V_D of lipophilic drugs
	↓ albumin	↑ free fraction of acidic drugs
	↑ a_1-acid glycoprotein	↓ free fraction of basic drugs
Metabolism	↓ hepatic flow	↓ drug clearance
	↓ phase 1 metabolism	↓ biotransformation
Excretion	↓ renal flow	↓ elimination
		↑ adverse drug reactions

Factors such as decreased renal plasma flow and GFR due to aging may affect the pharmacokinetics of a given drug by reducing elimination. These changes in metabolism contribute to the increased rate of adverse drug reactions noted in the elderly population.[10] Up to 40% of adverse drug reactions occur in older patients,[9] and the prevalence continues to rise.[10] Aging itself may only be a marker of co-morbidity rather than a risk factor for these adverse reactions.[10] Increased concentrations of drug may result from either decreased hepatic clearance or from decreased renal elimination.[16] Morphine-6-glucuronide, the active metabolite of glucuronidation of morphine by the liver, is renally excreted, but may in the older patient accumulate in cases of decreased renal function leading to prolonged duration of analgesia and adverse outcomes.[7,25] Adjustments in dosing for medications excreted by the kidneys should also be considered for drugs that will have prolonged half-lives, taking longer to reach steady state.[12]

A summary of the physiologic changes in pharmacokinetics due to aging can be seen in Table 7.1.

Endocrine

The endocrine system and its regulation is not excluded from changes due to aging. Diabetes is prevalent in the elderly population due to many of the metabolic changes associated with aging. It is estimated that about 20% of the population affected by diabetes will be those over the age of 75, with about half of all type 2 diabetics being over the age of 65.[26,27] The factors likely contributing to the higher prevalence of diabetes in the elderly include genetics, sarcopenia and changes in beta cell function, all culminating in glucose intolerance.[27,28] Genetics has been shown to play a role in the development of diabetes in those with a family history of the disease, especially in elderly men.[27] Environmental factors can contribute to the increase in insulin resistance by poor diet and decreased physical activity, compounding the physical changes of decreased muscle mass and increased fat distribution.[27,28] Decrease in beta cell activity, as well as reduced sensitivity of insulin at the tissue receptor contributes to the development of diabetes as well. Beta cell function can decline by up to 25% by the age of 85. In combination with decreased glucose uptake by noninsulin-mediated receptors, these changes may lead to an increase in glucose load for clearance by the renal system.[26-28] Renal clearance of glucose is reduced with aging, further increasing circulating levels of blood glucose.[26] Gluconeogeneis, a homeostatic process by which cells are provided glucose in times of stress or food deprivation, may be upregulated, causing an additional source of abnormally high blood glucose levels.[29]

Overall there may be a decrease in the levels and sensitivity to regulatory hormones in the elderly. Serum levels of thyroid stimulating hormone are reduced due to decreased secretion by the pituitary, contributing to decreased levels of free T3; however, free T4 levels remain unchanged.[30] Hypogonadism contributes to the reduced secretion of estrogen, testosterone and dehydroepiandrosterone (DHEA). Along with these changes, reduction in growth hormone may be the cause of comprehensive changes in body composition.[13]

Conclusions

Caring for the elderly patient, especially in the perioperative setting, can be challenging, with the numerous alterations of the metabolic systems of the body combined with co-morbid conditions often associated with aging. Caution must be used when creating an anesthetic plan for this subset of patients, as the functional reserve may not be preserved, particularly in the frail elderly patient. As discussed in this chapter, a comprehensive understanding of the basic metabolic changes will help with management of the different pharmacokinetic and pharmacodynamic alterations associated with aging, in order to minimize adverse outcomes.

References

1. Klotz U. Pharmacokinetics and drug metabolism in the elderly. *Drug Metab Rev.* 2009; 41(2):67–76.

2. Deiner S, Silverstein JH. Anesthesia for geriatric patients. *Minerva Anestesiol.* 2011; 77(2):180–189.

3. Sharma A, Mucino MJ, Ronco C. Renal functional reserve and renal recovery after acute kidney injury. *Nephron Clin Pract.* 2014; 127(1-4):94–100.

4. Sophie S. Anaesthesia for the elderly patient. *J Pak Med Assoc.* 2007; 57(4):196–201.

5. 2014 National Population Projections: summary tables. 2014; Available at: www.census.gov/population/projections/data/national/2014/summarytables.html. (Accessed July 5, 2017).

6. Tonner PH, Kampen J, Scholz J. Pathophysiological changes in the elderly. *Best Pract Res Clin Anaesthesiol.* 2003; 17(2):163–177.

7. McLachlan AJ, Bath S, Naganathan V, et al. Clinical pharmacology of analgesic medicines in older people: impact of frailty and cognitive impairment. *Br J Clin Pharmacol.* 2011; 71(3):351–364.

8. Grassi M, Petraccia L, Mennuni G, et al. Changes, functional disorders, and diseases in the gastrointestinal tract of elderly. *Nutr Hosp.* 2011; 26(4):659–668.

9. Steele AC, Meechan JG. Pharmacology and the elderly. *Dent Update.* 2010; 37(10):666–8, 670–2.

10. Hilmer SN, McLachlan AJ, Le Couteur DG. Clinical pharmacology in the geriatric patient. *Fundam Clin Pharmacol.* 2007; 21(3):217–230.

11. Butler JM, Begg EJ. Free drug metabolic clearance in elderly people. *Clin Pharmacokinet.* 2008; 47(5):297–321.

12. Crome P. Pharmacokinetics in older people. *Exp Lung Res.* 2005; 31(Suppl 1): 80–83.

13. Turnheim K. When drug therapy gets old: pharmacokinetics and pharmacodynamics in the elderly. *Exp Gerontol.* 2003; 38(8):843–853.

14. Vuyk J. Pharmacodynamics in the elderly. *Best Pract Res Clin Anaesthesiol.* 2003; 17(2):207–218.

15. Kazama T, Ikeda K, Morita K, *et al.* Relation between initial blood distribution volume and propofol induction dose requirement. *Anesthesiology.* 2001; 94(2):205–210.

16. Polasek TM, Patel F, Jensen BP, *et al.* Predicted metabolic drug clearance with increasing adult age. *Br J Clin Pharmacol.* 2013; 75(4):1019–1028.

17. Colloca G, Santoro M, Gambassi G. Age-related physiologic changes and perioperative management of elderly patients. *Surg Oncol.* 2010; 19(3):124–130.

18. Lamb EJ, O'Riordan SE, Delaney MP. Kidney function in older people: pathology, assessment and management. *Clin Chim Acta.* 2003; 334(1–2):25–40.

19. Buemi M, Nostro L, Aloisi C, *et al.* Kidney aging: from phenotype to genetics. *Rejuvenation Res.* 2005; 8(2):101–109.

20. Giannelli SV, Patel KV, Windham BG, *et al.* Magnitude of underascertainment of impaired kidney function in older adults with normal serum creatinine. *J Am Geriatr Soc.* 2007; 55(6):816–823.

21. El-Sharkawy AM, Sahota O, Maughan RJ, Lobo DN. The pathophysiology of fluid and electrolyte balance in the older adult surgical patient. *Clin Nutr.* 2014; 33(1):6–13.

22. Allison SP, Lobo DN. Fluid and electrolytes in the elderly. *Curr Opin Clin Nutr Metab Care.* 2004; 7(1):27–33.

23. Ferenczi E, Datta SS, Chopada A. Intravenous fluid administration in elderly patients at a London hospital: a two-part audit encompassing ward-based fluid monitoring and prescribing practice by doctors. *Int J Surg.* 2007; 5(6):408–412.

24. Luckey AE, Parsa CJ. Fluid and electrolytes in the aged. *Arch Surg.* 2003; 138(10):1055–1060.

25. Keita H, Tubach F, Maalouli J, Desmonts JM, Mantz J. Age-adapted morphine titration produces equivalent analgesia and adverse effects in younger and older patients. *Eur J Anaesthesiol.* 2008; 25(5):352–356.

26. Paolisso G. Pathophysiology of diabetes in elderly people. *Acta Biomed.* 2010; 81(Suppl 1):47–53.

27. Meneilly GS. Pathophysiology of type 2 diabetes in the elderly. *Clin Geriatr Med.* 1999; 15(2):239–253.

28. Geloneze B, de Oliveira Mda S, Vasques AC, Novaes FS, Pareja JC, Tambascia MA. Impaired incretin secretion and pancreatic dysfunction with older age and diabetes. *Metabolism.* 2014; 63(7):922–929.

29. Nin V, Chini CC, Escande C, Capellini V, Chini EN. Deleted in breast cancer 1 (DBC1) protein regulates hepatic gluconeogenesis. *J Biol Chem.* 2014; 289(9):5518–5527.

30. Peeters RP. Thyroid hormones and aging. *Hormones (Athens).* 2008; 7(1):28–35.

Chapter

8

Frailty and Functional Assessment

Dae Hyun Kim

Key Points

- Frailty is defined as a state of increased vulnerability to changes in health status due to decreased physiologic capacity to maintain homeostasis.
- The *frailty phenotype*, often known as physical frailty, is defined using five specific characteristics: weight loss, weak handgrip strength, exhaustion, slow gait and low physical activity. A score is generally given between 1 and 5.
- The *frailty index* is calculated as the count (or proportion) of "deficits" or abnormalities from a predetermined list of symptoms, signs, diagnoses and test abnormalities in medical, physical, psychological and social domains. This is a proportional score from 0 to 1.
- Frailty affects 10% of community-dwelling older adults, with higher prevalence in advanced age, increasing from 4% in 65–69 years to 26% in 85 years or older. The prevalence in surgical patients ranges from 10% in older adults undergoing elective major surgery up to 40–50% in those undergoing oncologic surgery or transcatheter aortic valve replacement.
- Preoperatively, a simple mobility assessment (e.g. TUG test or 5-meter walk test) appears to be the most practical and accurate test to detect frailty in older surgical patients.
- *Prehabilitation* is the process of identifying modifiable components of frailty, such as muscle weakness, mobility impairment, low activity and poor nutrition, and implementing changes that can enhance an individual's functional capacity prior to surgery. It appears that prehabilitation may yield beneficial effects on the length of stay and functional recovery after surgery.

Epidemiology of Frailty in the Aging Population

Frailty is defined as a state of increased vulnerability to changes in health status due to decreased physiologic capacity to maintain homeostasis. This occurs with age-related changes in multiple physiologic systems (brain, endocrine, immune, muscular, cardio-vascular, respiratory and renal) that are accelerated by cumulative effects of diseases interacting with genetic and environmental factors.[1] Frailty affects 10% of community-dwelling older adults, with higher prevalence in advanced age, increasing from 4% in 65–69 years to 26% in 85 years or older.[1] Frail individuals are at high risk of falls, disability, hospitalization, nursing home admission and death.[1]

With a rapidly expanding aging population and advances in surgical techniques, more people are undergoing surgery later in life. Frailty has been recently recognized as a major risk factor for poor outcomes in the older surgical population. The prevalence of frailty in these patients mainly depends on the age and type of surgery, ranging from 10% in older adults undergoing elective major surgery[2] up to 40–50% in those undergoing oncologic surgery[3] or transcatheter aortic valve replacement.[4] Frail individuals may lack physiologic reserves to tolerate the stress of the operation (e.g. anesthesia, hemodynamic change and surgery) as well as in the postoperative period (e.g. pain, polypharmacy, instrumentations, restricted mobility, undernutrition and hospital environment). As a result, these patients are predisposed to operative complications, prolonged hospitalization and postoperative functional decline. For example, 44% of frail older adults died or experienced functional decline over 6 months after transcatheter aortic valve replacement, compared with 15% in nonfrail adults.[5] In these patients, surgical success may not necessarily lead to improved quality of life.[6] To maximize the quality of life and functional independence in older surgical patients, a timely detection of frailty is crucial. Conventional preoperative assessments that focus on a single-organ system (e.g. cardiac or pulmonary risk) or rely on a subjective assessment (e.g. the American Society of Anesthesiologists Classification)[3,7] do not reliably identify frailty. Therefore, anesthesiologists and surgeons should become familiar with frailty assessment and its implications for surgical outcomes.

Emerging evidence suggests that frailty is potentially reversible.[8] Identification of frailty is possible using a validated instrument or a comprehensive geriatric assessment (CGA), which is composed of traditional medical assessment as well as evaluation of functional status, social support and disability (Table 8.1). Targeted multidisciplinary interventions based on CGA and exercise have proven effective in promoting functional gain and independence in community-dwelling and hospitalized populations.[9–13] A similar multidisciplinary approach involving anesthesiologists, surgeons and geriatricians can improve postoperative outcomes in this vulnerable population.

Frailty Assessment in Older Surgical Patients

An Overview of Frailty Assessment

Geriatricians have developed several instruments to assess frailty in clinical and research settings. Although no uniform operationalized definition exists, there are two widely accepted approaches to define frailty: *frailty index*[14] and *frailty phenotype*.[15] The *frailty index* is calculated as the count (or proportion) of "deficits" or abnormalities from a predetermined list of symptoms, signs, diagnoses and test abnormalities in medical, physical, psychological and social domains.[14] These deficits can be flexibly chosen from the available information in clinical and research databases (e.g. medical records or surveys), as long as they are acquired conditions that increase in prevalence with age. The *frailty index* can be also constructed based on CGA (Table 8.1).

The *frailty phenotype*, often known as physical frailty, is defined using five specific characteristics that are obtained via self-report or objective measurements: weight loss, weak handgrip strength, exhaustion, slow gait and low physical activity.[15] As each characteristic is potentially amenable to interventions, the *frailty phenotype* may allow immediate clinical translation. Therefore, the *frailty phenotype* is considered to be a specific medical syndrome of physical frailty within a broader context of frailty.[16] However, the *frailty index* enables better discrimination of outcome risks than the *frailty phenotype*.[17]

Table 8.1 Components of comprehensive geriatric assessment

Domains	Components	How to Measure*	Administration Time
Medical	Multimorbidity	Count of selected diagnoses	N/A (medical record)
		Charlson Comorbidity Index ≥3	N/A (medical record)
	Polypharmacy	Taking five medications	N/A (medical record)
	Malnutrition	Weight loss >10 lbs in the last year	≤0.5 min
		Mini-Nutritional Assessment–Short Form score <8 points	≤3 min
		Serum albumin ≤3.3 g/dl	N/A (laboratory test)
Psychological	Cognitive impairment	History of dementia	N/A (medical record)
		Mini-Cog test (3-item recall and clock-drawing test) score ≤3 points	3 min
		Mini-Mental State Examination score <24 points	5–10 min
	Depression	Self-reported depressed mood	≤1 min
		Geriatric Depression Scale (Short Form) >5 points	≤5 min
	Exhaustion	Positive response (≥3–4 days/week) to any of the following two statements: "I felt that everything I did was an effort." "I could not get going."	≤1 min
Physical	Mobility impairment	Fall within the past 6 months	≤0.5 min
		Timed Up and Go test >15 seconds	≤1 min
		5-meter timed walk in the lowest 20th percentile of the population Men: if height ≤173 cm, time ≥7 seconds if height >173 cm, time ≥6 seconds Women: if height ≤159 cm, time ≥7 seconds if height >159 cm, time ≥6 seconds	≤1 min

(cont.)

Table 8.1 (cont.)

Domains	Components	How to Measure*	Administration Time
	Muscle weakness	Dominant grip strength (kg) in the lowest 20th percentile of the population Men: if BMI ≤24.0 kg/m², grip strength ≤29 kg if BMI 24.1–26.0 kg/m², grip strength ≤30 kg if BMI 26.1–28.0 kg/m², grip strength ≤31 kg if BMI >28.0 kg/m², grip strength ≤32 kg Women: if BMI ≤23.0 kg/m², grip strength ≤17 kg if BMI 23.1–26.0 kg/m², grip strength ≤17.3 kg if BMI 26.1–29.0 kg/m², grip strength ≤18 kg if BMI >29.0 kg/m², grip strength ≤21 kg	≤2 min
	Low activity	Activity level (kcal/week) using the short version of the Minnesota Leisure Time Physical Activity Questionnaire in the lowest 20th percentile of the population Men: physical activity level <383 kcal/week Women: physical activity level <270 kcal/week	≤5 min
Social	Limited support	Lack of informal support from family or friends Lack of access to formal support or care resources	≤1 min
Disability	ADL dependence	Needing assistance with toileting, dressing, eating, transferring, grooming, bathing and walking	≤5 min
	IADL dependence	Needing assistance with housekeeping, meal preparation, shopping, transportation, managing money, telephone and taking medications	≤5 min
	Nagi scale	Difficulty with pulling or pushing a large object; bending over, crouching, or kneeling; raising arms over head; picking up or handling small objects with fingers; lifting 10 lbs; walking up or down a flight of stairs; walking a mile	≤5 min

Abbreviations: ADL, activity of daily living; BMI, body mass index; IADL, instrumental activity of daily living.
*Definitions used in validated frailty instruments for older surgical populations.

Several alternative frailty instruments are available. They are variations of these two approaches or a subset of the components (e.g. gait speed, malnutrition).[18-20]

Frailty Assessment in the Preoperative Setting

The main purpose of preoperative frailty assessment is twofold: (i) improve risk stratification for short-term and long-term postoperative outcomes and (ii) optimize postoperative outcomes through individualized perioperative interventions for high-risk patients. Although preoperative CGA can serve both purposes, it is not practical to administer CGA to every older patient undergoing surgery. CGA is time-consuming and requires a geriatrician or trained member of staff who is capable of performing CGA and formulating treatment plans. Therefore, a more practical approach is to use a simple screening test to identify older adults at high risk for adverse postoperative outcomes, and refer them to a geriatrician who performs CGA for risk stratification and delivers perioperative and follow-up care to optimize health status (Figure 8.1).

Surgical Risk Stratification

Frailty assessment can identify older adults at high risk for adverse postoperative outcomes.[21-24] It seems to outperform conventional risk assessments (e.g. the American Society of Anesthesiologists Classification) that fail to capture frailty and geriatric conditions in risk prediction.[3,7] However, published instruments include different measures of frailty instead

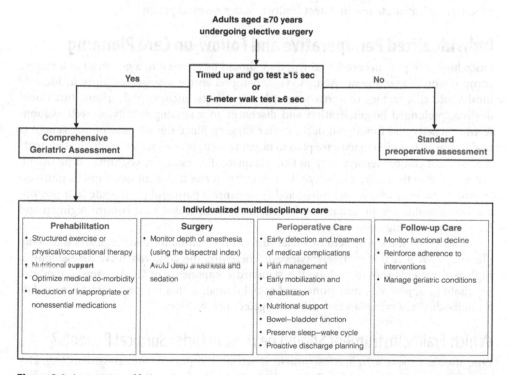

Figure 8.1 An overview of frailty assessment and individualized multidisciplinary care in older surgical patients.

of a standard set of CGA components, and very few instruments have been validated in the population other than the one in which the instrument was developed (Table 8.2).

The current evidence consistently shows that a mobility assessment is a simple, practical test to predict 30-day adverse events as well as 1-year mortality after major surgery. The Timed Up and Go (TUG) test is a simple test that measures the time for a patient to stand from a chair without using their arms, walk 10 feet, return to the chair and sit back down.[25] Robinson *et al.* reported that patients who took 15 seconds or longer on TUG test had a five- to sixfold increased risk of adverse events at 30 days and a six- to ninefold increased risk of mortality at 1 year after colorectal or cardiac surgery.[20] Similarly, poor performance on the 5-meter gait speed[26,27] and 6-minute walk distance[28,29] was associated with short-term and long-term adverse outcomes in older adults undergoing cardiac surgery. When mobility assessment is not feasible, a simple disability questionnaire, such as activity of daily living, instrumental activity of daily living and Nagi scales (see definitions in Table 8.1), can be used to predict adverse outcomes after cardiac surgery.[27,30]

Multicomponent frailty instruments, despite their comprehensiveness, do not consistently provide better risk prediction than a single mobility assessment (Table 8.2). Because mobility impairment is correlated with other characteristics of frailty,[31] assessing additional domains of frailty may add little to risk prediction. A TUG test of ≥6 seconds had 100% sensitivity and of ≥15 seconds had 100% specificity in detecting frailty or a prefrail state.[31] Gait speed measurement seems as good as TUG test in detecting frailty.[31] The 6-minute walk distance may not be practical in a routine clinical setting.

In summary, any frailty assessment can identify individuals at high risk for poor outcomes. A mobility assessment (e.g. TUG test or 5-meter walk test) appears to be a simple, practical and accurate test to detect frailty in older surgical patients.

Individualized Perioperative and Follow-up Care Planning

Once high-risk patients are identified, they should be referred to a geriatrician for more comprehensive assessment. At this stage, comprehensive assessment aims to identify modifiable risk factors of short-term adverse events, including delirium, functional decline, prolonged hospitalization and discharge to a nursing facility, as well as long-term mortality and functional decline after surgery. Since the purpose of assessment is to develop an individualized care plan to target reversible risk factors, frailty instruments that are not comprehensive may not be adequate. For example, cognitive impairment, not assessed in the *frailty phenotype*, is an important risk factor for delirium. Cognitively impaired patients who have limited ability to express pain and participate in a postoperative rehabilitation program may benefit from a scheduled pain control regimen and frequent prompting from carers.

In addition, the assessment of social support is essential for discharge and follow-up planning, but it is not routinely assessed. Therefore, the comprehensive assessment in high-risk patients should include the standard components of CGA, namely, medical, psychological, physical, nutritional and social domains, that are necessary to formulate an individualized care plan and deliver targeted interventions.

Which Frailty Instrument Should be Used in Older Surgical Patients?

One should choose a frailty instrument based on the purpose of assessment (e.g. risk stratification versus care planning) and the amount of effort and resource needed to

Table 8.2 Validated frailty instruments for surgical risk stratification in older adults

Frailty Instruments	Assessment Domain					Surgery Population	30-Day Adverse Events			1-Year Mortality		
	Medical	Psych	Physical	Nutrition	Social		C-statistic	Relative Risk[a]	Absolute Risk[a]	C-statistic	Relative Risk[a]	Absolute Risk[a]
Timed Up and Go test[20]			√			Colorectal	0.78	5.8	13%/77%	–	9.2	3%/31%
Administration time: ≤1 min						Cardiac	0.68	4.6	11%/52%	–	6.4	2%/12%
Category: ≤10/11–14/≥15 s												
5-Meter walk test[26,27]			√			Cardiac	0.64	2.6	13%/35%	–	–	–
Administration time: ≤1 min												
Category: <6/≥6 s												
6-Minute walk test distance[28,29]			√			Cardiac	–	–	–	–	3.6	3%/8%
Administration time: 7 min						TAVR	–	–	–	–	2.8	9%/25%
Category: ≥300/<300 m (cardiac) ≥182/<182 m (TAVR)												
ADL/IADL disability scale[2,30]			√			Cardiac	0.54	1.2 (per 1 point)	–	–	–	–
Administration time: 5 min						TAVR	–	1.6	24%/39%	–	2.7	24%/56%
Category: independent/ dependent												
Nagi scale[27]			√			Cardiac	0.65	1.3 (per 1 point)	–	–	–	–
Administration time: 5 min												
Category: 0–7 continuous												
Frailty phenotype[8,52]		√	√	√		Major	0.70[b]	3.2[b]	20%/44%	–	–	–
Administration time: 10–15 min						Cardiac	0.60	1.4 (per 1 point)	–	–	–	–
No of components: 5						TAVR	–	–	–	–	3.1	–
Category: 0–1/2–3/4–5 (major) 0–5 continuous (cardiac) 0–2/3–5 (TAVR)												

(cont.)

Table 8.2 (cont.)

Frailty Instruments	Assessment Domain					Surgery Population	30-Day Adverse Events			1-Year Mortality		
	Medical	Psych	Physical	Nutrition	Social		C-statistic	Relative Risk[a]	Absolute Risk[a]	C-statistic	Relative Risk[a]	Absolute Risk[a]
Edmonton Frail Scale[53] Administration time: 5 min No of components: 10 Category: 0–7/8–17	√	√	√	√	√	Noncardiac	–	5.0	20%/56%	–	–	–
CGA-Frailty Index–Robinson[54] Administration time: 5 min No of components: 7 Category: 0–1/2–3/4–7	√	√	√	√		Colorectal	0.70	2.8	21%/58%	–	–	–
						Cardiac	0.71	3.4	17%/56%	–	–	–
CGA-Frailty Index–Kim[7] Administration time: 30 min No of components: 9 Category: 0–5/6–15	√	√	√	√		Noncardiac	0.73	4.5	6%/19%	0.82	8.1	2%/22%

Abbreviations: ADL, activity of daily living; CGA, comprehensive geriatric assessment; IADL, instrumental activity of daily living; TAVR, transcatheter aortic valve replacement.

[a] Relative risk and absolute risk comparing frail versus robust category are presented, unless specified otherwise.

[b] Derived from the model that includes frailty phenotype and American Society of Anesthesiologists class.

gather information to measure frailty status (e.g. existing medical records versus in-person assessment by a trained professional). Compared with a simple mobility assessment, a more time-consuming and resource-intensive multicomponent assessment does not provide additional gain in global surgical risk stratification. Given the practicality and high sensitivity, TUG or gait speed measurement is an appropriate screening test to identify frail individuals at high risk for poor surgical outcomes. Among the multicomponent frailty instruments for risk stratification, the *frailty index* that covers more comprehensive health domains may be more useful than the *frailty phenotype* that represents physical frailty in predicting a wide range of postoperative outcomes, such as cardiac and pulmonary complications and delirium.[32] Once a patient is identified as being high risk, a CGA by a geriatrician is recommended to develop an individualized perioperative and follow-up care plan to optimize the patient's outcomes.

Interventions for Frail Older Patients Undergoing Surgery

An Overview of Interventions for Frail Older Patients

The information from frailty assessment and preoperative CGA can be used to design interventions to optimize reversible components of frailty before surgery, prevent and manage complications during the hospitalization, and promote long-term functional gain (Figure 8.1). Although numerous randomized controlled trials have shown a positive impact of CGA and targeted interventions on long-term functional status, nursing home admission, and mortality in older adults living at home or admitted to hospital,[9–11] the effects of preoperative CGA on postoperative outcomes have not been extensively studied.[33] Most evidence comes from single-center-based, pre- and postintervention comparison studies in a small number of patients. Nonetheless, several interventions can be recommended to prevent postoperative complications, reduce the length of stay, and facilitate functional recovery in frail older adults undergoing surgery. Some interventions that have not been evaluated in older surgical patients are also mentioned, according to best practice guidelines.[34]

Considerations in Anesthesia and Sedation for Surgery

Frail older adults with limited physiologic reserve may be prone to the adverse effects of anesthesia, such as hypotension, bradycardia, respiratory depression, aspiration pneumonia and cognitive impairment. Due to the multifactorial nature of most postoperative complications, it remains poorly understood to what extent such outcomes are attributable to the mode and depth of anesthesia. There is inconsistent evidence on the effect of regional versus general anesthesia on postoperative complications. In hip fracture patients, regional anesthesia was associated with lower early mortality, deep vein thrombosis and postoperative confusion compared with general anesthesia.[35] In patients undergoing total hip arthroplasty, postoperative complications did not differ between regional and general anesthesia.[36] There was no difference by the mode of anesthesia in the incidence of delirium and postoperative cognitive dysfunction.[37,38] However, the depth of anesthesia seems to influence the risk of cognitive outcomes. In patients receiving general anesthesia, intraoperative monitoring using the bispectral index (BIS) and maintaining BIS levels between 40 and 60 (versus lower levels) reduced delirium and postoperative cognitive dysfunction by 20–30%.[39,40] Similarly, in patients receiving regional anesthesia, a light sedation protocol of maintaining BIS levels at 80 or higher reduced delirium by 50% compared with deep sedation.[41] Modifying the depth of anesthesia and sedation is an important intervention by anesthesiologists that can potentially improve the surgical outcomes of frail older adults.

Prehabilitation and perioperative care

Optimization of modifiable components of frailty, such as muscle weakness, mobility impairment, low activity and poor nutrition, can enhance an individual's functional capacity prior to surgery so that one can better tolerate the physiologic stress related to the surgery. This process, often called "prehabilitation," appears to yield beneficial effects on the length of stay and functional recovery after surgery (Table 8.3). A randomized controlled trial evaluated a multidisciplinary program that is composed of structured exercise and nutritional support in the preoperative period, combined with proactive pain management and an early rehabilitation program during hospitalization for adults undergoing spinal surgery.[42] The prehabilitation group had better functional status at the time of the surgery, as well as faster recovery after surgery compared with the routine care group. Another trial evaluated a structured exercise program involving a stationary bike and strengthening versus walking and breathing exercises in older adults undergoing colorectal surgery.[43] Unexpectedly, more individuals in the light exercise group had a meaningful improvement in the 6-minute walk test distance than those in the structured exercise group, partly due to low adherence to the structured program. The functional change during the prehabilitation period was an important determinant of postoperative functional recovery.[44]

Other pre- and postintervention comparison studies showed positive results on postoperative complications, functional status, length of stay and frailty (Table 8.3). While most studies focus on prehabilitation, it is noteworthy that the Proactive Care of Older People Undergoing Surgery program includes multidisciplinary prehabilitation, hospital care and postdischarge follow-up care.[45] A modified version of the Hospital Elder Life Program that was originally developed to prevent delirium in hospitalized older adults appears to reduce frailty after surgery.[46] However, simply informing the surgical team of the CGA findings without targeted interventions did not seem to improve health-related quality of life after surgery.[47] A hospital care model in which both geriatricians and surgeons have shared responsibility for perioperative care showed greater reduction in length of stay compared with consultation-based models in older adults undergoing hip fracture surgery.[48]

Based on the available evidence, several important lessons can be learned about delivering effective prehabilitation and perioperative interventions. Most prehabilitation interventions included exercise and nutritional support, and the duration of intervention was 5–8 weeks. Light exercise programs, such as daily 30-minute exercise of walking and breathing, can be more effective than vigorous exercise programs that are difficult to adhere to.[43] Nutritional support is provided in the form of high-energy, protein-rich drinks, dietetics referral or education. During hospitalization, adequate postoperative pain management, early mobilization and nutritional support were shared components of the effective interventions. Although the supporting evidence in the perioperative setting is lacking, the following interventions can be considered: providing assistive devices (e.g. hearing aids, eyeglasses, dentures), optimizing medical co-morbidities, discontinuing potentially inappropriate or nonessential medications, paying attention to bowel and bladder function,

Table 8.3 Prehabilitation and perioperative interventions for older adults undergoing surgery

Interventions	Intervention Domain					Comparison	Surgery Population	Main Findings
	Medical	Psych	Physical	Nutrition	Social			
Randomized controlled trials								
Carli 2010[43] Prehabilitation (8 weeks) – Bike/strengthening 20-45 min/day			✓			Walk/breathing exercises 30 min/day	Colorectal surgery (mean age 60 years)	Improvement in 6-minute walk test distance (>20 m) at 10 weeks was higher in the comparison group than intervention group (41% versus 11%)
Nielsen 2010[42] Prehabilitation (6-8 weeks) – Structured exercise 30 min/day – Nutritional support Hospital care – Pain management – Early rehabilitation	✓		✓	✓		Routine care by surgery team and no prehabilitation	Orthopedic surgery (mean age 50 years)	Length of stay was shorter in the intervention group than control group (5 days versus 7 days). Functional status and recovery were also better
Pre–post comparison studies								
Chen 2014[46] *Modified Hospital Elder Life Program ("modified HELP")* Hospital care – Early mobilization – Nutritional support – Orienting communications		✓	✓	✓		Routine care before intervention	Abdominal surgery (mean age 73 years)	Frailty was reduced in the intervention phase than preintervention phase at hospital discharge (19% versus 65%) and at 3 months (17% versus 23%)
Ellis 2012[55] Prehabilitation – Referrals to physical and occupational therapy, dietetics, social work, fall prevention team, general practice, and nursing or support services	✓		✓	✓	✓	Routine care before intervention	Orthopedic, urological or gastrointestinal surgery (age ≥65 years)	Surgery cancellation was reduced in the intervention phase than preintervention phase (5% versus 18%). Length of stay (5 days versus 9 days) and complications (2% versus 9%) also improved

(cont.)

Table 8.3 (cont.)

Interventions	Intervention Domain					Comparison	Surgery Population	Main Findings
	Medical	Psych	Physical	Nutrition	Social			
Harari 2007[45] *Proactive Care of Older People Undergoing Surgery ("POPS")* Prehabilitation (1–4 clinic visits) – Treatment of medical co-morbidity – Physical and occupational therapy – Social work for discharge planning – Education – Hospital care – Treatment of complications – Pain management – Early mobilization – Bowel–bladder function – Nutritional support – Discharge planning Follow-up care – Home and clinic visits	✓	✓	✓	✓	✓	Routine care before intervention	Orthopedic surgery (mean age 75 years)	Length of stay was shorter in the intervention phase than preintervention phase (12 days versus 16 days). Medical complications also decreased
Li 2013[56] Prehabilitation (5 weeks) – Exercise 30 min x 3/week – Nutritional support – Relaxation techniques		✓	✓	✓		Routine care before intervention	Colorectal surgery (mean age 67 years)	Improvement in 6-minute walk test distance above baseline at 8 weeks was higher in the intervention phase than preintervention phase (81% versus 40%)
Richter 2005[47] Preoperative assessment – Inform the surgical team of the assessment results, without actual targeted interventions	✓					Routine care before intervention	Pelvic floor surgery (mean age 72 years)	Change in health-related quality of life did not differ between the intervention phase and preintervention phase.

and preserving sleep–wake cycles. These interventions can effectively reduce delirium in hospitalized older adults.[49,50] Even when adequate prehabilitation is not feasible (i.e. non-elective surgery), collaborative care between surgery and geriatrics should be considered.

Follow-up Care After Hospital Discharge

Considering that many frail individuals experience long-term functional decline or worsening of other co-morbidities after surgery, it is important to provide follow-up care beyond hospitalization to monitor functional status, reinforce adherence to interventions and manage co-existing geriatric conditions. As mentioned in the previous section, most published studies (Table 8.3) discontinued interventions at the time of or immediately after hospital discharge, overlooking the ongoing geriatric care needs of frail individuals. To maximize the benefits of surgery and help them live independently, the information from preoperative frailty assessment and CGA should also be used to inform community-based, long-term follow-up care after discharge. Systematic reviews concluded that older adults who received CGA and multidisciplinary interventions at home or in the hospital were more likely to live at home and less likely to die or experience functional decline.[9-11] The benefit of multidisciplinary interventions is generally larger when the intervention plan for identified problems is actively implemented, compared with when such a plan is simply recommended. Multidisciplinary home-visit programs[11] and fall prevention programs[51] in older adults were more effective when there were multiple follow-up visits and active interventions were provided. Therefore, preoperative frailty screening and CGA should be considered as an opportunity to begin comprehensive care of vulnerable older adults.

Areas of Uncertainty

Surgery may reverse frailty in some individuals by correcting the underlying pathologic condition, while surgery should not be offered to others because of frailty. It is not known whether there is a threshold in the frailty spectrum beyond which surgery becomes futile. Without a consensus on how to measure frailty, defining the threshold is challenging. Such decision-making should be viewed in the context of an individual's goals of care and personal values. In addition, numerous frailty instruments have been developed for surgical risk stratification, but further research is needed to compare their performance in independent patient populations before clinical application. Finally, the effects of preoperative CGA on short-term postoperative outcomes, as well as long-term functional decline should be evaluated more rigorously in a randomized controlled trial.

Conclusion

Perioperative care of older surgical patients is a rapidly evolving field in clinical medicine. Recent research findings highlight that previously ignored frailty and geriatric conditions are important determinants of surgical outcomes in older adults. Anesthesiologists and surgeons can administer a simple test of mobility, such as TUG or gait speed, to screen for frail older adults who are at high risk for postoperative complications, functional decline and mortality. These individuals can benefit from individualized multidisciplinary interventions that comprise prehabilitation to enhance functional reserve, avoiding deep anesthesia and sedation during the surgery, and targeted interventions to prevent complication and treat geriatric conditions.

References

1. Clegg A, Young J, Iliffe S, Rikkert MO, Rockwood K. Frailty in elderly people. *Lancet*. 2013; 381(9868):752–762.

2. Makary MA, Segev DL, Pronovost PJ, *et al.* Frailty as a predictor of surgical outcomes in older patients. *J Am Coll Surg*. 2010; 210(6):901–908.

3. Kristjansson SR, Nesbakken A, Jordhoy MS, *et al.* Comprehensive geriatric assessment can predict complications in elderly patients after elective surgery for colorectal cancer: a prospective observational cohort study. *Crit Rev Oncol Hematol*. 2010; 76(3):208–217.

4. Green P, Woglom AE, Genereux P, *et al.* The impact of frailty status on survival after transcatheter aortic valve replacement in older adults with severe aortic stenosis: a single-center experience. *JACC Cardiovasc Interv*. 2012; 5(9):974–981.

5. Schoenenberger AW, Stortecky S, Neumann S, *et al.* Predictors of functional decline in elderly patients undergoing transcatheter aortic valve implantation. *Eur Heart J*. 2013; 34(9):684–692.

6. Kim CA, Rasania SP, Afilalo J, *et al.* Functional status and quality of life after transcatheter aortic valve replacement: a systematic review. *Ann Intern Med*. 2014; 160(4):243–254.

7. Kim SW, Han HS, Jung HW, *et al.* Multidimensional frailty score for the prediction of postoperative mortality risk. *JAMA Surg*. 2014; 149(7):633–640.

8. Gill TM, Gahbauer EA, Allore HG, Han L. Transitions between frailty states among community-living older persons. *Arch Intern Med*. 2006; 166(4):418–423.

9. Ellis G, Whitehead MA, Robinson D, O'Neill D, Langhorne P. Comprehensive geriatric assessment for older adults admitted to hospital: meta-analysis of randomised controlled trials. *BMJ*. 2011; 343:d6553.

10. Beswick AD, Rees K, Dieppe P, *et al.* Complex interventions to improve physical function and maintain independent living in elderly people: a systematic review and meta-analysis. *Lancet*. 2008; 371(9614):725–735.

11. Stuck AE, Egger M, Hammer A, Minder CE, Beck JC. Home visits to prevent nursing home admission and functional decline in elderly people: systematic review and meta-regression analysis. *JAMA*. 2002; 287(8):1022–1028.

12. de Vries NM, van Ravensberg CD, Hobbelen JS, *et al.* Effects of physical exercise therapy on mobility, physical functioning, physical activity and quality of life in community-dwelling older adults with impaired mobility, physical disability and/or multi-morbidity: a meta-analysis. *Ageing Res Rev*. 2012; 11(1):136–149.

13. Forster A, Lambley R, Hardy J, *et al.* Rehabilitation for older people in long-term care. *Cochrane Database Syst Rev*. 2009(1):CD004294.

14. Rockwood K, Mitnitski A. Frailty in relation to the accumulation of deficits. *J Gerontol A Biol Sci Med Sci*. 2007; 62(7):722–727.

15. Fried LP, Tangen CM, Walston J, *et al.* Frailty in older adults: evidence for a phenotype. *J Gerontol A Biol Sci Med Sci*. 2001; 56(3):M146–M156.

16. Morley JE, Vellas B, van Kan GA, *et al.* Frailty consensus: a call to action. *J Am Med Dir Assoc*. 2013; 14(6):392–397.

17. Rockwood K, Andrew M, Mitnitski A. A comparison of two approaches to measuring frailty in elderly people. *J Gerontol A Biol Sci Med Sci*. 2007; 62(7):738–743.

18. Woo J, Leung J, Morley JE. Comparison of frailty indicators based on clinical phenotype and the multiple deficit approach in predicting mortality and physical limitation. *J Am Geriatr Soc*. 2012; 60(8):1478–1486.

19. Ensrud KE, Ewing SK, Taylor BC, *et al.* Comparison of 2 frailty indexes for prediction of falls, disability, fractures, and death in older women. *Arch Intern Med*. 2008; 168(4):382–389.

20. Robinson TN, Wu DS, Sauaia A, *et al.* Slower walking speed forecasts increased postoperative morbidity and 1-year mortality across surgical specialties. *Ann Surg.* 2013; 258(4):582–588; discussion 588–590.

21. Beggs T, Sepehri A, Szwajcer A, Tangri N, Arora RC. Frailty and perioperative outcomes: a narrative review. *Can J Anaesth.* 2015; 62(2):143–157.

22. Sepehri A, Beggs T, Hassan A, *et al.* The impact of frailty on outcomes after cardiac surgery: a systematic review. *J Thorac Cardiovasc Surg.* 2014; 148(6):3110–3117.

23. Partridge JS, Harari D, Dhesi JK. Frailty in the older surgical patient: a review. *Age Ageing.* 2012; 41(2):142–147.

24. Hubbard RE, Story DA. Patient frailty: the elephant in the operating room. *Anaesthesia.* 2014; 69(Suppl 1):26–34.

25. Podsiadlo D, Richardson S. The timed "Up & Go": a test of basic functional mobility for frail elderly persons. *J Am Geriatr Soc.* 1991; 39(2):142–148.

26. Afilalo J, Eisenberg MJ, Morin JF, *et al.* Gait speed as an incremental predictor of mortality and major morbidity in elderly patients undergoing cardiac surgery. *J Am Coll Cardiol.* 2010; 56(20):1668–1676.

27. Afilalo J, Mottillo S, Eisenberg MJ, *et al.* Addition of frailty and disability to cardiac surgery risk scores identifies elderly patients at high risk of mortality or major morbidity. *Circ Cardiovasc Qual Outcomes.* 2012; 5(2):222–228.

28. de Arenaza DP, Pepper J, Lees B, *et al.* Preoperative 6-minute walk test adds prognostic information to Euroscore in patients undergoing aortic valve replacement. *Heart* 2010; 96(2):113–117.

29. Mok M, Nombela-Franco L, Urena M, *et al.* Prognostic value of exercise capacity as evaluated by the 6-minute walk test in patients undergoing transcatheter aortic valve implantation. *J Am Coll Cardiol.* 2013; 61(8):897–898.

30. Puls M, Sobisiak B, Bleckmann A, *et al.* Impact of frailty on short- and long-term morbidity and mortality after transcatheter aortic valve implantation: risk assessment by Katz Index of activities of daily living. *EuroIntervention* 2014; 10(5):609–619.

31. Savva GM, Donoghue OA, Horgan F, O'Regan C, Cronin H, Kenny RA. Using timed up-and-go to identify frail members of the older population. *J Gerontol A Biol Sci Med Sci.* 2013; 68(4):441–446.

32. Kristjansson SR, Ronning B, Hurria A, *et al.* A comparison of two pre-operative frailty measures in older surgical cancer patients. *J Geriatr Oncol.* 2012; 3:1–7.

33. Partridge JS, Harari D, Martin FC, Dhesi JK. The impact of pre-operative comprehensive geriatric assessment on postoperative outcomes in older patients undergoing scheduled surgery: a systematic review. *Anaesthesia.* 2014; 69(Suppl 1):8–16.

34. Chow WB, Rosenthal RA, Merkow RP, *et al.* Optimal preoperative assessment of the geriatric surgical patient: a best practices guideline from the American College of Surgeons National Surgical Quality Improvement Program and the American Geriatrics Society. *J Am Coll Surg.* 2012; 215(4):453–466.

35. Luger TJ, Kammerlander C, Gosch M, *et al.* Neuroaxial versus general anaesthesia in geriatric patients for hip fracture surgery: does it matter? *Osteoporos Int.* 2010; 21(Suppl 4):S555–572.

36. Macfarlane AJ, Prasad GA, Chan VW, Brull R. Does regional anesthesia improve outcome after total knee arthroplasty? *Clin Orthop Relat Res.* 2009; 467(9):2379–2402.

37. Bryson GL, Wyand A. Evidence-based clinical update: general anesthesia and the risk of delirium and postoperative cognitive dysfunction. *Can J Anaesth.* 2006; 53(7):669–677.

38. Newman S, Stygall J, Hirani S, Shaefi S, Maze M. Postoperative cognitive dysfunction after noncardiac surgery: a systematic review. *Anesthesiology.* 2007; 106(3):572–590.

39. Radtke FM, Franck M, Lendner J, *et al.* Monitoring depth of anaesthesia

in a randomized trial decreases the rate of postoperative delirium but not postoperative cognitive dysfunction. *Br J Anaesth*. 2013; 110(Suppl 1):i98–i105.

40. Chan MT, Cheng BC, Lee TM, Gin T, Group CT. BIS-guided anesthesia decreases postoperative delirium and cognitive decline. *J Neurosurg Anesth*. 2013; 25(1):33–42.

41. Sieber FE, Zakriya KJ, Gottschalk A, *et al.* Sedation depth during spinal anesthesia and the development of postoperative delirium in elderly patients undergoing hip fracture repair. *Mayo Clin Proc*. 2010; 85(1):18–26.

42. Nielsen PR, Jorgensen LD, Dahl B, Pedersen T, Tonnesen H. Prehabilitation and early rehabilitation after spinal surgery: randomized clinical trial. *Clin Rehabil*. 2010; 24(2):137–148.

43. Carli F, Charlebois P, Stein B, *et al.* Randomized clinical trial of prehabilitation in colorectal surgery. *Br J Surg*. 2010; 97(8):1187–1197.

44. Mayo NE, Feldman L, Scott S, *et al.* Impact of preoperative change in physical function on postoperative recovery: argument supporting prehabilitation for colorectal surgery. *Surgery*. 2011; 150(3):505–514.

45. Harari D, Hopper A, Dhesi J, *et al.* Proactive care of older people undergoing surgery ('POPS'): designing, embedding, evaluating and funding a comprehensive geriatric assessment service for older elective surgical patients. *Age Ageing*. 2007; 36(2):190–196.

46. Chen CC, Chen CN, Lai IR, *et al.* Effects of a modified Hospital Elder Life Program on frailty in individuals undergoing major elective abdominal surgery. *J Am Geriatr Soc*. 2014; 62(2):261–268.

47. Richter HE, Redden DT, Duxbury AS, *et al.* Pelvic floor surgery in the older woman: enhanced compared with usual preoperative assessment. *Obstet Gynecol*. 2005; 105(4):800–807.

48. Grigoryan KV, Javedan H, Rudolph JL. Orthogeriatric care models and outcomes in hip fracture patients: a systematic review and meta-analysis. *J Orthop Trauma*. 2014; 28(3):e49–e55.

49. Inouye SK, Bogardus ST Jr., Charpentier PA, *et al.* A multicomponent intervention to prevent delirium in hospitalized older patients. *N Engl J Med*. 1999; 340(9):669–676.

50. Inouye SK, Bogardus ST Jr., Baker DI, Leo-Summers L, Cooney LM Jr. The Hospital Elder Life Program: a model of care to prevent cognitive and functional decline in older hospitalized patients. Hospital Elder Life Program. *J Am Geriatr Soc*. 2000; 48(12):1697–1706.

51. Gillespie LD. Preventing falls in older people: the story of a Cochrane review. *Cochrane Database Syst Rev*. 2013(2):ED000053.

52. Ewe SH, Ajmone Marsan N, Pepi M, *et al.* Impact of left ventricular systolic function on clinical and echocardiographic outcomes following transcatheter aortic valve implantation for severe aortic stenosis. *Am Heart J*. 2010; 160(6):1113–1120.

53. Dasgupta M, Rolfson DB, Stolee P, Borrie MJ, Speechley M. Frailty is associated with postoperative complications in older adults with medical problems. *Arch Gerontol Geriatr*. 2009; 48(1):78–83.

54. Robinson TN, Wu DS, Pointer L, *et al.* Simple frailty score predicts postoperative complications across surgical specialties. *Am J Surg*. 2013; 206(4):544–550.

55. Ellis G, Spiers M, Coutts S, Fairburn P, McCracken L. Preoperative assessment in the elderly: evaluation of a new clinical service. *Scott Med J*. 2012; 57(4):212–216.

56. Li C, Carli F, Lee L, *et al.* Impact of a trimodal prehabilitation program on functional recovery after colorectal cancer surgery: a pilot study. *Surg Endos*. 2013; 27(4):1072–1082.

Chapter

9

The Surgeon's Perspective

Cynthia E. Weber, Anthony J. Baldea and
Fred A. Luchette

Key Points

- Chronological age alone should not be an absolute contraindication to surgery as this segment of the population demonstrates significant heterogeneity.
- There are a multitude of factors that should be considered when evaluating an elderly patient for surgery: co-morbidities, degree of independence, baseline cognitive and psychological status, extent of polypharmacy and overall general fitness should all be regarded carefully.
- The Hopkins Frailty Score defines the frailty phenotype based on five factors: shrinking (unintentional weight loss), weakness (decreased grip strength), exhaustion, slowness (gait speed) and low activity. Using this instrument, patients are classified as "not frail," "intermediately frail" or "frail."
- The ACS NSQIP database identified that patients older than 90 years of age who present in septic shock, with an ASA class of V, a dependent baseline functional status and an abnormal white blood cell count have <10% chance of survival; surgeons should consider a discussion about futility with the patient and their family.
- There is a definite role for laparoscopic surgery in elderly patients and studies have repeatedly demonstrated superior outcomes compared to open procedures and confirmed its safety, even in extremely elderly patients.
- While elderly patients tend to fare well after elective procedures, they tend to fare poorly following emergency surgery compared to their younger counterparts.

Introduction

Currently more than half of all operations in the US annually are performed on elderly patients.[1] Furthermore, as the "baby boomer" segment of the US population ages, the proportion of surgical patients classified as elderly (≥65 years of age) and extreme elderly (≥80 years of age) will continue to increase. In 2000, the elderly represented 12.4% of the US population, or 35.1 million people. By 2050, it is projected that 20.2%, or 85.5 million Americans will be 65 years of age or older.[2] A thorough understanding and appreciation of the unique needs and physiology of the elderly surgical patient is necessary to provide safe perioperative care. Numerous studies have demonstrated that elderly patients suffer a disproportionately higher percentage of postoperative complications and higher 30-day mortality rates than their younger counterparts.[3-5] In addition, it has been shown that elderly patients are less resilient; the prevention of the first postoperative complication is of utmost importance perioperatively to prevent an acute deterioration in health status.[6,7]

Chronological age alone, however, should not be an absolute contraindication to surgery, as this segment of the population demonstrates significant heterogeneity. Rather, the surgeon, with the assistance of the patient's primary physician or geriatrician, should attempt to determine the individual's specific perioperative risks. There are multiple tools to assess the degree of frailty, or multidimensional functional reserve of the elderly patient, which can be used to determine the likelihood that they will be able to withstand the stress of a surgical procedure. Some of these measures are either impractical or are confounded by the presence of an acute surgical disease process, further complicating the preoperative assessment of an elderly patient in need of an emergent operation. Thus, the surgeon is often confronted with a difficult task when asked to counsel an elderly patient and their family about the risks and benefits of surgery. Perhaps an even more important, albeit challenging, role of the surgeon is to determine when surgery would be a futile endeavor due to the underlying frail condition of the elderly patient.

The Surgeon's Role in Preoperative Assessment of the Elderly Patient

When confronted with an elderly patient suffering from a surgical disease process, the determination of whether or not to offer surgery ultimately rests with the surgeon. In the elective setting, preoperative consultation can be requested from the patient's primary care physician, who has a more complete and historical understanding of the patient's co-morbidities and overall fitness for surgery. In addition, the patient can undergo preoperative cardiac testing, preoperative pulmonary function testing and a preoperative assessment by an anesthesiologist. However, the final decision "to operate" or "not to operate" falls into the hands of the surgeon.

There are a multitude of factors that should be considered when evaluating an elderly patient for surgery. The patient's co-morbidities, degree of independence, baseline cognitive and psychological status, extent of polypharmacy and overall general fitness should all be regarded carefully. The goal of the perioperative assessment is to provide an educated prognosis with regards to the patient's perioperative risks of morbidity and mortality that is as accurate as possible based on the available information in order to guide decision-making and encourage productive conversation with the surgeon. The importance of appropriate counseling of elderly patients and their families prior to consenting for an elective surgery cannot be overemphasized.

In 2012, the American College of Surgeons published *Best Practices Guidelines: Optimal Preoperative Assessment of the Geriatric Surgical Patient*, which suggests that in addition to a complete history and physical, the surgeon assesses the patient's cognitive ability, functional status, nutritional status and baseline frailty.[8] It also recommends screening the patient for alcohol and substance abuse, taking an accurate medication history, identifying risk factors for postoperative delirium and obtaining appropriate preoperative cardiac/pulmonary evaluations, as well as diagnostic tests needed before surgery. These guidelines advocate determining the patient's capacity to understand the upcoming surgery, the patient's treatment goals and expectations, and the family and social support system. Finally, screening for depression is recommended.[8] Multiple studies have demonstrated that depression among the elderly is under-recognized and is associated with higher rates of postoperative complications, in-hospital mortality and discharge to a skilled nursing facility.[9] Preoperative anxiety is also an independent risk factor of mortality and major morbidity.[10]

The concept of "frailty" has emerged in recent literature as an attempt to quantify what is otherwise an often subjective decision. The goal is to accurately and reliably identify patients at risk for poor postoperative outcomes and avoid the practice of *ageism* (denying older patients necessary surgery based on chronological age alone).[5,11-21] In addition, with the ever-increasing life expectancies, a patient in their mid 60s has the potential to live another 20–30 years after a major surgical procedure. While there is no standard operational definition of frailty, the general principle is that there are multisystem impairments, separate from the normal process of aging, that result in diminished physiologic and functional reserve. Thus, a frail individual, due to accumulated deficits, possesses limited ability to respond to stressors, such as a major surgical procedure. Inherent in frailty is an increased vulnerability to the development of disability and in the perioperative setting, length of stay, increased rates of discharge to skilled nursing facilities and higher 30-day mortality rates.[9,11,14,17,19]

There are multiple scoring instruments, of varying degrees of complexity and ease of administration, available to help quantify preoperative frailty. These models have repeatedly proven more predictive than common risk assessment tools such as the American Society of Anesthesiologists (ASA) Physical Status Classification System. The Hopkins Frailty Score, also referred to as the Fried Frailty Criteria, defines the frailty phenotype based on five factors: shrinking (unintentional weight loss), weakness (decreased grip strength), exhaustion, slowness (gait speed) and low activity. Using this instrument, patients are classified as "not frail," "intermediately frail," or "frail."[17,19] In one study that compared patient and surgeon perceptions of frailty with objective ratings, the authors demonstrated that surgeons have a tendency to overemphasize the patient's age in their subjective assessment of the patient, and conversely, elderly patients have a tendency to overestimate their ability to tolerate surgery, potentially creating unrealistic expectations.[16] Another definition of frailty that has evolved from prospective studies at the Denver Veteran's Affairs Medical Center encompasses seven factors: Timed Up and Go (time needed to stand from a chair, walk 10 feet, return to chair and sit), Katz Index (measured independence of activities of daily living), Mini-Cog (measures cognition using a paired three-item recall and clock-drawing test), Charlson Index (measures burden of disease based on co-morbidities), anemia (defined as hematocrit <35%), poor nutrition (defined as albumin <3.4 g/dl) and geriatric syndrome of falls (how many falls in 6 months prior to surgery). In this scoring system, "nonfrail" is defined as 0 to 1 traits, "pre-frail" is defined as 2 to 3 traits, and "frail" is defined as 4 or more traits.[13-15]

In the Acute Care Surgery realm, the Modified Frailty Index is an 11-item frailty index that has been validated as predictive of outcome in emergency general surgery and vascular surgery in elderly patients.[5,18] The Modified Frailty Index was created by comparing the Canadian Study of Health and Aging, Clinical Frailty Index (a 70-item scale based on "accumulating deficits" or parameters obtained by history, physical examination and capability) with the American College of Surgeons (ACS) National Surgical Quality Improvement Program (NSQIP) database.[5] Finally, as one study argues, there is probable utility in risk-stratifying elderly patients immediately postoperatively, as the acute stress of surgery might serve as the impetus to move a patient from subclinical frailty that would not be detected preoperatively into frailty because of their diminished underlying reserve. This study identified the Braden Scale, a validated tool already routinely documented by nurses to predict pressure ulcer risk, as a potential predictive perioperative tool. They demonstrated that a lower Braden Scale was associated with an increased risk of postoperative complication, longer length of stay and predictive of discharge to a skilled nursing facility.[22]

Elective Versus Emergent Surgery

The rate of postoperative morbidity and mortality after elective noncardiac surgery in elderly patients generally falls into a range of acceptable risk for both patient and surgeon. Most studies report overall morbidity somewhere in the 15–30% range and postoperative mortality rates of 4–7%.[4] Ideally, with appropriate preoperative risk stratification and medical optimization, the majority of elderly patients will return to normal baseline function postoperatively. Unfortunately, the same cannot be said of the outcomes after emergency surgery in the elderly. Depending on the exact definition of "elderly" used, morbidity rates after emergency general surgery have been reported to range between 27% and 70% and mortality rates from 15% to upwards of 44%.[3,4,23,24] Numerous studies have demonstrated that octogenarians and nonagenarians have the highest propensity to suffer major life-altering complications and death.[3,23-25]

This disparity in outcomes between the elective and emergent settings is likely multifactorial, as the surgeon has limited time to assess the patient's baseline frailty and optimize the existing co-morbidities in the acute setting. In addition, the ability to effectively communicate with an elderly patient's primary care physician is substantially hindered on nights and weekends. A number of the frailty assessments outlined previously are too time-consuming or the results are confounded by the presence of an acute surgical disease process, thus limiting the accuracy of the frailty estimation. For example, many of the frailty indices require functional testing and in the acute setting, an untrained observer in nonstandardized conditions will produce unreliable results. In addition, as is frequently the case in patients presenting with an acute abdomen, there is a large amount of variation in the severity and reversibility of the underlying disease process contributing to the acute deterioration. Lastly, in the elective setting, there is often a window of time available to optimize the patient medically or modify patient-specific risk factors.

Various models have been created to attempt to predict factors that are associated with a higher preoperative risk of a poor outcome, especially in the extremely elderly population where the rates are very high. A major factor that has arisen in recent literature is not only the prevention of the first postoperative complication, but also the importance of a timely and effective rescue of the elderly patient at the first sign of a complication. It has been shown that the in-hospital mortality rate after the development of a postoperative complication is significantly higher in elderly surgical patients than in their younger counterparts.[6,7,24] The underlying factors that play a role in failure-to-rescue rates, which have been shown to vary vastly between hospitals, are likely related to hospital resource availability and utilization, as well as the safety culture at the institutional level.[7] These factors are potentially modifiable and represent a very real way to improve elderly postoperative mortality rates if they are identified and corrected in the lower-performing hospitals.

One study identified that a preoperative hypoalbuminemia (<3.5 mg/dl), a positive blood culture and the presence of panperitonitis were negative prognostic indicators in the setting of emergent laparotomy.[25] Hypoalbuminemia, which has been found to correlate with postoperative morbidity and mortality, is somewhat controversial to interpret because it is likely not a direct measurement of the patient's underlying nutritional status in the acute setting, but rather serves as a marker of the degree of underlying inflammatory catabolism.[25-27] Several models have found both ASA class and chronological age to be significant independent predictive variables, but this is not a uniform finding across the literature.[3,23,24] Other factors implicated with postoperative outcome in the emergency setting include baseline functional status and sarcopenia (severe skeletal muscle depletion).[3,11,28] Of note, a study that examined sarcopenia as a predictive factor found that ASA score and sarcopenia were independently predictive of outcome and likely represent separate patient-specific factors (ASA score – cardiopulmonary status; sarcopenia – nutritional/functional status).[28] It is also postulated that the wide variation in morbidity and mortality might be attributable, at least in part, to age-specific processes of care such as the overall aggressiveness of care and end-of-life decision-making.[4]

Laparoscopic Surgery in the Elderly

The last 25 years have seen major advances in minimally invasive and laparoscopic surgical techniques. For example, 95% of cholecystectomies currently are performed laparoscopically. Among some surgeons, however, there remains concern regarding the ability of elderly patients to tolerate the pneumoperitoneum required for laparoscopic surgery. Insufflation of the abdomen with CO_2 can produce hypercarbia, leading to a significant acidosis, especially in patients with underlying cardiopulmonary disease. In addition, the increased intra-abdominal pressure may result in elevated peak airway pressures, decreased pulmonary compliance, decreased venous return, decreased cardiac output and can potentially worsen gastro-esophageal reflux and aspiration risk in vulnerable patients.[29]

A combination of this feared intolerance of pneumoperitoneum as well as higher rates of co-morbidities, a history of more prior abdominal surgeries and the increased severity of acute cholecystitis among elderly patients has led to a significant disparity between elderly and nonelderly in the use of laparoscopy for cholecystectomy.[30] One study, utilizing the ACS NSQIP database for 2005–2008, found that laparoscopic cholecystectomy was underused in the elderly population (80% versus 85% in nonelderly), despite the fact that it is associated with fewer complications, shorter length of stay and a lower mortality rate when compared with open cholecystectomy.[31] Thus, although the rate of conversion to an open procedure is higher among the elderly (6% versus 5%), many studies have demonstrated that most elderly patients, including the extreme elderly (>80 years of age), tolerate laparoscopic cholecystectomy very well, including no added cardiopulmonary risk from pneumoperitoneum. Gallbladder disease is the most common indication for abdominal surgery in the elderly population, because the incidence of gallstones and the severity of disease increases with age; efforts should focus on educating primary care physicians and surgeons about the safety and efficacy of laparoscopic cholecystectomy in the elderly surgical patient to prevent delay in care.[30-33]

Studies have also demonstrated a decreased risk of postoperative complications and lower 30-day mortality rates in elderly patients undergoing laparoscopic colorectal surgery compared to open colorectal surgery. In addition, the commonly cited benefits of laparoscopy (decreased postoperative pain, earlier return of bowel function, shorter hospital stay, more rapid return to baseline function, etc.) may even be more pronounced in elderly patients compared to their younger counterparts. The general consensus is that laparoscopic colorectal surgery is safe and beneficial for the majority of the elderly population.[34]

In the postoperative period, the elderly are prone to develop delirium, an altered mental state characterized by fluctuating changes in level of awareness and cognition. For some, this acute change in cognitive function can persist for weeks to months after surgery and manifest as issues with attention and memory as well as executive dysfunction. When the symptoms are more persistent postoperatively, it is commonly referred to as postoperative cognitive dysfunction (POCD).[35,36] Surgeons have postulated that laparoscopic surgery, which when compared to open surgery often represents a lesser stress on the patient and enables a quicker return to their home environment and baseline activities, might be protective against the development of POCD. However, preliminary data have been unsuccessful in supporting this notion.[37,38]

This is an area that warrants further investigation. The incidence of POCD in elderly surgery patients at about 3 months postoperatively is estimated to be around 10–15%,[35,39] and an elderly community-dwelling patient who suffers POCD may experience the devastating loss of their independence. The potential causal link between general anesthesia, surgery and the onset of cognitive decline in elderly patients is controversial and has prompted extensive research on the topic. Some studies have shown a correlation between the use of inhalational general anesthetics, such as sevoflurane, and postoperative cognitive dysfunction, whereas other studies have failed to demonstrate a significant correlation between route or type of anesthetic.[35,36,39] However, the role of the anesthetic regimen in the development of postoperative cognitive decline has not been fully elucidated, and continues to be an active area of research.

Frailty Versus Futility

A very difficult, but often necessary, decision to make, for the surgeon as well as the patient and their family, is the decision not to proceed with surgery for a theoretically curable surgical disease process if the patient's underlying risk factors are too prohibitive. The conclusion that an attempt at an operation would be futile in an elderly patient can potentially save the patient unneeded suffering and can save the health care system substantial cost. One study, utilizing the ACS NSQIP database, examined the outcomes of 37,553 patients after emergency laparotomy to create predictive models for 30-day mortality. They identified that patients older than 90 years of age who present in septic shock, with an ASA class of V, a dependent baseline functional status and an abnormal white blood cell count have <0% chance of survival.[3] Surgeons can make use of these objective results when discussing possible outcomes with an ill extremely elderly patient and their family in the acute setting.

Globally, according to the Organization for Economic Cooperation and Development, the US spends more on health care than any other industrialized country (17.7% of GDP or $8,508 per capita, compared to an average of 9.3% or about $3,322 per capita worldwide).[40] The percentage of health care funds spent on the elderly in their final years or weeks of life is staggering.[41] One study that examined the 1.8 million deaths that occurred in 2008 among Medicare elderly beneficiaries showed that 32% of patients underwent an inpatient surgical procedure during the last year of life, 18% in the last month of life and 8% in the last week of life. There was regional variation and the proportion of patients undergoing surgical procedures was less amongst the extreme elderly.[42] With the aging US population increasing, the importance of appropriate allocation of health care resources and funds will likely garner more national attention.

Conclusion

In conclusion, from the surgeon's perspective, the perioperative care of the elderly demands a careful appreciation for the unique needs and vulnerabilities of this heterogeneous segment of the population. No patient should be denied surgery based on chronological age alone, but rather the patient's underlying physiologic reserve and co-morbidities should be prudently investigated. There is a definite role for laparoscopic surgery in elderly patients and studies have repeatedly demonstrated superior outcomes compared to open procedures and confirmed its safety, even in extremely elderly patients. Finally, while elderly patients tend to fare well after elective procedures, the same does not necessarily apply in the acute setting. Thus, surgeons need to be trained how to have realistic conversations with the elderly patient and their family as to the appropriate expectations from an emergency surgery and know when to advise against a futile operation.

References

1. American Geriatrics Society. *Geriatric Review Syllabus – A Core Curriculum in Geriatric Medicine, 6th edn.* New York, American Geriatrics Society, 2006.

2. Halaweish I, Alam HB. Changing demographics of the American population. *Surg Clin North Am.* 2015; 95:1–10.

3. Al-Temimi MH, Griffee M, Enniss TM, *et al.* When is death inevitable after emergency laparotomy? Analysis of the American College of Surgeons National Surgical Quality Improvement Program database. *J Am Coll Surg.* 2012; 215:503–511.

4. Ingraham AM, Cohen ME, Raval MV, Ko CY, Nathens AB. Variation in quality of care after emergency general surgery procedures in the elderly. *J Am Coll Surg.* 2011; 212:1039–1048.

5. Farhat JS, Velanovich V, Falvo AJ, *et al.* Are the frail destined to fail? Frailty index as predictor of surgical morbidity and mortality in the elderly. *J Trauma Acute Care Surg.* 2012; 72:1526–1530.

6. Sheetz KH, Krell RW, Englesbe MJ, *et al.* The importance of the first complication: understanding failure to rescue after emergent surgery in the elderly. *J Am Coll Surg.* 2014; 219:365–370.

7. Sheetz KH, Waits SA, Krell RW, *et al.* Improving mortality following emergent surgery in older patients requires focus on complication rescue. *Ann Surg.* 2013; 258:614–617.

8. Chow WB, Rosenthal RA, Merkow RP, *et al.* Optimal preoperative assessment of the geriatric surgical patient: a best practices guideline from the American College of Surgeons National Surgical Quality Improvement Program and the American Geriatrics Society. *J Am Coll Surg.* 2012; 215:453–466.

9. Kim S, Brooks AK, Groban L. Preoperative assessment of the older surgical patient: honing in on geriatric syndromes. *Clin Interv Aging.* 2015; 10:13–27.

10. Williams JB, Alexander KP, Morin JF, *et al.* Preoperative anxiety as a predictor of mortality and major morbidity in patients aged >70 years undergoing cardiac surgery. *Am J Cardiol.* 2013; 111:137–142.

11. Saxton A, Velanovich V. Preoperative frailty and quality of life as predictors of postoperative complications. *Ann Surg.* 2011; 253:1223–1229.

12. Kim SW, Han HS, Jung HW, *et al.* Multidimensional frailty score for the prediction of postoperative mortality risk. *JAMA Surg.* 2014; 149:633–640.

13. Robinson TN, Eiseman B, Wallace JI, et al. Redefining geriatric preoperative assessment using frailty, disability and co-morbidity. *Ann Surg.* 2009; 250:449–455.

14. Robinson TN, Wallace JI, Wu DS, et al. Accumulated frailty characteristics predict postoperative discharge institutionalization in the geriatric patient. *J Am Coll Surg.* 2011; 213:37–42.

15. Robinson TN, Wu DS, Pointer L, et al. Simple frailty score predicts postoperative complications across surgical specialties. *Am J Surg.* 2013; 206:544–550.

16. Revenig LM, Canter DJ, Henderson MA, et al. Preoperative quantification of perceptions of surgical frailty. *J Surg Res.* 2015; 193:583–589.

17. Revenig LM, Canter DJ, Taylor MD, et al. Too frail for surgery? Initial results of a large multidisciplinary prospective study examining preoperative variables predictive of poor surgical outcomes. *J Am Coll Surg.* 2013; 217:665–670 e1.

18. Karam J, Tsiouris A, Shepard A, Velanovich V, Rubinfeld I. Simplified frailty index to predict adverse outcomes and mortality in vascular surgery patients. *Ann Vasc Surg.* 2013; 27:904–908.

19. Makary MA, Segev DL, Pronovost PJ, et al. Frailty as a predictor of surgical outcomes in older patients. *J Am Coll Surg.* 2010; 210:901–908.

20. Amrock LG, Neuman MD, Lin HM, Deiner S. Can routine preoperative data predict adverse outcomes in the elderly? Development and validation of a simple risk model incorporating a chart-derived frailty score. *J Am Coll Surg.* 2014; 219:684–694.

21. Soreide K, Desserud KF. Emergency surgery in the elderly: the balance between function, frailty, fatality and futility. *Scand J Trauma Resusc Emerg Med.* 2015; 23:10.

22. Cohen RR, Lagoo-Deenadayalan SA, Heflin MT, et al. Exploring predictors of complication in older surgical patients: a deficit accumulation index and the Braden Scale. *J Am Geriatr Soc.* 2012; 60:1609–1615.

23. Wilson I, Paul Barrett M, Sinha A, Chan S. Predictors of in-hospital mortality amongst octogenarians undergoing emergency general surgery: a retrospective cohort study. *Int J Surg.* 2014; 12:1157–1161.

24. Merani S, Payne J, Padwal RS, et al. Predictors of in-hospital mortality and complications in very elderly patients undergoing emergency surgery. *World J Emerg Surg.* 2014; 9:43.

25. Park SY, Chung JS, Kim SH, et al. The safety and prognostic factors for mortality in extremely elderly patients undergoing an emergency operation. *Surg Today.* 2016; 46(2):241–247.

26. Daley J, Khuri SF, Henderson W, et al. Risk adjustment of the postoperative morbidity rate for the comparative assessment of the quality of surgical care: results of the National Veterans Affairs Surgical Risk Study. *J Am Coll Surg.* 1997; 185:328–340.

27. Khuri SF, Daley J, Henderson W, et al. Risk adjustment of the postoperative mortality rate for the comparative assessment of the quality of surgical care: results of the National Veterans Affairs Surgical Risk Study. *J Am Coll Surg.* 1997; 185:315–327.

28. Du Y, Karvellas CJ, Baracos V, et al. Sarcopenia is a predictor of outcomes in very elderly patients undergoing emergency surgery. *Surgery.* 2014; 156:521–527.

29. Bates AT, Divino C. Laparoscopic surgery in the elderly: a review of the literature. *Aging Dis.* 2015; 6:149–155.

30. Antoniou SA, Antoniou GA, Koch OO, Pointner R, Granderath FA. Meta-analysis of laparoscopic vs open cholecystectomy in elderly patients. *World J Gastroenterol.* 2014; 20:17626–17634.

31. Tucker JJ, Yanagawa F, Grim R, Bell T, Ahuja V. Laparoscopic cholecystectomy is safe but underused in the elderly. *Am Surg.* 2011; 77:1014–1020.

32. Lee SI, Na BG, Yoo YS, Mun SP, Choi NK. Clinical outcome for laparoscopic cholecystectomy in extremely elderly patients. *Ann Surg Treat Res.* 2015; 88:145–151.

33. Weber DM. Laparoscopic surgery: an excellent approach in elderly patients. *Arch Surg.* 2003; 138:1083–1088.

34. Seishima R, Okabayashi K, Hasegawa H, *et al.* Is laparoscopic colorectal surgery beneficial for elderly patients? A systematic review and meta-analysis. *J Gastrointest Surg.* 2015; 19:756–765.

35. Shoair OA, Grasso Ii MP, Lahaye LA, *et al.* Incidence and risk factors for postoperative cognitive dysfunction in older adults undergoing major noncardiac surgery: a prospective study. *J Anaesthesiol Clin Pharmacol.* 2015; 31:30–36.

36. Kotekar N, Kuruvilla CS, Murthy V. Postoperative cognitive dysfunction in the elderly: a prospective clinical study. *Indian J Anaesth.* 2014; 58:263–268.

37. Tan CB, Ng J, Jeganathan R, *et al.* Cognitive changes after surgery in the elderly: does minimally invasive surgery influence the incidence of postoperative cognitive changes compared to open colon surgery? *Dement Geriatr Cogn Disord.* 2015; 39:125–131.

38. Gameiro M, Eichler W, Schwandner O, *et al.* Patient mood and neuropsychological outcome after laparoscopic and conventional colectomy. *Surg Innov.* 2008; 15:171–178.

39. Hussain M, Berger M, Eckenhoff RG, Seitz DP. General anesthetic and the risk of dementia in elderly patients: current insights. *Clin Interv Aging.* 2014; 9:1619–1628.

40. OECD. Health at a glance 2013: OECD indicators. OECD Publishing, 2013. Available at: www.oecd.org/els/health-systems/Health-at-a-Glance-2013.pdf (Accessed July 7, 2017).

41. Barnet CS, Arriaga AF, Hepner DL, *et al.* Surgery at the end of life: a pilot study comparing decedents and survivors at a tertiary care center. *Anesthesiology.* 2013; 119:796–801.

42. Kwok AC, Semel ME, Lipsitz SR, *et al.* The intensity and variation of surgical care at the end of life: a retrospective cohort study. *Lancet.* 2011; 378:1408–1413.

Chapter 10

Geriatric Cardiac Procedures

John D. Mitchell

Key Points

- Mortality following coronary artery bypass grafting (CABG) and aortic valve replacement (AVR) is higher in patients over the age of 80 years compared to younger cohorts, and in general age remains an important predictor of outcome for cardiac procedures.
- Meticulous care of the octogenarian and avoidance of complications is essential to attain the best possible outcomes following cardiac procedures.
- Noninvasive or less invasive cardiac procedures such as percutaneous coronary intervention (PCI) may offer some benefit to older patients, with improved short-term benefits, but benefits are not always sustained long term. More research in this area is merited.
- Aortic valve disease occurs in over 10% or patients over 80 years of age and the degree of aortic calcification is a significant risk factor for adverse embolic events following aortic valve replacement.
- Transcatheter aortic valve replacement (TAVR) is less invasive than traditional surgical AVR (SAVR) and may offer benefits to the very elderly patient.
- Assessment of frailty – using known scales, muscle mass or walking speed is becoming an important part of the preoperative risk assessment for the older cardiac patient.

Introduction

With the number of elderly patients steadily increasing, there are more patients developing cardiovascular and valvular diseases each year.[1–5] Patients with cardiovascular disease tend to be in their sixth through eighth decades of life at baseline, but most early studies were on the younger subgroup of these patients. Newer data have emerged on the management of patients over the age of 80, demonstrating that they are a distinct, if heterogeneous population. We will focus on this cohort in order to differentiate management from that offered traditionally. Unless otherwise noted, this chapter will reference considerations for this older population of cardiac surgical patients. Our objectives will be to discuss new procedural options for the elderly cardiovascular patient, understand risks of surgery for those of advanced age, and briefly touch on frailty and other approaches to risk-stratifying cardiac surgical patients.

Overall Risk of Cardiac Procedures in the Elderly

Historically, patients over the age of 80 were deemed poor surgical candidates and offered limited or no interventional options. In 2000, Alexander's group looked at outcomes in a subgroup of 4743 octogenarians as compared to nearly 68,000 total patients. They demonstrated that procedural risks were higher for CABG, CABG with AVR and CABG with MVR (Table 10.1).

While the mortality rates were elevated for octogenarians, given the high mortality of medical management, they were felt to be acceptable in some patients, especially for those undergoing CABG or CABG with AVR. Furthermore, they noted that the same predictors of risk could be used to triage out older patients, including age, gender, previous CABG, COPD, vascular disease, renal failure or dysfunction, and MI prior to surgery. Despite an overall more encouraging impression of cardiac surgery in select patients over 80, age was still found to be the top predictor of mortality, both overall and in both age-defined subgroups, tempering enthusiasm.[8–12]

In 2004, Srinivasan led a group investigating outcomes in cardiac surgical patients over age 75 and found a 5-year survival of 71.7%. While seemingly low, this was found to be no different from the age- and gender-matched population on the whole, and was thus an encouraging finding.[9,10,13–15]

Likosky and colleagues explored long-term survival in patients undergoing CABG. They split their cohort into three age groups: less than 80, 80–84 and 85 or older. Not surprisingly, the median years of survival were lower as age increased and the incidence of death was higher. Of note, the oldest group had more female patients, more emergency procedures and more co-morbidities at baseline (Table 10.2).

Table 10.1 Procedural outcomes for patients over age 80

	Mortality 80+	Mortality <80
CABG	8.1%	3.0%
+ AVR	10.1%	7.8%
+ MVR	19.6%	12.2%

Adapted from Alexander, 2000[6–8]

Table 10.2 Long-term survival for elderly patients after coronary artery bypass grafting

Age	Median Survival (Years)	Incidence of Death
<80	14.4	4.2%
80–84	7.4	10.3%
85+	5.8	13.7%

Adapted from Likosky, 2008[2,16–18]

Zingone and colleagues looked at 355 consecutive octogenarians for cardiac surgery in 2009. They stratified patients into those who had complications and those who did not. They examined results both for all patients and a subgroup that eliminated in-hospital deaths. In both subgroups, survival was markedly higher in those patients who did not have any perioperative complications, highlighting the need for both meticulous perioperative care and careful patient selection.[1,7,19,20]

Saxena examined Australian patients over age 80 as compared both to those less than 80 and also age-matched controls.[9,13] While morbidity and mortality were higher in patients over 80 who had surgery, they did not differ from age-matched controls in terms of 5-year mortality.

Taken together, these data opened the door for cardiac surgical procedures in patients over the age of 80, but emphasized:

1. The need for careful patient selection based on predictive modeling.
2. The need for meticulous perioperative care.
3. Selection of appropriate procedures based on patient age and other factors.
4. Comparison of outcomes to age-matched general population cohorts instead of younger patients having the same procedure.
5. The need for more research and alternative techniques.

These elements help frame the discussion as we consider each type of cardiovascular procedure for patients over age 80.

Cardiac Risks and Outcomes by Procedure Type

Coronary Interventions

We have already summarized the baseline data for CABG outcome in elderly patients. We will now explore how these rates compare with those for percutaneous coronary interventions (PCI) or off-pump (OP) techniques.

CABG versus PCI

In large, retrospective database evaluations of octogenarians, PCI has shown lower short-term mortality, but higher long-term mortality (Figure 10.1).[1,4,10,21,22] Most of this early mortality effect is attributable to the higher risks of the initial surgical procedure over percutaneous intervention.

CABG versus OP-CABG

It has been suggested that off-pump CABG may be beneficial in older patients by reducing the risks of atheroemboli secondary to aortic manipulation or effects of cardiopulmonary bypass itself. The two major areas of exploration have been neurological outcomes and mortality.

Stroke Rates/Neurocognitive Outcomes

Multiple meta-analyses and nonrandomized studies of patients over 80 suggested substantially reduced stroke rates with off-pump CABG,[11,14,17,23,24] but a randomized controlled trial was unable to demonstrate cognitive benefits of OP-CABG.[1,3,5] This may be due to equivalence in techniques, but could be confounded by nonstandard definitions of

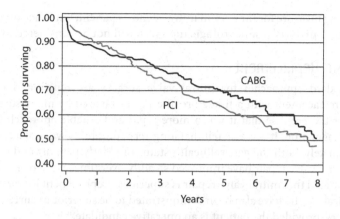

Figure 10.1 2-year survival for PCI versus CABG.

Number of patients at risk by year – 2-vessel disease

	At Procedure	At Year							
		1	2	3	4	5	6	7	8
PCI	532	387	321	248	170	130	96	61	35
CABG	443	335	273	198	142	114	75	52	28

neurocognitive deficits, short durations of follow-up or negative effects of decreased cerebral perfusion during periods of relative hypotension during OP-CABG procedures.[2,4,6,7]

Mortality Data: RCT Versus Case Series Data and Emerging Data Trends

When compared to on-pump CABG in patients over age 80, off-pump CABG appeared to have a lower operative mortality,[6,7,9,11] and benefits in survival[9–11,13,14] in several early meta-analyses. OP-CABG was therefore felt to be a good option for patients in this age group. Propensity-matched, nonrandomized data also supported a reduced mortality in this age group, with a mortality reduction from 12.2% to 1.3% (range 4.6–5.9%).[2,10,13,16] Unfortunately, meta-analysis of randomized controlled trials shows similar in-hospital mortality between techniques.[7,19] While many surgeons do not select OP-CABG as routine for octogenarians, it may be preferable in scenarios where the aorta is severely calcified or has substantial atheroma burdens near the sites of potential cross clamp or cannulation. Chest CT and epiaortic ultrasound may help provide information to aid in this decision tree.

Mitral Valve

Mitral valve regurgitation and stenosis are present in many patients over the age of 80 and may either present as the dominant issue driving symptoms or be discovered as part of the workup for concomitant coronary artery disease. There are several standard options for procedures and other emerging approaches that deserve brief mention. Commisurotomy is a temporizing measure for the very ill mitral stenosis patient, but lacks long-term durability and carries high risks of neurologic injury, so will not be considered in depth here.

Repair Versus Replacement

The two standard approaches for mitral valve surgery are repair and replacement. Historically, replacement with a tissue prosthesis was favored by many surgeons in the elderly, under the premise that it was a more rapid and reliable approach that did not require anticoagulation. It was also felt that long-term durability was not a concern in the elderly. Fortunately, both the general health status of elderly patients and surgical techniques for mitral valve repair have improved steadily over time. More recent assessments have demonstrated that mitral valve repair is superior to replacement for outcomes in the elderly; surgical repairs have also been demonstrated to be superior to current percutaneous approaches, provided the patient is an operative candidate.[10,12]

Minimally Invasive Versus Open

Minimally invasive options for mitral valve surgery were at one time considered too complex for application in elderly patients. Recent studies have demonstrated that they provide similar postoperative outcomes to standard approaches and are associated with both a shorter hospital stay and a faster return to activity.[10] They may also be preferable for patients who have already had a sternotomy, as a thoracotomy incision avoids the need for a redo sternotomy.

MitraClip

Percutaneous approaches to mitral valve repair have become increasingly more plausible. MitraClip allows for the placement of a clip that tethers the mid portion of the A2 scallop to the mid portion of the P2 scallop, effectively acting as an Alfieri repair of the mitral valve and creating two smaller orifices for flow between the atria and ventricle.[4,17,22] This techniques requires real-time 3D TEE and fluoroscopy for positioning of the clip and assessment of the expected residual mitral regurgitation, and so requires close collaboration between cardiovascular anesthesiologists and cardiologists. It has been approved in Europe for patients with symptomatic severe mitral regurgitation and in the United States for patients with prohibitive risk and degenerative mitral regurgitation.[1,11,14,17,23,24] A 2015 meta-analysis of almost 900 patients with a median follow-up of 9 months demonstrated a significant reduction in severe or moderate mitral regurgitation (95% to 11%) and New York Heart Association Classification III/IV symptoms (90% to 19%). Complication rates were 26% with a mortality of 15% in a population of patients deemed nonsurgical candidates (Figure 10.2).[2,4] Unfortunately, the patients in these trials were in their 70s, so further assessment needs to be done to evaluate the utility of this approach in patients over age 80. Given a demonstrated 30-day mortality across studies of less than 5%,[1,4,7] it will likely find broader applications soon.

Transcatheter Mitral Valves

Transcatheter mitral valves are entering testing phases and case reports are emerging.[10,23] They may be deployed either via a transapical approach through the left ventricle, requiring surgical intervention, or via a trans-septal, percutaneous approach.[3] Applications

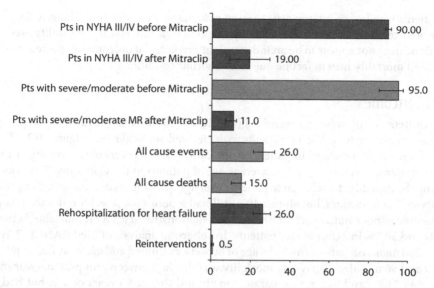

Figure 10.2 MitraClip outcomes.
From D'ascenzo, 2015.

Table 10.3 Mortality

Age Group	1-Year Mortality (%)	3-Year Mortality (%)
60–69	6	16
70–79	10	27
80–89	13	39

Created with data from reference 16.

described thus far have been for deployment "in-valve" for failed replacements, but reports are starting to emerge for use in degenerative disease as well. They are currently only used for nonoperative candidates. Human studies are underway, and further assessment will be required to determine risk profiles and patients ideally suited to this approach.[6]

Aortic Valve

Aortic valve disease is common in the elderly, and is present in nearly 10% of patients older than 80.[9] The extent of aortic valve calcification increases with age. Mortality approaches 50% within 2 years without surgical intervention.[9,13] Surgical aortic valve replacement (SAVR) represents the mainstay of therapy, but evolving percutaneous approaches have expanded the pool of candidates eligible for intervention.

Primary SAVR outcomes

Outcomes for primary aortic valve surgery for patients over the age of 80 have been reasonable, though 1- and 3-year mortality are both more than twice as high as for patients aged 60–69 (Table 10.2).[16]

Patients with low or intermediate surgical risk, based on a Society of Thoracic Surgeons Score of lower than 8% predicted mortality, respond well and have low mortality overall.[25] Age alone does not appear to be an independent predictor of outcomes in some series, so increased mortality may in fact be due to co-morbid conditions.[19]

TAVR Outcomes

Transcatheter aortic valve interventions (TAVR) are commercially available and provide a viable alternative to SAVR for patients with elevated surgical risks (Figure 10.3). These valves were originally tested in patients with >50% risk of irreversible morbidity or mortality ("extreme surgical risk"). The average age of patients in the CoreValve Trial was 84, making the data directly relevant to patients over age 80. Patients demonstrated improved quality-of-life indicators, but almost 40% still had a poor outcome. Of note, age was not a predictor of poor outcome.[26,27] Other studies demonstrated a TAVR mortality between 16.6% and 30.7% in extreme-risk patients. In subgroup analysis of the FRANCE-2 Trial, over 2,200 high-risk patients over the age of 80 were examined and age stratified as 80–84, 85–89 and 90 or older. Thirty-day mortality was similar between groups. One-year mortality was 23.8% and began to separate, mostly splitting at 85 years of age, but had no significantly detectable differences.[8,28] As the risk profiles were acceptable in multiple studies, TAVR has become a viable option the elderly.

Redo AVR

Redo sternotomy for aortic valve replacement in patients over 80 has been accomplished with a reasonable survival profile (90% at 1 year for AVR and 85% for AVR and CABG) and so deserves consideration in appropriate candidates.[8,29] Other studies have also shown similar results.[15,30]

Mini-Sternontomy AVR

Some groups advocate the use of mini-sternotomy in the elderly to enhance recovery and improve outcomes.[18,31] While feasible and promising in case series, randomized studies are needed.

TAVR Versus Open AVR

These percutaneous valves are now approved for use in high-surgical-risk patients, as predicted by scoring systems, making direct comparisons possible in high-risk patients.

A randomized multicenter trial of TAVR versus SAVR for nearly 800 high-risk patients (30-day predicted mortality between 15% and 50%) explored both all-cause mortality and a composite endpoint of death or stroke over 2 years. TAVR showed lower all-cause death, major adverse cardiac outcomes and stroke rates than AVR. It also demonstrated a trend toward higher valve areas and lower mean gradients.[20,32]

The average age of patients in this study was 83. Of note, while patients younger than 85 had a mortality benefit from TAVR, the subgroup of patients over age 85 showed no mortality benefit.[32,33]

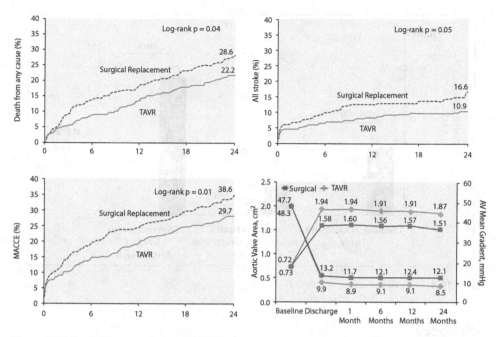

Figure 10.3 Surgical repair compared with TAVR.

Patient Selection Strategies

There is some controversy over whether scoring systems overestimate the risk of surgical outcomes.[21,22,34] Nonetheless, with comparable or better outcomes in high-risk patients, TAVR should be considered in context. Gallo and colleagues described a potential triage strategy focusing on life expectancy and predicted morbidity. They suggested that lowest-risk, longest-life-expectancy patients should be triaged to SAVR, whereas higher-risk patients with good life expectancy should be considered for TAVR. Importantly their plan emphasizes the value of counseling for patients with low life expectancy even in the setting of low morbidity.[11,14,24,35]

Frailty and Risk Stratification

The concept of frailty and functional status will be covered more fully elsewhere in this text, so we will briefly touch only on the points relevant to the assessment of patients for cardiovascular interventions.

Frailty Relationship to CAD

The prevalence of cardiovascular disease is significantly higher in frail patients as compared to nonfrail patients across multiple cohort studies (Figure 10.4).[5,36] It is unclear whether one causes the other or if they are simply co-morbid, but work is underway examining this important issue.

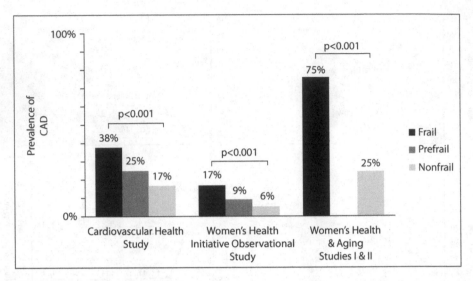

Figure 10.4 Frailty compared to nonfrailty.

Gait Speed

It has also been demonstrated that slow gait speed correlates well with elevated Society for Thoracic Surgery (STS) database prediction of morbidity and mortality.[7,37]

Muscle Mass

Muscle mass is being evaluated as a simple way to estimate frailty in patients. Radiologic studies have correlated the size of psoas and paraspinous muscles with odds of frailty.[11,38] Work is ongoing to establish bedside techniques such as paraspinous muscle ultrasound to evaluate frailty, but results are not yet conclusive on this approach. Nonetheless, having a simple bedside tool to evaluate for frailty would be a tremendous asset in efforts to risk stratify patients and provide accurate risk assessments for different types of interventions. Any risk stratification system should take into account frailty, disability (inability to complete activities of daily living) and co-morbid medical conditions.[14,36,39]

Conclusion

There are many procedural options available to the geriatric cardiac patient. Patients over 80 have elevated, but acceptable risks for all types of cardiac interventions. Functional outcomes are usually improved with interventions, and while higher than in younger patients, risks track along with elevated mortality in age-matched controls. Minimally invasive approaches may improve outcomes in the elderly, but more studies are needed. There are a number of newer percutaneous interventions that offer additional options for the sickest patients, many of whom are over the age of 80. Current and future research is focused on randomized controlled assessment of outcomes in the elderly and will allow for improved decision-making. Age in general is not a strong predictor of outcome in multivariate analyses, but functional status and frailty are more significant factors to consider; risk modeling should seek ways to factor these elements in and assess them consistently.

References

1. Philip F, Athappan G, Tuzcu EM, Svensson LG, Kapadia SR. MitraClip for severe symptomatic mitral regurgitation in patients at high surgical risk: a comprehensive systematic review. *Catheter Cardiovasc Interv.* 2014; 84(4):581–590.

2. Meco M, Biraghi T, Panisi P, *et al.* Aortocoronary bypass grafting in high-risk patients over 75 years. Propensity score analysis of on versus off-pump, early and midterm results. *J Cardiovasc Surg (Torino).* 2007; 48(3):339–347.

3. Buzzatti N, Taramasso M, Latib A, *et al.* Transcatheter mitral repair and replacement: state of the art and future directions. *J Heart Valve Dis.* 2014; 23(4):492–505.

4. D'ascenzo F, Moretti C, Marra WG, *et al.* Meta-analysis of the usefulness of Mitraclip in patients with functional mitral regurgitation. *Am J Cardiol.* 2015; 116(2):325–331.

5. Jensen BØ, Hughes P, Rasmussen LS, Pedersen PU, Steinbrüchel DA. Health-related quality of life following off-pump versus on-pump coronary artery bypass grafting in elderly moderate to high-risk patients: a randomized trial. *Eur J Cardiothorac Surg.* 2006; 30(2):294–299.

6. Maisano F, Alfieri O, Banai S, *et al.* The future of transcatheter mitral valve interventions: competitive or complementary role of repair vs. replacement? *Eur Heart J.* 2015; 36(26):1651–1659.

7. Raja SG. Myocardial revascularization for the elderly: current options, role of off-pump coronary artery bypass grafting and outcomes. *Curr Cardiol Rev.* 2012; 8(1):26–36.

8. Alexander KP, Anstrom KJ, Muhlbaier LH, *et al.* Outcomes of cardiac surgery in patients > or = 80 years: results from the National Cardiovascular Network. *J Am Coll Cardiol.* 2000; 35(3):731–738.

9. Rashedi N, Otto CM. Aortic stenosis: changing disease concepts. *J Cardiovasc Ultrasound.* 2015; 23(2):59–69.

10. Nicolini F, Agostinelli A, Vezzani A, *et al.* The evolution of cardiovascular surgery in elderly patient: a review of current options and outcomes. *BioMed Res Int.* 2014:1–10.

11. Panesar SS, Chikwe J, Mirza SB, *et al.* Off-pump coronary artery bypass surgery may reduce the incidence of stroke in patients with significant left main stem disease. *Thorac Cardiovasc Surg.* 2008; 56(5):247–255.

12. Seco M, Edelman JJ, Forrest P, *et al.* Geriatric cardiac surgery: chronology vs. biology. *Heart Lung Circ.* 2014; 23(9):794–801.

13. Kodali SK, Williams MR, Smith CR, *et al.* Two-year outcomes after transcatheter or surgical aortic-valve replacement. *N Engl J Med.* 2012; 366(18):1686–1695.

14. Cheng DC, Bainbridge D, Martin JE, Novick RJ; Evidence-Based Perioperative Clinical Outcomes Research Group. Does off-pump coronary artery bypass reduce mortality, morbidity, and resource utilization when compared with conventional coronary artery bypass? A meta-analysis of randomized trials. *Anesthesiology.* 2005; 102(1):188–203.

15. Srinivasan AK, Oo ΛY, Grayson AD, *et al.* Mid-term survival after cardiac surgery in elderly patients: analysis of predictors for increased mortality. *Interact Cardiovasc Thorac Surg.* 2004; 3(2):289–293.

16. Thourani VH, Myung R, Kilgo P, *et al.* Long-term outcomes after isolated aortic valve replacement in octogenarians: a modern perspective. *Ann Thorac Surg.* 2008; 86(5):1458–1465.

17. Denti P, Maisano F, Alfieri O. Devices for mitral valve repair. *J Cardiovasc Transl Res.* 2014; 7(3):266–281.

18. Likosky DS, Dacey LJ, Baribeau YR, *et al.* Long-term survival of the very elderly undergoing coronary artery bypass grafting. *Ann Thorac Surg.* 2008; 85(4):1233–1237.

19. Abel NJ, Rogal GJ, Burns P, Saunders CR, Chamberlain RS. Aortic valve replacement with and without coronary artery bypass graft surgery in octogenarians: is it safe and feasible? *Cardiology.* 2013; 124(3):163–173.

20. Zingone B, Gatti G, Rauber E, *et al.*
Early and late outcomes of cardiac
surgery in octogenarians. *ATS.* 2009;
87(1):71–78.

21. Dacey LJ, Likosky DS, Ryan TJ Jr.,
et al. Long-term survival after surgery
versus percutaneous intervention
in octogenarians with multivessel
coronary disease. *Ann Thorac Surg.* 2007;
84(6):1904–1911.

22. Sheridan BC, Stearns SC, Rossi JS, *et al.*
Three-year outcomes of multivessel
revascularization in very elderly acute
coronary syndrome patients. *ATS.* 2010;
89(6):1889–1895.

23. Coylewright M, Cabalka AK, Malouf
JA, *et al.* Percutaneous mitral valve
replacement using a transvenous,
transseptal approach: transvenous mitral
valve replacement. *J Am Coll Cardiol Intv.*
2015; 8(6):850–857.

24. Athanasiou T, Al-Ruzzeh S, Kumar P, *et al.*
Off-pump myocardial revascularization
is associated with less incidence of
stroke in elderly patients. *ATS.* 2004;
77(2):745–753.

25. Rashedi N, Otto CM. When should we
operate in asymptomatic severe aortic
stenosis? 2015. Available from:
www.acc.org/latest-in-cardiology
/articles/2015/02/04/14/49/when-should-
we-operate-in-asymptomatic-severe-
aortic-stenosis (Accessed July 19, 2017).

26. Wiedemann D, Bernhard D, Laufer G,
Kocher A. The elderly patient and cardiac
surgery: a mini-review. *Gerontology.* 2010;
56(3):241–249.

27. Osnabrugge RL, Arnold SV, Reynolds
MR, *et al.* Health status after transcatheter
aortic valve replacement in patients at
extreme surgical risk: results from the
CoreValve U.S. Trial. *J Am Coll Cardiol
Intv.* 2015; 8(2):315–323.

28. Yamamoto M, Mouillet G, Meguro K,
et al. Clinical results of transcatheter
aortic valve implantation in octogenarians
and nonagenarians: insights from
the FRANCE-2 Registry. *ATS.* 2014;
97(1):29–36.

29. Timek TA, Turfe Z, Hooker RL, *et al.*
Aortic valve replacement in octogenarians
with prior cardiac surgery. *ATS.* 2015;
99(2):518–523.

30. Maganti M, Rao V, Armstrong S, *et al.*
Redo valvular surgery in elderly patients.
ATS. 2009; 87(2):521–525.

31. Kaneko T, Loberman D, Gosev I, *et al.*
Reoperative aortic valve replacement in
the octogenarians: minimally invasive
technique in the era of transcatheter valve
replacement. *J Thoracic Cardiovasc Surg.*
2014; 147(1):155–162.

32. Reardon MJ, Adams DH, Kleiman NS,
et al. 2-year outcomes in patients
undergoing surgical or self-expanding
transcatheter aortic valve replacement.
J Am Coll Cardiol. 2015; 66(2):113–121.

33. Saxena A, Dinh DT, Yap CH, *et al.* Critical
analysis of early and late outcomes
after isolated coronary artery bypass
surgery in elderly patients. *ATS.* 2011;
92(5):1703–1711.

34. Grossi EA, Schwartz CF, Yu P-J, *et al.*
High-risk aortic valve replacement: are
the outcomes as bad as predicted? *Ann
Thorac Surg.* 2008; 85(1):102–107.

35. Gallo M, Gerosa G. Multiparameter
approach to evaluate elderly patients
undergoing aortic valve replacement.
J Thoracic Cardiovasc Surg. 2014;
148(4):1749–1751.

36. Afilalo J, Karunananthan S, Eisenberg MJ,
Alexander KP, Bergman H. Role of frailty
in patients with cardiovascular disease.
Am J Cardiol. 2009; 103(11):1616–1621.

37. Afilalo J, Eisenberg MJ, Morin JF, *et al.*
Gait speed as an incremental predictorof
mortality and major morbidity in elderly
patients undergoing cardiac surgery. *J Am
Coll Cardiol.* 2010; 56(20):1668–1676.

38. Canvasser LD, Mazurek AA, Cron DC,
et al. Paraspinous muscle as a predictor
of surgical outcome. *Surg Res.* 2014;
192(1):76–81.

39. Englesbe MJ, Terjimanian MN, Lee JS,
et al. Morphometric age and surgical risk.
J Am Coll Surg. 2013; 216(5):976–985.

The Aging Valve

Mario E. Montealegre, Rabya S. Saraf and
Robina Matyal

Key Points

- The prevalence of valvular heart disease (VHD) is approximately 2.5% in the United States, with a notable increase after the age of 65 (from <2% to 13%). This likely represents an underestimation of true prevalence, as VHD is often asymptomatic.
- Aortic stenosis (AS) is the most common VHD, occurring in approximately 2% of the population aged 70–80 years, and increasing even more after age 80. The prevalence of aortic sclerosis, characterized by leaflet calcification and thickening without restriction in leaflet opening, is approximately 25–30%.
- Surgical valve replacement and transcatheter aortic valve replacement (TAVR) are the only conclusive treatments for severe AS and are recommended as a course of action for symptomatic patients, asymptomatic patients with severe AS undergoing cardiac surgery for other reasons, and asymptomatic patients with severe AS and left ventricular ejection fraction ≤50%.
- Mitral stenosis (MS) due to calcification of the mitral annulus is more common in the older age group, as opposed to MS secondary to rheumatic fever.
- The prevalence of mitral regurgitation (MR) increases proportionally with age. In elderly patients, the most common causes of severe MR requiring surgery are ischemic heart disease and mitral valve prolapse secondary to fibroelastic deficiency.
- Patients with prosthetic valves, heart transplant recipients and those with a previous history of infective endocarditis should receive preoperative antibiotic prophylaxis for selected procedures.

Introduction

During the past few decades, the aging of the population has led to an increased number of patients with valvular heart disease (VHD).[1-3] Currently, the prevalence of VHD is approximately 2.5% in the United States, with no significant difference between genders, and a notable increase after the age of 65 (from <2% to 13%).[1,4,5] These numbers may be an underestimation of the problem, since VHD is frequently asymptomatic.[1,2,6] VHD can be classified by severity (Table 11.1) based on physical examination and transthoracic echo-cardiography (TTE).[7,8] In some cases, additional testing such as transesophageal echocardiography, stress testing, catheterization and computerized tomography may be used.[6-10] The management of severe, symptomatic VHD has been traditionally limited to surgical valve replacement. Recent advances in surgical valvuloplasty and repair techniques, as well as transcatheter valve implantation, have allowed treatment of patients who were

Table 11.1 Perioperative management of valvular heart disease for noncardiac surgery[11,16–20]

Preoperative Evaluation[27]

Preoperative echocardiography should be performed for patients with clinically suspected moderate or greater degrees of stenosis or regurgitation within 1 year or there is significant change in the clinical status or physical examination since the last evaluation

Valve repair or replacement is indicated before elective noncardiac surgery in patients that meet standard indications for intervention on the basis of symptoms and severity of stenosis or regurgitation

Disease- Specific Management[3]

	Frequent underlying valvular abnormalities	Echocardiographic criteria of severe disease	Additional features in severe disease	Perioperative management
AS	Calcification of tri-leaflet AV Calcification of congenital bicuspid AV Rheumatic changes with commissural fusion (usually in association with rheumatic MV disease)	Aortic $V_{max} \geq 4$ m/s Mean gradient ≥ 40 mmHg AV area ≤ 1 cm^2 (or ≤ 0.6 cm^2/m^2)	*Asymptomatic:* LV diastolic dysfunction Mild LV hypertrophy Normal or ↓ LV ejection fraction *Symptomatic:* Significant LV hypertrophy with diastolic dysfunction Exertional dyspnea, ↓ exercise tolerance, angina or syncope Patients with poor LV function may have low gradients (i.e. low-gradient/low-flow AS) Patients with severe LV hypertrophy with small LV chambers may have low gradient despite preserved LV ejection fraction (i.e. paradoxical low-flow AS)	Sinus rhythm and atrial contraction are important for filling of poorly compliant LV Atrial contraction can account for 30–40% of LV filling in these patients Avoid tachycardia, which ↓ diastolic time and can ↓ perfusion of hypertrophic LV Avoid bradycardia due to ↓ cardiac output Preserve afterload ↓ in afterload (e.g. during neuraxial anesthesia) may significantly ↓ coronary perfusion Avoid vasodilation Vasoconstrictors to treat hypotension
AR	Calcified AV (bicuspid or tri-leaflet) Dilated aortic sinuses or ascending aorta Rheumatic changes Previous infective endocarditis with leaflet perforation	Jet width > 65% of LV outflow tract Vena contracta > 0.6 cm Holodiastolic flow reversal in proximal abdominal aorta Regurgitant fraction ≥ 50% ERO ≥ 0.3 cm^2	*Asymptomatic:* Evidence of LV dilation *Symptomatic:* Moderate to severe LV dilation May occur with normal or ↓ LV ejection fraction Exertional angina, dyspnea, and/or other heart failure symptoms	Modest ↑ in heart rate (↓ diastolic period, therefore ↓ regurgitation) ↓ in diastolic period also ↓ LV end diastolic pressure and may result in ↑ coronary perfusion Afterload reduction ↓ regurgitant volume

MS	Rheumatic MV changes with commissural fusion and diastolic doming of leaflets	MV area ≤ 1.5 cm² Very severe if MV area ≤ 1 cm²	*Asymptomatic:* Severe LA enlargement ↑ PASP > 30 mmHg *Symptomatic:* Severe LA enlargement ↑ PASP > 30 mmHg ↓ exercise tolerance and/or exertional dyspnea	Maintain ↑ LA pressure to increase LV filling Avoid ↑ preload, which may generate LA distension and AF Avoid tachycardia, which ↓ diastolic time and LV filling Avoid bradycardia due to fixed stroke volume If patient has baseline sinus rhythm, acute AF may significantly ↓ LV filling (consider cardioversion)
Primary MR	MV prolapse Loss of coaptation or flail leaflet Rheumatic MV changes with leaflet restriction Prior infective endocarditis Leaflet thickening with radiation therapy	Central MR jet > 40% LA or holosystolic eccentric MR jet Vena contracta > 0.7 cm Regurgitant fraction ≥ 50% ERO ≥ 0.4 cm²	*Asymptomatic:* Moderate to severe LA enlargement LV enlargement Pulmonary hypertension at rest or with exercise *Symptomatic:* Moderate to severe LA enlargement LV enlargement Pulmonary hypertension present ↓ exercise tolerance and/or exertional dyspnea	↓ afterload to improve antegrade flow MR may appear less severe when evaluated in patients under anesthesia due to decreased afterload
Secondary MR	LV dilation or regional wall motion abnormalities Severe tethering of MV leaflets Mitral annular dilation with loss of central leaflet coaptation	ERO ≥ 0.2 cm² Regurgitant fraction ≥ 50%	*Asymptomatic:* May have LV systolic dysfunction May present with LV dilation Symptoms may be present due to coronary ischemia or heart failure but respond to revascularization and medical therapy *Symptomatic:* LV dilation and/or systolic dysfunction Heart failure symptoms due to MR persist after revascularization and optimized medical therapy ↓ exercise tolerance and/or exertional dyspnea	Similar to primary MR Patients with ischemic MR are at increased risk for myocardial ischemia

(cont.)

Table 11.1 (cont.)

	Frequent underlying valvular abnormalities	Echocardiographic criteria of severe disease	Additional features in severe disease	Perioperative management
TR	Flail or grossly distorted leaflets Severe dilation of the tricuspid annulus Marked leaflet tethering	Central jet area > 10 cm^2 Vena contracta > 0.7 cm Systolic flow reversal in hepatic veins	*Asymptomatic:* Dilated RA/RV/IVC ↓ respiratory variation of IVC ↑ RA pressure Diastolic flattening of the interventricular septum Symptoms related to left heart or pulmonary vascular disease *Symptomatic:* Dilated RA/RV/IVC ↓ respiratory variation of IVC ↑ RA pressure Diastolic flattening of the interventricular septum ↓ RV systolic function in late phase Fatigue, palpitations, dyspnea, abdominal bloating, anorexia, edema	Avoid ↑ in pulmonary vascular resistance (hypoxia, hypercarbia, acidosis) Avoid mechanical ventilation with high airway pressures, which may result in ↓ RV filling

Abbreviations: AS, aortic stenosis; AR, aortic regurgitation; MS, mitral stenosis; MR, mitral regurgitation; TR, tricuspid regurgitation; AV, aortic valve; MV, mitral valve; ERO, effective regurgitant orifice; LV, left ventricle; LA, left atrium; PASP, pulmonary artery systolic pressure; RA, right atrium; RV, right ventricle; IVC, inferior vena cava; AF, atrial fibrillation once deemed poor surgical candidates due to co-morbidities and/or advanced age.[7,9,11-15] In this chapter we will discuss valvulopathies, especially those affecting the elderly population, as well as their medical and surgical treatment.

A summary of the specific types of VHD and their perioperative management is presented in Table 11.1.

Specific Types of Valvular Heart Disease

Aortic Stenosis

Aortic stenosis (AS) is the most common VHD in developed countries,[21-23] occurring in approximately 2% of the population aged 70–80 years, and increasing even more after age 80.[10,24,25] Additionally, the prevalence of leaflet calcification and thickening without restriction in leaflet opening (i.e. aortic sclerosis) is approximately 25–30%.[11,14,26-28] Severe symptomatic AS is associated with a high morbidity and mortality, although this can be reduced with appropriate management.[22,29]

In AS, progressive leaflet degeneration results in narrowing of the valve orifice, which in turn produces an outflow obstruction of the left ventricle.[11,30] This narrowing is commonly due to calcification of the leaflet and commissural fusion, which lead to restricted leaflet motion.[6,31]

In normal patients, the aortic valve area is approximately 3–4 cm^2, and when it decreases to <1 cm^2, the patient usually becomes symptomatic.[23,30,32,33] Early calcification of the aortic valve can occur secondary to congenital abnormalities (e.g. bicuspid valve), but age-related calcification usually occurs in the setting of an anatomically normal valve.[24,30] Age-related aortic valve calcification occurs gradually, often spanning decades before patients begin to demonstrate symptoms, at which point, the AS is likely to be severe.[27,28,30,34] AS shares similar risk factors with atherosclerosis, leading to a simultaneous occurrence of the two diseases.[6,27,34-36] The major clinical risk factors for degenerative aortic valve disease include age, male gender, smoking, dyslipidemia and a history of arterial hypertension.[36-40]

AS has a pathophysiology similar to other degenerative cardiovascular diseases, such as atherosclerosis. It typically starts as inflammation of the leaflet tissue in the setting of increased leaflet stress or flow abnormalities, with foam cell and lipid accumulation. This subsequently progresses to fibrosis and valvular thickening, eventually leading to calcification.[30,34] One proposed mechanism for this calcification is that stress activates the interstitial cells in the aortic valve resulting in cell proliferation, osteogenesis and calcification.[34,41]

Although rheumatic valve disease is no longer a major cause of aortic stenosis in developed countries, it remains a significant risk factor for aortic valve disease in developing countries.[30,42] In rheumatic AS, commissural fusion occurs as a consequence of the inflammatory response. This renders the valve susceptible to further damage, greatly increasing the development and progression of fibrosis and calcification.[16,30,35,43] Rheumatic aortic stenosis rarely occurs in isolation, and is frequently associated with mitral stenosis.

Diagnosis and Clinical Manifestations

The three classic symptoms of AS are syncope, angina and dyspnea on exertion.[30,34] Symptoms of AS and their severity are directly associated with mortality. An asymptomatic patient with severe stenosis has a better prognosis than one that is symptomatic.[22,44,45]

Echocardiography can help establish the presence and severity of the disease.[30,34] The gold standard for diagnosis AS is two-dimensional Doppler echocardiography, which can be used to determine aortic valve velocities, pressure gradients and valve area. However, there is a chance of underestimating the severity of AS with Doppler echocardiography when left ventricular function is impaired (i.e. low ejection fraction), since aortic valve velocities and gradients can be decreased, despite a severe stenosis.[30,46] This is commonly referred to as low-flow, low-gradient severe AS and can be confirmed using a dobutamine stress test.[20,30] Other factors that may affect the diagnosis of severe AS include uncontrolled systemic hypertension, concomitant aortic insufficiency and high-output state such as severe anemia and hemodialysis.[30,47,48] If noninvasive imaging is unsuccessful in helping determine the presence and/or severity of the disease, cardiac catheterization is the recommended diagnostic tool.[30,47]

Medical Management

The American College of Cardiology (ACC) and American Heart Association (AHA) recommend that asymptomatic patients with mild AS undergo a TTE examination every 3–5 years, those with moderate AS every 1–2 years and one every 6–12 months in patients with severe AS.[30,49,50] Exercise stress testing can be performed on asymptomatic patients with severe AS, but is not routinely recommended for symptomatic patients.[30,50] Severe AS progression cannot be managed through medical therapy alone, and requires surgical intervention to relieve the obstruction and improve prognosis. On the other hand, in the case of mild or moderate AS, medical treatment, specifically heart failure therapies, such as ACE inhibitors, beta-blockers, angiotensin receptor blockers and aldosterone receptor antagonists should be used. Additionally, in such patients, existing co-morbidities should be appropriately treated.[30,51]

Surgical Management

Balloon Aortic Valvotomy

Although it is a fairly simple procedure, balloon aortic valvotomy is the least effective surgical approach to deal with AS.[16,52] This percutaneous procedure consists of passing a balloon through a stenotic aortic valve and inflating it inside the valve orifice. The results are often short-lived, and the risk of periprocedural complications is high.[50,52] Therefore, balloon aortic valvotomy is performed either if patients are unsuitable candidates for aortic valve replacement or as a temporary palliative measure for those that will be undergoing aortic valve replacement in the near future.[52-54]

Surgical or Transcatheter Aortic Valve Replacement

Transcatheter aortic valve replacement (TAVR) was performed for the first time in humans in 2002. This procedure has become increasingly popular, with about half of the high-risk patients with severe AS benefiting from it.[17] Surgical valve replacement and TAVR are the only conclusive treatments for severe AS and are recommended as a course of action for symptomatic patients, asymptomatic patients with severe AS undergoing cardiac surgery for other reasons and asymptomatic patients with severe AS and left ventricular ejection fraction ≤50%.[3,30,47-49,55]

Outcome of Surgery

Age is an important factor determining the outcome of aortic valve surgery, and elderly patients have increased postoperative mortality rates. In one study, patients older than

80 years of age were shown to have a higher mortality than patients aged 65–75 years (14% versus 4% mortality).[56,57] Age-related calcification of the valve also contributes to poor outcomes in elderly patients and makes surgery difficult and high risk.[53,57-59] If an additional procedure (e.g. coronary artery bypass) is performed in association with aortic valve replacement, the mortality rate increases significantly.[50,57]

Different types of prosthetic valves are available in the market, but in general they can be divided into bioprosthetic and mechanical valves. Mechanical valves have a significantly longer duration than bioprosthetic valves, but are limited by the need for chronic anticoagulation.[57,59-61] Bioprosthetic valves are frequently recommended for elderly patients, since their functional life is much longer than the patient's life expectancy.[58-60,62] Furthermore, only bioprosthetic TAVR devices are currently available for clinical use.

Aortic Regurgitation

Aortic regurgitation (AR) can occur secondary to degeneration of a bicuspid or tricuspid aortic valve degeneration (frequently co-existing with AS), or secondary to dilation of the aortic root.[8,60,61,63,64] AR is more commonly a slowly progressive disease, resulting in left ventricular volume overload, with dilation and hypertrophy.[8,60,61,65] Aortic valve repair is the preferred method of treatment for isolated AR, especially in younger patients.[66-68] This procedure does not require long-term anticoagulation therapy, it preserves the integrity of the aortic root physiology and function, and the lack of a prosthetic material lowers the risk of bacterial endocarditis.[59,67] However, the long-term durability is low, and significant expertise is required for a successful procedure.[51,67]

Mitral Stenosis

Mitral stenosis (MS) is most commonly caused by rheumatic heart disease.[60,69,70] With the widespread use of antibiotic therapy, the incidence of rheumatic MS has significantly decreased in developed countries.[60,61,69-71] Although rheumatic MS is not frequent in elderly patients, MS due to calcification of the mitral annulus is more common in this age group. In one study, of patients aged >62 years with mitral annular calcification, up to 6% had associated MS.[60,65,72,73]

Rheumatic MS is a slowly progressive disease often taking years to become clinically significant.[8,74-76] Clinical features of MS include dyspnea on exertion, palpitations, chest pain, dizziness, fatigue and pulmonary hypertension.[63,69-71,74] TTE can provide important information regarding disease progression and pulmonary artery systolic pressures.[8,73,74,77]

MS also increases the likelihood of associated atrial arrhythmias (e.g. atrial fibrillation), which frequently require heart rate control and anticoagulation to prevent left atrial appendage thrombi formation.[8,78-80]

A suitable and effective choice to treat MS is percutaneous mitral valve balloon valvuloplasty.[81,82] The average age of the population undergoing mitral valvuloplasty has been increasing over the last few decades, especially in developed countries.[3,74,82,83] The success of valvuloplasty depends upon strict selection criteria, such as age and co-morbidities.[82,84] Complication rates increase with age, since elderly patients frequently have large rotated hearts, increased atrial size and increased vessel tortuosity.[79,82] The best outcomes for percutaneous valvuloplasty are obtained when the valve is mobile, not calcified, and has no significant thickening.[8,20,54,83] Outcome is also affected by such factors as age, presence or absence of atrial fibrillation, and heart failure classification[3,7,8,83] If there is significant thickening of the valve and fibrosis of the subvalvular apparatus, then surgical valve replacement is preferred.[8,74,85,86] Patients with severe MS who are undergoing cardiac surgery other than for MS are recommended for concomitant mitral valve replacement.[8,87] In general, it is recommended to withhold intervention unless symptoms are seen. Considerations for selecting mechanical or bioprosthetic replacements are similar to those for AS.

Mitral Regurgitation

The prevalence of mitral regurgitation (MR) increases proportionately with age.[20,86,88] In elderly patients, the most common causes of severe MR requiring surgery are ischemic heart disease and mitral valve prolapse secondary to fibroelastic deficiency.[1,7,88] Mitral regurgitation may be caused due to excessive or restricted leaflet motion, or may occur in anatomically normal leaflets (e.g. secondary to mitral annular dilation). Ischemic compromise of the papillary muscles may also result in MR.[8,89] Additional causes of MR include infective endocarditis, rheumatic heart disease, previous radiation treatment, cleft mitral valve and connective tissue disorders.[8,90]

TTE is commonly used in patients with MR to assess left and right ventricular function, pulmonary artery pressure and to evaluate the mechanism of regurgitation.[8,79] In cases where TTE is not conclusive, transesophageal echocardiography may be used to clarify the diagnosis, due to its greater ability to visualize the mitral valve and exclude left atrial appendage thrombi.[1,3,8,91,92]

Surgical intervention for MR in the elderly is reserved for highly symptomatic patients, although younger asymptomatic patients with left ventricular dysfunction may also undergo surgery.[1,86,93-95] Patients with ischemic MR tend to have a higher operative mortality than patients with MR due to other causes.[1,29,96,97]

In chronic secondary MR due to coronary artery or idiopathic myocardial disease, regurgitation is one of many components of the disease; thus solely treating MR will not solve the underlying cause. Rather, a more holistic approach is necessary.[1,3,5,8,92,98] Patients that have heart failure with reduced ejection fraction tend to develop chronic secondary MR. In such cases, the standard medical therapy should be given (diuretics, beta-blockers, ACE inhibitors and aldosterone antagonists).[8,94,99] In cases where patients are symptomatic, cardiac resynchronization therapy may be necessary.[8,9,21,98] Patients that are undergoing coronary artery bypass graft or aortic valve replacement and have chronic severe secondary MR are excellent candidates for concomitant mitral valve surgery (repair or replacement).[7,8,10,18,99] For severely symptomatic patients whose symptoms do not subside despite medical treatment, it is recommended that mitral valve repair or replacement be performed.

Mitral valve repair is a lower-risk alternative for valve replacement in patients suffering from MR, results in improvement of left ventricular function and is associated with a lower mortality.[6-9,14] Mitral valve repair avoids the problems associated with the use of a prosthetic valve, such as bacterial endocarditis, need for anticoagulation and risk of thrombosis.[8,9,11,19,21]

Tricuspid Regurgitation

Tricuspid valve disease has traditionally been underappreciated, and some have referred to the tricuspid as "the forgotten valve." Despite this, tricuspid regurgitation (TR) is a common valvular disease, occurring in roughly 74% of men and 86% of women over the age of 70.[10,11,18,24,88] TR may be caused by disease of the leaflets or subvalvular parts such as tricuspid valve prolapse or flail leaflet. Functional TR may be due to left-sided heart disease or pulmonary hypertension. Isolated TR is associated with atrial fibrillation and aging, and frequently occurs secondary to right ventricular dilation.[9,11,14,27,88] TR may also present due to right ventricular pacing-induced dyssynchrony, or delayed activation of the right ventricle due to alteration in right ventricular geometry. TR is medically treated through the use of diuretics, along with handling any correlated left-sided heart or pulmonary disease.[11,19,27–29,88]

Additional Factors to Consider in Patients with Valvular Heart Disease

Anticoagulation

Heart disease in general, and atrial fibrillation in particular, can result in thrombi formation and embolic stroke. Anticoagulation therapy in high-risk patients can decrease the rate of embolic events from 5–10% to 2%.[3] Patients with mechanical prosthetic valves should receive long-term anticoagulation with a vitamin K antagonist with a goal to prevent thromboembolic complications.[17] In these patients, the target International Normalized Ratios are between 2.5 and 3.5. In patients with bioprosthetic valves, short-term anticoagulation with vitamin K antagonists and aspirin therapy is started soon after implantation.[17] Anticoagulation can then be discontinued 3 months after valve replacement unless the patient has another indication for anticoagulation (e.g. atrial fibrillation).[17]

In patients undergoing noncardiac surgery with a low hemorrhagic risk, anticoagulation may be continued throughout the perioperative period. In patients with a higher hemorrhagic risk, vitamin K antagonists should be discontinued 2–3 days before surgery and the patient anticoagulated either with unfractionated or low-molecular-weight heparin.[17]

Endocarditis prophylaxis

Patients with prosthetic valves, heart transplant recipients and those with previous history of infective endocarditis should receive preoperative antibiotic prophylaxis for selected procedures.[6,8,11,24,40] Among these procedures are dental surgery (if there is gingival manipulation or perforation of the oral mucosa) and invasive procedures of the respiratory tract that involve a mucosal incision or biopsy. Prophylaxis is not recommended for routine bronchoscopy (unless there is a mucosal incision), gastrointestinal or urinary tract procedures. Elderly patients at risk for infective endocarditis should maintain good oral health and schedule regular dental appointments.

Conclusion

In the last few decades, major advances have allowed physicians to better manage and treat various types of VHD. Increased life expectancy has resulted in a higher prevalence of VHD in the geriatric patient. The geriatric population has specific characteristics that necessitate specific treatments that may vary from those needed by a younger population. Different medical and surgical interventions have shown to be very beneficial in not only attenuating the consequences of the underlying disease, but also in improving the life expectancy of individuals living with VHD.

References

1. Bach DS, Deeb GM, Bolling SF. Accuracy of intraoperative transesophageal echocardiography for estimating the severity of functional mitral regurgitation. *Am J Cardiol.* 1995; 76(7):508–512.

2. Iung B, Vahanian A. Epidemiology of acquired valvular heart disease. *Can J Cardiol.* 2014; 30(9):962–970.

3. Khabbaz KR, Mahmood F, Shakil O, *et al.* Dynamic 3-dimensional echocardiographic assessment of mitral annular geometry in patients with functional mitral regurgitation. *Ann Thorac Surg.* 2013; 95(1): 105–110.

4. Iung B, Baron G, Butchart EG. A prospective survey of patients with valvular heart disease in Europe: the Euro Heart Survey on Valvular Heart Disease. *Eur Heart J.* 2003; 24(13):1231–1243.

5. Grewal KS, Malkowski MJ, Piracha AR, *et al.* Effect of general anesthesia on the severity of mitral regurgitation by transesophageal echocardiography. *Am J Cardiol.* 2000; 85(2):199–203.

6. Gorman JH, Jackson BM, Enomoto Y, Gorman RC. The effect of regional ischemia on mitral valve annular saddle shape. *ATS.* 2004; 77(2):544–548.

7. Hahn RT, Abraham T, Adams MS, *et al.* Guidelines for performing a comprehensive transesophageal echocardiographic examination: recommendations from the American Society of Echocardiography and the Society of Cardiovascular Anesthesiologists. *J Am Soc Echocardiogr.* 2013; 26(9):921–964.

8. Nishimura RA, Otto CM, Bonow RO, *et al.* 2014 AHA/ACC Guideline for the Management of Patients with Valvular Heart Disease: a report of the American College of Cardiology/ American Heart Association Task Force on Practice Guidelines. *Circulation* 2014; 129(23):e650.

9. Kocica MJ, Gorman JH, Corno AF, *et al.* Annuloplasty ring selection for chronic ischemic mitral regurgitation: lessons from the ovine model. *Ann Thorac Surg.* 2003; 76(5):1556–63.

10. Lancellotti P, Moura L, Piérard LA, *et al.* European Association of Echocardiography recommendations for the assessment of valvular regurgitation. Part 2: mitral and tricuspid regurgitation (native valve disease). *Eur J Echocardiogr.* 2010; 11(4):307–332.

11. Warraich HJ, Chaudary B, Maslow A, *et al.* Mitral annular nonplanarity: correlation between annular height/ commissural width ratio and the nonplanarity angle. *J Cardiothorac Vasc Anesth.* 2012; 26(2):186–190.

12. Bonow RO, Carabello B, de Leon AC Jr., *et al.* Guidelines for the management of patients with valvular heart disease: executive summary. A report of the American College of Cardiology/ American Heart Association Task Force on Practice Guidelines (Committee on Management of Patients with Valvular Heart Disease). *Circulation.* 1998; 98(18):1949–1984.

13. Smith CR, Leon MB, Mack MJ, *et al.* Transcatheter versus surgical aortic-valve replacement in high-risk patients. *N Engl J Med.* 2011; 364(23):2187–2198.

14. Marsan NA, Westenberg JJM, Ypenburg C, *et al.* Quantification of functional mitral regurgitation by real-time 3D echocardiography: comparison with 3D velocity-encoded cardiac magnetic resonance. *JACC Cardiovasc Imaging.* 2009; 2(11):1245–1252.

15. Leon MB, Smith CR, Mack M, *et al.* Transcatheter aortic-valve implantation for aortic stenosis in patients who cannot undergo surgery. *N Engl J Med.* 2010; 363(17):1597–1607.

16. Grewal J, Mankad S, Freeman WK, *et al.* Real-time three-dimensional transesophageal echocardiography in the intraoperative assessment of mitral valve disease. *J Am Soc Echocardiogr.* 2009; 22(1):34–41.

17. Fleisher LA, Fleischmann KE, Auerbach AD, et al. 2014 ACC/AHA Guideline on perioperative cardiovascular evaluation and management of patients undergoing noncardiac surgery: a report of the American College of Cardiology/ American Heart Association Task Force on Practice Guidelines. *Circulation*. 2014; 130(24):2215–2245.

18. Vergnat M, Levack MM, Jassar AS, et al. The influence of saddle-shaped annuloplasty on leaflet curvature in patients with ischaemic mitral regurgitation. *Eur J Cardiothorac Surg*. 2012; 42(3):493–499.

19. Wang W, Lin Q, Wu W, et al. Quantification of mitral regurgitation by general imaging three-dimensional quantification: feasibility and accuracy. *J Am Soc Echocardiogr*. 2014; 27(3):268–276.

20. Bartels K, Thiele RH, Phillips-Bute B, et al. Dynamic indices of mitral valve function using perioperative three-dimensional transesophageal echocardiography. *J Cardiothorac Vasc Anesth*. 2014; 28(1):18–24.

21. Hien MD, Rauch H, Lichtenberg A, et al. Real-time three-dimensional transesophageal echocardiography: improvements in intraoperative mitral valve imaging. *Anesth Analg*. 2013; 116(2):287–295.

22. Carabello BA, Paulus WJ. Aortic stenosis. *Lancet*. 2009; 373(9667):956–966.

23. La Canna G, Arendar I, Maisano F, et al. Real-time three-dimensional transesophageal echocardiography for assessment of mitral valve functional anatomy in patients with prolapse-related regurgitation. *Am J Cardiol*. 2011; 107(9):1365–1374.

24. Hung J, Lang R, Flachskampf F, et al. 3D echocardiography: a review of the current status and future directions. *J Am Soc Echocardiogr*. 2007; 20(3): 213–233.

25. Lindroos M, Kupari M, Heikkilä J, Tilvis R. Prevalence of aortic valve abnormalities in the elderly: an echocardiographic study of a random population sample. *J Am Coll Cardiol*. 1993; 21(5):1220–1225.

26. Otto CM, Lind BK, Kitzman DW, Gersh BJ, Siscovick DS. Association of aortic-valve sclerosis with cardiovascular mortality and morbidity in the elderly. *N Engl J Med*. 1999; 341(3):142–147.

27. Mahmood F, Warraich HJ, Shahul S, et al. En face view of the mitral valve: definition and acquisition. *Anesth Analg*. 2012; 115(4):779–784.

28. Kwan J, Yeom BW, Jones M, et al. Acute geometric changes of the mitral annulus after coronary occlusion: a real-time 3D echocardiographic study. *J Korean Med Sci*. 2006; 21(2):217–223.

29. Kwan J, Qin JX, Popović ZB, et al. Geometric changes of mitral annulus assessed by real-time 3-dimensional echocardiography: becoming enlarged and less nonplanar in the anteroposterior direction during systole in proportion to global left ventricular systolic function. *J Am Soc Echocardiogr*. 2004; 17(11):1179–1184.

30. Czarny MJ, Resar JR. Diagnosis and management of valvular aortic stenosis. *Clin Med Insights Cardiol*. 2014; 8(Suppl 1):15–24.

31. Cary T, Pearce J. Aortic stenosis: pathophysiology, diagnosis, and medical management of nonsurgical patients. *Crit Care Nurse*. 2013; 33(2):58–72.

32. Kuppahally SS, Paloma A, Craig Miller D, Schnittger I, Liang D. Multiplanar visualization in 3D transthoracic echocardiography for precise delineation of mitral valve pathology. *Echocardiography*. 2008; 25(1):84–87.

33. Thavendiranathan P, Phelan D, Thomas JD, Flamm SD, Marwick TH. Quantitative assessment of mitral regurgitation: validation of new methods. *J Am Coll Cardiol*. 2012; 60(16): 1470–1483.

34. Anyanwu AC, Adams DH. Etiologic classification of degenerative mitral valve disease: Barlow's disease and fibroelastic deficiency. *Semin Thorac Cardiovasc Surg*. 2007; 19(2):90–96.

35. Eriksson MJ, Bitkover CY, Omran AS, *et al.* Mitral annular disjunction in advanced myxomatous mitral valve disease: echocardiographic detection and surgical correction. *J Am Soc Echocardiogr.* 2005; 18(10):1014–1022.

36. Stewart BF, Siscovick D, Lind BK, *et al.* Clinical factors associated with calcific aortic valve disease. Cardiovascular Health Study. *J Am Coll Cardiol.* 1997; 29(3):630–634.

37. Carmo P, Andrade MJ, Aguiar C, *et al.* Mitral annular disjunction in myxomatous mitral valve disease: a relevant abnormality recognizable by transthoracic echocardiography. *Cardiovasc Ultrasound.* 2010; 8:53.

38. Hutchins GMG, Moore GWG, Skoog DKD. The association of floppy mitral valve with disjunction of the mitral annulus fibrosus. *N Engl J Med.* 1986; 314(9):535–540.

39. Filsoufi F, Carpentier A. Principles of reconstructive surgery in degenerative mitral valve disease. *Semin Thorac Cardiovasc Surg.* 2007; 19(2):103–110.

40. Barlow JB, Pocock WA. Billowing, floppy, prolapsed or flail mitral valves? *Am J Cardiol.* 1985 Feb 1; 55(4):501–502.

41. Rajamannan NM, Bonow RO, Rahimtoola SH. Calcific aortic stenosis: an update. *Nat Clin Pract Cardiovasc Med.* 2007; 4(5):254–262.

42. Maffessanti F, Marsan NA, Tamborini G, *et al.* Quantitative analysis of mitral valve apparatus in mitral valve prolapse before and after annuloplasty: a three-dimensional intraoperative transesophageal study. *J Am Soc Echocardiogr.* 2011; 24(4):405–413.

43. Carpentier A, Chauvaud S, Fabiani JN, *et al.* Reconstructive surgery of mitral valve incompetence: ten-year appraisal. *J Thoracic Cardiovasc Surg.* 1980; 79(3):338–348.

44. Chandra S, Salgo IS, Sugeng L, *et al.* Characterization of degenerative mitral valve disease using morphologic analysis of real-time three-dimensional echocardiographic images: objective insight into complexity and planning of mitral valve repair. *Circ Cardiovasc Imaging.* 2011; 4(1):24–32.

45. Addetia K, Mor-Avi V, Weinert L, *et al.* A new definition for an old entity: improved definition of mitral valve prolapse using three-dimensional echocardiography and color-coded parametric models. *J Am Soc Echocardiogr.* 2014; 27(1):8–16.

46. Zakkar M, Patni R, Punjabi PP. Mitral valve regurgitation and 3D echocardiography. *Future Cardiol.* 2010; 6(2):231–242.

47. Biaggi P, Jedrzkiewicz S, Gruner C, *et al.* Quantification of mitral valve anatomy by three-dimensional transesophageal echocardiography in mitral valve prolapse predicts surgical anatomy and the complexity of mitral valve repair. *J Am Soc Echocardiogr.* 2012; 25(7):758–765.

48. Mahmood F, Gorman JH, Subramaniam B, *et al.* Changes in mitral valve annular geometry after repair: saddle-shaped versus flat annuloplasty rings. *Ann Thorac Surg.* 2010; 90(4):1212–1220.

49. Ahmed S, Nanda NC, Miller AP, *et al.* Usefulness of transesophageal three-dimensional echocardiography in the identification of individual segment/scallop prolapse of the mitral valve. *Echocardiography.* 2003; 20(2):203–209.

50. Agricola E, Oppizzi M, Pisani M, *et al.* Ischemic mitral regurgitation: mechanisms and echocardiographic classification. *Eur J Echocardiogr.* 2007; 9(2): 207–221.

51. Silbiger JJ. Mechanistic insights into ischemic mitral regurgitation: echocardiographic and surgical implications. *J Am Soc Echocardiogr.* 2011; 24(7):707–719.

52. Otto CM, Mickel MC, Kennedy JW, *et al.* Three-year outcome after balloon aortic valvuloplasty: insights into prognosis of valvular aortic stenosis. *Circulation.* 1994; 89(2):642–650.

53. Macnab A, Jenkins NP, Bridgewater BJM, *et al.* Three-dimensional echocardiography is superior to multiplane transoesophageal echo in the

assessment of regurgitant mitral valve morphology. *Eur J Echocardiogr*. 2004; 5(3):212–222.

54. Carpentier A. Cardiac valve surgery: the "French correction." *J Thorac Cardiovasc Surg*. 1983; 86(3):323–337.

55. Pepi M, Tamborini G, Maltagliati A, *et al*. Head-to-head comparison of two- and three-dimensional transthoracic and transesophageal echocardiography in the localization of mitral valve prolapse. *J Am Coll Cardiol*. 2006; 48(12): 2524–2530.

56. Looi J-L, Lee AP-W, Wan S, *et al*. Diagnosis of cleft mitral valve using real-time 3-dimensional transesophageal echocardiography. *Int J Cardiol*. 2013; 168(2):1629–1630.

57. Olsson M, Granström L, Lindblom D, Rosenqvist M, Rydén L. Aortic valve replacement in octogenarians with aortic stenosis: a case-control study. *J Am Coll Cardiol*. 1992; 20(7):1512–1516.

58. Levine RA, Glasson JR, Handschumacher MD, *et al*. Three-dimensional echocardiographic reconstruction of the mitral valve, with implications for the diagnosis of mitral valve prolapse. *Circulation*. 1989; 80(3):589–598.

59. Gaasch WH, Meyer TE. Left ventricular response to mitral regurgitation: implications for management. *Circulation*. 2008; 118(22):2298–2303.

60. Silbiger JJ. Anatomy, mechanics, and pathophysiology of the mitral annulus. *Am Heart J*. 2012; 164(2):163–176.

61. Piérard LA, Carabello BA. Ischaemic mitral regurgitation: pathophysiology, outcomes and the conundrum of treatment. *Eur Heart J*. 2010; 31(24):2996–3005.

62. Hammermeister K, Sethi GK, Henderson WG, *et al*. Outcomes 15 years after valve replacement with a mechanical versus a bioprosthetic valve: final report of the Veterans Affairs randomized trial. *J Am Coll Cardiol*. 2000; 36(4): 1152–1158.

63. Salgo IS, Gorman JH, Gorman RC, *et al*. Effect of annular shape on leaflet curvature in reducing mitral leaflet stress. *Circulation*. 2002; 106(6):711–717.

64. Silbiger JJ, Bazaz R. Contemporary insights into the functional anatomy of the mitral valve. *Am Heart J*. 2009; 158(6): 887–895.

65. Otsuji Y, Levine RA, Takeuchi M, Sakata R, Tei C. Mechanism of ischemic mitral regurgitation. *J Cardiol*. 2008; 51(3):145–156.

66. Burkhoff D, Flaherty JT, Yue DT, *et al*. *In vitro* studies of isolated supported human hearts. *Heart Vessels*. 1988; 4(4):185–196.

67. Mangini A, Contino M, Romagnoni C, *et al*. Aortic valve repair: a ten-year single-centre experience. *Interact CardioVasc Thorac Surg*. 2014; 19(1):28–35.

68. Cohn JN, Ferrari R, Sharpe N. Cardiac remodeling: concepts and clinical implications: a consensus paper from an international forum on cardiac remodeling. *J Am Coll Cardiol*. 2000; 35(3):569–582.

69. Ranganathan N, Lam JHC, Wigle ED, Silver MD. Morphology of the human mitral valve: II. The valve leaflets. *Circulation*. 1970; 41(3):459–467.

70. Turi ZG. Cardiology patient page: mitral valve disease. *Circulation*. 2004; 109(6):e38–e41.

71. Otsuji Y, Handschumacher MD, Schwammenthal E, *et al*. Insights from three-dimensional echocardiography into the mechanism of functional mitral regurgitation: direct *in vivo* demonstration of altered leaflet tethering geometry. *Circulation*. 1997; 96(6):1999–2008.

72. Aronow WS, Kronzon I. Correlation of prevalence and severity of mitral regurgitation and mitral stenosis determined by Doppler echocardiography with physical signs of mitral regurgitation and mitral stenosis in 100 patients aged 62 to 100 years with mitral anular calcium. *Am J Cardiol*. 1987; 60(14):1189–1190.

73. Yiu SF, Enriquez-Sarano M, Tribouilloy C, Seward JB, Tajik AJ. Determinants of the degree of functional mitral regurgitation in patients with systolic left ventricular

dysfunction: a quantitative clinical study. *Circulation.* 2000; 102(12):1400–1406.

74. Agricola E, Oppizzi M, Maisano F, *et al.* Echocardiographic classification of chronic ischemic mitral regurgitation caused by restricted motion according to tethering pattern. *Eur J Echocardiogr.* 2004; 5(5):326–334.

75. Watanabe N, Ogasawara Y, Yamaura Y, *et al.* Geometric differences of the mitral valve tenting between anterior and inferior myocardial infarction with significant ischemic mitral regurgitation: quantitation by novel software system with transthoracic real-time three-dimensional echocardiography. *J Am Soc Echocardiogr.* 2006; 19(1):71–75.

76. Kwan J, Shiota T, Agler DA, *et al.* Geometric differences of the mitral apparatus between ischemic and dilated cardiomyopathy with significant mitral regurgitation: real-time three-dimensional echocardiography study. *Circulation* 2003; 107(8):1135–1140.

77. Victor S, Nayak VM. Definition and function of commissures, slits and scallops of the mitral valve: analysis in 100 hearts. *Asia Pacific J Thoracic Cardiovasc Surg.* 1994; 3(1):10–16.

78. Yamauchi T, Taniguchi K, Kuki S, *et al.* Evaluation of the mitral valve leaflet morphology after mitral valve reconstruction with a concept "coaptation length index." *J Card Surg.* 2005; 20(5):432–435.

79. Tibayan FA, Wilson A, Lai DTM, *et al.* Tenting volume: three-dimensional assessment of geometric perturbations in functional mitral regurgitation and implications for surgical repair. *J Heart Valve Dis.* 2007; 16(1):1–7.

80. Messas E, Bel A, Szymanski C, *et al.* Relief of mitral leaflet tethering following chronic myocardial infarction by chordal cutting diminishes left ventricular remodeling. *Circ Cardiovasc Imag.* 2010; 3(6):679–686.

81. Lai DT, Tibayan FA, Myrmel T, *et al.* Mechanistic insights into posterior mitral leaflet inter-scallop malcoaptation during

acute ischemic mitral regurgitation. *Circulation.* 2002; 106(12 Suppl 1):I40–I45.

82. Chmielak Z, Kłopotowski M, Demkow M, *et al.* Percutaneous mitral balloon valvuloplasty beyond 65 years of age. *Cardiol J.* 2013; 20(1):44–51.

83. Nesta F, Otsuji Y, Handschumacher MD, *et al.* Leaflet concavity: a rapid visual clue to the presence and mechanism of functional mitral regurgitation. *J Am Soc Echocardiogr.* 2003; 16(12):1301–1308.

84. Donal EE, Levy FF, Tribouilloy CC. Chronic ischemic mitral regurgitation. *J Heart Valve Dis.* 2006; 15(2):149–157.

85. Bothe W, Miller DC, Doenst T. Sizing for mitral annuloplasty: where does science stop and voodoo begin? *Ann Thorac Surg.* 2013; 95:1475–1483.

86. Mihalatos DG, Mathew ST, Gopal AS, *et al.* Relationship of mitral annular remodeling to severity of chronic mitral regurgitation. *J Am Soc Echocardiogr.* 2006; 19(1):76–82.

87. Kim K, Kaji S, An Y, *et al.* Mechanism of asymmetric leaflet tethering in ischemic mitral regurgitation: 3D analysis with multislice CT. *JACC Cardiovasc Imag.* 2012; 5(2):230–232.

88. Singh JP, Evans JC, Levy D, *et al.* Prevalence and clinical determinants of mitral, tricuspid, and aortic regurgitation (the Framingham Heart Study). *Am J Cardiol.* 1999; 83(6):897–902.

89. Song J-M, Kihara T, Fukuda S, *et al.* Value of mitral valve tenting volume determined by real-time three-dimensional echocardiography in patients with functional mitral regurgitation. *Am J Cardiol.* 2006; 98(8):1088–1093.

90. Kwan J, Gillinov MA, Thomas JD, Shiota T. Geometric predictor of significant mitral regurgitation in patients with severe ischemic cardiomyopathy, undergoing Dor procedure: a real-time 3D echocardiographic study. *Eur J Echocardiogr.* 2007; 8(3):195–203.

91. Enriquez-Sarano M, Akins CW, Vahanian A. Mitral regurgitation. *Lancet.* 2009; 373(9672):1382–1394.

92. Kaplan SR, Bashein G, Sheehan FH, *et al.* Three-dimensional echocardiographic assessment of annular shape changes in the normal and regurgitant mitral valve. *Am Heart J.* 2000; 139(3): 378–387.

93. Olson LJ, Subramanian R, Ackermann DM, Orszulak TA, Edwards WD. Surgical pathology of the mitral valve: a study of 712 cases spanning 21 years. *Mayo Clin Proc.* 1987; 62(1):22–34.

94. Lawrie GM. Structure, function, and dynamics of the mitral annulus: importance in mitral valve repair for myxamatous mitral valve disease. *Methodist Debakey Cardiovasc J.* 2010; 6(1):8–14.

95. Shiran A, Merdler A, Ismir E, *et al.* Intraoperative transesophageal echocardiography using a quantitative dynamic loading test for the evaluation of ischemic mitral regurgitation. *J Am Soc Echocardiogr.* 2007; 20(6):690–697.

96. Grewal J, Suri R, Mankad S, *et al.* Mitral annular dynamics in myxomatous valve disease: new insights with real-time 3-dimensional echocardiography. *Circulation.* 2010; 121(12):1423–1431.

97. Grossi EA, Zakow PK, Sussman M, *et al.* Late results of mitral valve reconstruction in the elderly. *Ann Thorac Surg.* 2000; 70(4):1224–1226.

98. Biner S, Rafique A, Rafii F, *et al.* Reproducibility of proximal isovelocity surface area, vena contracta, and regurgitant jet area for assessment of mitral regurgitation severity. *JACC Cardiovasc Imag.* 2010; 3(3):235–243.

99. Lee AP-W, Fang F, Jin C-N, *et al.* Quantification of mitral valve morphology with three-dimensional echocardiography. *Circ J.* 2014; 78(5):1029–1037.

Thoracic Surgery in the Elderly

Elifce Cosar and Stephanie Cintora

Key Points

- Most of the aging-associated changes in the respiratory system evolve from a decrease in chest wall compliance, a reduction in static elastic recoil of the lungs and decreasing strength of the respiratory muscles. These changes alter tests of pulmonary function, respiratory mechanics and gas exchange.
- According to current guidelines developed by the American College of Chest Physicians, the preoperative physiologic assessment of pulmonary function in patients of any age should begin with a cardiovascular evaluation, spirometry to measure FEV_1, diffusion capacity for carbon monoxide (DLCO) and room arterial blood gas (ABG) analysis.
- Elderly individuals exhibit impaired pharyngeal function, seen as abnormal swallowing, and tracheal aspiration. Oropharyngeal dysphagia is an important etiologic factor for pneumonia in elderly individuals.
- The focus of intraoperative ventilation during thoracotomy has shifted towards a more protective approach by using individualized ventilator settings focused on open-lung ventilation strategy.
- Goal-directed fluid therapy (GDFT) involves the monitoring of hemodynamic parameters and rational fluid administration based on the information obtained to optimize tissue perfusion, and is an important tool in fluid management of thoracic surgery patients.
- In post-thoracotomy patients, thoracic epidural analgesia has been shown to decrease splinting, reduce dynamic pain scores and improve mucociliary clearance, thereby improving postoperative respiratory mechanics, and decreasing postoperative respiratory complications.

Introduction

As the world enters the twenty-first century, most developed nations face a progressive and sustained shift in their demographics with a greater percentage of the older population. By 2035 more than 1.1 billion people, 13% of the population, will be above the age of 65.[1] The American population is also getting older, with the current life expectancy in the United States at 78.7 years and increasing.[2]

Lung cancer is the most frequently diagnosed cancer, the second most common cancer in both men and women and is by far the leading cause of cancer death among both men and women, accounting for about 27% of all cancer deaths.[1] Approximately 80% of all the lung cancers diagnosed in 2012 fall into the category of non-small-cell lung cancer (NSCLC).[3] The peak incidence of lung cancer, as with other cancers, has "aged," with diagnosis now usually being made between the ages of 70 and 75 years;[3] 30% of all lung cancers are diagnosed in patients older than 70 and 14% in patients over 80 years.[3]

In an analysis of the incidence of common surgical procedures, patients over 65 accounted for 58% of operations compared with other age groups, and when broken down by specialty, this age group accounted for the majority of cardiothoracic and ophthalmologic procedures.[4] Treatment options for lung cancer frequently include surgery; this is not benign and may result in serious morbidity and mortality in elderly patients.[5] Even in the absence of cancer, the elderly population is particularly susceptible to pulmonary disease, and lower respiratory disease is the third leading cause of death and a significant source of disability in patients older than 65 years.[6] This further increases surgical risk in the older patient and in-hospital mortality rates are increased in elderly patients, especially those with compromised respiratory functions. Thus, anesthetic management has to incorporate the impact of acute and chronic pulmonary diseases as well as age-related physiological changes.

The Effect of the Aging Process on Respiratory Function

The lungs develop throughout life, with maximal functional status achieved in the early part of the third decade.[7] There is minimal change in function from ages 20 to 35, but subsequently an age-related decline is noted. Aging impacts the upper airways and the control of breathing, but much of the clinically significant functional changes are related to a decrease in the static elastic recoil of the lung, a decrease in the chest wall compliance and a decrease in respiratory muscle strength.[8]

Structural Age-Related Changes

Changes to the Lung Parenchyma

Structural changes in the lung parenchyma occur with age (Table 12.1), leading to a reduction in parenchymal elasticity. This in turn causes a loss of elastic recoil and subsequent increase in lung compliance.[9] Mean bronchiolar diameter also decreases significantly after the age of 40.[10] This reduction in airway size due to alterations in supporting

Table 12.1 Age-related structural changes in the respiratory system

Decreased alveolar–capillary surface area, due to diminished intra-alveolar fenestration
Decreased number of alveoli, number of lung capillaries
Decreased elastic recoil, causing easier collapse of peripheral airways
Decreased negative intrapleural pressure
Increased interstitial connective tissue
Enlarged respiratory bronchioles and alveolar ducts (ductectasis)
Smaller airway diameter, due to destruction of supporting connective tissue
Increased proteolysis of elastin, reduced elastin/collagen ratio, reduced/ altered surfactant
Stiffer chest wall due to calcification and fibrosis of ribs and vertebral joints
Loss of respiratory accessory muscle mass

connective tissue results in premature closure of small airways, and causes air trapping and hyperinflation, sometimes called "senile emphysema."[8] Although the term "senile emphysema" has been used to describe these age-related changes because of the functional similarities with classic emphysema, in fact the age-related changes are associated with a homogeneous dilation of air spaces without destruction of tissue, so the term "senile lung" may be more accurate.[11]

As stated, with aging there is a homogeneous degeneration of the elastic fibers around the alveolar duct starting around 50 years of age. This air-space enlargement (ductectasis) is not due to alveolar wall destruction, but most likely to a decrease in elastic tissue and an increase in collagen with age.[12]

The lungs' ability to clear particles from small airways also appears to decrease with age. This is due to the combined effects of sarcopenia-induced reduction in cough strength and the aging-induced dysfunction of the mucociliary escalator of both the upper and lower airway.[13]

Changes to the Chest Wall and Respiratory Muscles

Chest wall compliance decreases with age due to structural changes of the intercostal muscles, and the joints and calcification of the costal cartilage. Stiffening of the thoracic cage reduces its ability to expand during inspiration. These changes, as well as contractures of intercostal muscles, result in rigidity and reduced rib cage mobility.[14] This shifts the breathing muscle-use pattern from thoracic muscles to the diaphragm and abdomen.

In addition to structural changes of the chest wall, there are age-related changes in the intrinsic function of the muscles. Overall muscle function in the body decreases by 2% annually in adults.[15] It is well known that the diaphragm is the most important respiratory muscle and plays an essential role in inspiration. However there is limited information on the effect of aging on the contractile properties of the diaphragm. It does appear that the diaphragm becomes weakened and the strength is thought to be reduced by approximately 10–20% in healthy elderly individuals compared to younger individuals. Maximum inspiratory and expiratory pressures are reduced by more than 50%.[16] The age-related atrophy of type II fast-twitch muscle fibers may also explain part of the reduced inspiratory and expiratory muscle strength in the elderly.

Pulmonary Blood Vessels

Beyond the age of 30–35 years, there is a gradual increase in the stiffness of the pulmonary vasculature. This structural remodeling can lead to incremental increases in pulmonary arterial pressure.[17]

Airway

Elderly individuals exhibit an impaired pharyngeal function and sensitivity, seen as an increased frequency of misdirected swallowing and tracheal aspiration.[18] Loss of muscular pharyngeal support due to atrophy of the hypopharygeal and genioglossal muscles also disposes elderly patients to upper airway obstruction. Ossification of the laryngeal skeleton can be seen in elderly patients. This can result in incomplete glottal closure secondary to bowing of the vocal folds.[19]

Overall the deterioration of protective mechanisms of cough and swallowing in the elderly lead to ineffective clearance of secretions and increased susceptibility to aspiration.[18]

Physiologic Age-Related Changes

The pulmonary physiologic changes that occur with age are best described in terms of their effect on lung volumes, gas exchange and respiratory effort. The pulmonary physiologic changes observed with age are summarized in Table 12.2.

Table 12.2 Pulmonary physiologic changes with age

Variable	Type of Change
Lung volumes and flows	
Total lung capacity	Unchanged
Functional residual capacity	Increased
Vital capacity	Reduced
Forced vital capacity	Reduced
Inspiratory capacity	Reduced
Residual volume	Increased
Closing volume	Increased
FEV$_1$	Reduced
Peak expiratory flow	Decreased
Gas exchange	
Shunt	Increased
Diffusing capacity for carbon monoxide	Reduced
PaO$_2$	Reduced
PaCO$_2$	Unchanged
Maximum oxygen consumption	Reduced
Pulmonary vascular resistance	Increased
Dead-space ventilation	Increased
Respiratory drive	
Central ventilatory control	Decreased
Peripheral chemoreceptor	Decreased mechanoreceptor signaling
Response to hypoxemia	Reduced
Response to hypercarbia	Reduced
Central sleep apnea	Increased
Secretory and immune	
Mucociliary function	Decreased
Protective airway reflexes	Decreased
Innate immunity	Decreased
Adaptive immunity	Decreased

Pulmonary Function and Gas Exchange

Most of the aging-associated changes in the respiratory system evolve from a decrease in chest wall compliance, a reduction in static elastic recoil of the lungs and decreasing strength of the respiratory muscles. These changes alter tests of pulmonary function, respiratory mechanics and gas exchange.

Total lung capacity (TLC) remains fairly constant throughout life.[8]

Residual volume (RV), the volume of gas remaining in the lung after a maximal forced expiration, increases with age along with the ratio RV/TLC. RV is determined by two factors:

1. The strength of the expiratory muscles that oppose outward chest wall recoil at low thoracic volumes.

2. Collapse of small airways and trapping of gas in alveoli during forced expiration.[20]

With loss of expiratory muscle strength, outward chest recoil is less opposed, resulting in increase in RV by approximately 50%. Vital capacity is reduced by 25% between the ages of 20 and 70 years.[7]

Functional residual capacity (FRC), the volume of gas at the end of normal tidal expiration when the respiratory muscles are relaxed, increases with age, by 1–3% per decade, along with the FRC/TLC ratio. Elderly subjects breathe at higher lung volumes than younger subjects.[21]

Other markers of dynamic lung function decrease with age, including forced vital capacity (FVC), a maximal expiratory flow rate and forced expiratory flow rate over 1 second (FEV_1). The estimated rate of decline in FEV_1 is 25–35 ml/year starting at ages 35–40 years and can double to 60 ml/year after age 70 years.[7]

Closing volume (CV), the lung volume at which small airways begin to close during forced expiration, increases. CV can exceed FRC, in which case airway closure is present and alveoli may be underventilated in dependent areas of the lung. The overall effect is less efficient matching of lung ventilation and perfusion (VA/Q mismatch, or inequality).[22]

Arterial oxygenation progressively declines with aging, whereas CO_2 elimination remains unaffected despite an increase in dead-space ventilation.[22] The linear deterioration of the PaO_2 that occurs with aging (about 0.3% per year) is estimated by the equation $PaO_2 = 109 - (0.43 \times age)$.[23] After age 75, the PaO_2 level of healthy nonsmokers is stable at about 83 mmHg.

The efficiency of alveolar gas exchange decreases progressively with age. Factors responsible for the reduction include loss of alveolar surface area, decreased capillary blood volume and decreased surface area for alveolar–capillary gas diffusion.

Alveolar surface area decreases from 75 m² at the age of 30 to about 60 m² at age of 70, a reduction of 0.27 m²/year.[21]

Regulation of Breathing

With aging, the ventilatory response to hypoxia and hypercarbia is blunted, most likely due to combination of a reduced neural output to respiratory muscles, disturbances of chemosensory function and structural changes in lung and chest wall that reduce motor performance.

Aging also is associated with decreased self-perception of dyspnea and bronchoconstriction,[24] as well as a decreased ability to clear mucus from the lungs. This is due to reduced cough strength and alterations in the body's ability to clear particles from the airway.[25]

Immunologic Age-Related Pulmonary Changes

Aging is associated with systemic immune dysfunction sometimes called "inflamm-aging"; often manifesting as increased levels of tissue and circulating proinflammatory cytokines.[26] Heightened levels of these cytokines in the absence of an immunologic threat or infectious target may play a role in the age-related destruction of lung parenchyma with advanced age.[27] Related to inflamm-aging, there is a blunted immune response, following a pathogenic threat or tissue injury known as " immunosenescence."[26]

The immunologic changes observed with age affect both the innate and adaptive immunological systems. Innate immune response is the critical first line of defense for the lungs such as pathogen recognition, chemotaxis and phagocytosis, and is decreased with age. Adaptive immune (acquired) response is responsible for antibody-mediated cytotoxity.

A thorough preoperative assessment of patients prior to thoracic surgery is imperative to determine whether a patient is an appropriate surgical candidate and to predict and avoid postoperative complications. Age-related changes occur at different rates in different individuals and are not necessarily reflected in chronological age, and the physiologic age of a person will be more important when planning antineoplastic surgery.

Preoperative Pulmonary Evaluation

According to current guidelines developed by the American College of Chest Physicians the preoperative assessment of pulmonary function in patients contemplating thoracic surgery of any age should begin with a cardiovascular evaluation, spirometry to measure FEV_1, diffusion capacity for carbon monoxide (DLCO) and room arterial blood gas (ABG) analysis.[28]

Predicted postoperative (PPO) lung functions can be calculated. If the PPO FEV_1 and PPO DLCO values are both >60%, the patient is considered at low risk for anatomic lung resection, and no further testing is needed. If either of these tests is between 30% and 60% predicted, a low-technology exercise test such as stair climbing, shuttle walk or 6-minute walk test (6MWT) should be performed as a screening test. In patients with either PPO FEV_1 <30% or PPO DLCO <30%, predicted performance of a formal cardiopulmonary exercise testing (CPET) with measurement of maximal oxygen consumption (VO_{2max}) is recommended.

Howewer, while exercise testing is a potentially powerful tool, it is not always applicable in the geriatric population due to the presence of co-morbidities that limit mobility, independent of VO_{2max}. Although age has been traditionally considered a risk factor, the most recent European Respiratory Society/European Society of Thoracic Surgeons (ERS-ESTS) guidelines have emphasized that age alone is not a contraindication to surgery and the cardiopulmonary fitness of elderly cancer patients should be fully evaluated without any prejudice regarding chronological age.[29]

Factors such as tumor stage, patient life expectancy, performance status and presence of underlying co-morbidities should be taken into account in the surgical decision-making process. In the elderly population, it is also important to consider cognitive and geriatric assessment. The Comprehensive Geriatric Assessment (CGA) includes an evaluation of cognitive functions, mood and depression, nutritional status, activities of daily living, co-morbidities, polypharmacy, the presence of geriatric syndromes and social support.[30]

Intraoperative Management

Anesthetic requirements in elderly patients are significantly reduced. Minimum alveolar concentration (MAC) decreases with age, 6–8% per decade after 40 years. Similarly, the dose of intravenous anesthetic induction agents and opioids should be decreased by 25%. Although elderly patients show increased sensitivity to anesthetic drugs, desflurane and sevoflurane may have protective effects such as attenuating the release of alveolar mediators and decreasing the expression of systemic proinflammatory cytokines.[31]

Elderly individuals exhibit impaired pharyngeal function, seen as abnormal swallowing, and tracheal aspiration. Oropharyngeal dysphagia is an important etiologic factor for pneumonia in elderly individuals.[32] Partial neuromuscular block in healthy elderly individuals also causes an increased incidence of pharyngeal dysfunction.[33] Thus, it is very important to reverse neuromuscular blockers before extubation. There are age-dependent differences in rocuronium potency, which are related to decreased elimination in the elderly.[34] Cisatracurium has been recommended as a neuromuscular blocker of choice in the elderly.

Ventilation

Anesthesia in thoracic surgery conventionally involves one-lung ventilation (OLV) to isolate and protect the lungs, and provides optimum surgical operating conditions. Arterial hypoxemia is still a serious complication of OLV, and this complication is seen in elderly patients with poor pulmonary function.[35] Due to degeneration of the respiratory system and decreasing respiratory function, elderly patients have increased risk of hypoxemia.[36] However, its incidence has decreased significantly over the years, likely due to the increased use of fiberoptic bronchoscopy for confirmation of lung isolation and the use of anesthetic agents with less effect on hypoxic pulmonary vasoconstriction (HPV).[37]

The focus of intraoperative ventilation during thoracotomy has shifted towards a more protective approach by using individualized ventilator settings focused on open-lung ventilation strategy (OV). The concept of OV initially originated in the intensive care literature and is an evolution of the management of patients with acute respiratory distress syndrome (ARDS). It consists of avoidance of cycling recruitment and derecruitment for lung injury prevention.[38] OV uses low (physiologic) tidal volume (Vt), low respiratory rate (RR), low concentration of inspired oxygen (FiO2) and a high level of continuous positive airway pressure (CPAP), which allow optimization of the intraoperative lung mechanics and gas exchange. In essence, the OV strategy is designed to maintain alveoli open and functional throughout the ventilatory cycle.

A recent phase I pilot study showed that using OV strategy during elective lung resection surgery can prevent intraoperative atelectasis. This may have a beneficial effect on the postoperative course of patients who are high risk for developing pulmonary complications, such as the very elderly.[39] Additionally, evidence suggests that only a single alveolar recruitment maneuver (ARM) 30 cm H_2O followed by sufficient positive endexpiratory pressure (PEEP) application 5 cm H_2O is required to reduce the amount of atelectasis by 60%.[40]

There are few trials that look at intraoperative ventilation in geriatric patients, however Lin *et al.* were able to show pressure control ventilation (PCV) during OLV had some advantages in elderly patients with poor pulmonary function (FEV$_1$ <1.5 L).[41]

Although further studies are lacking at this point, the following can be recommended for intraoperative ventilation of geriatric patients[42]:

1. Ventilation targeting tidal volumes 6 ml/kg based on ideal body weight.
2. Adjust respiratory rate to keep exhaled CO_2 40–45 mmHg. Avoid hypocarbia, as reduced cerebral blood flow is associated with postoperative cognitive dysfunction.
3. Minimum inspired oxygen (FiO_2) to maintain oxygen saturation (SpO_2).
4. Remember recruitment maneuvers.
5. PEEP or CPAP 10–20 cmH_2O initially, then reduce amount needed to maximize compliance.

Perioperative Fluid Management

Perioperative fluid management is a key component of anesthetic management during thoracic surgery.

Damage to the lung either directly by surgical manipulation or mechanical ventilation, or indirectly by alveolar epithelial damage, can lead to acute lung injury (ALI) or ARDS. In both cases, inflammation, cytokine and chemokine release are thought to be the main culprits of the damage. The inflammatory cascade leads to breakdown of the alveolar–capillary membrane resulting in alveolar flooding, hyaline membrane formation and fibrosis.[43] The alveolar–capillary membrane is maintained primarily by three factors: capillary hydrostatic pressure, oncotic pressure and alveolar–capillary permeability.

Hydrostatic pressure can be reduced primarily by fluid restriction. The goal should be for a slightly negative to even fluid balance for the intraoperative period and up to the first 48 hours after surgery.[44] Recent studies indicate that postoperative lung complications (ALI, edema, pneumonia) are more likely when infusion rates exceed 6 ml/kg/h, or >2500 ml for the duration of the operation.[44] Restricted fluid infusion should continue for 48 hours postoperatively so as to decrease the likelihood of pulmonary edema.[44,45]

Controversy remains about the role of colloid infusions in increasing oncotic pressure. Evidence on whether to use colloid versus crystalloid infusions remains equivocal with regard to fluid resuscitation in critical care and in anesthesia. Studies have shown that there does not appear to be a mortality benefit to using colloid over crystalloid in ALI/ARDS patients, although in all studies avoiding volume overload is a primary goal.[46]

Finally, preventing increasing alveolar permeability is a potential target for improved postoperative outcomes. ALI is often seen in the dependent lung and not in the operative lung. This suggests a correlation between ventilation strategy and lung injury. It is known that mechanical ventilation and one-lung ventilation at higher tidal volumes can cause alveolar trauma by causing overdistension, tensile strain and shear stress.[43] Lung protective ventilation strategies (low tidal volume and application of PEEP), pressure limited ventilation and pressure control ventilation is preferred to other ventilation settings.

Goal-directed fluid therapy (GDFT) involves the monitoring of hemodynamic parameters and rational fluid administration based on the information obtained to optimize tissue perfusion. There are several techniques and devices that can be used to guide fluid management. In pulmonary resection surgery, the use of transesophageal Doppler and pulse pressure (PPV)/stroke volume variation (SVV) monitoring was examined in several studies.[47,48] Esophageal Doppler was able to detect low cardiac output during lung surgery, and PPV was able to predict fluid responsiveness during protective OLV, but not conventional OLV.[47] Both techniques use the heart–lung interaction during mechanical ventilation to assess fluid responsiveness. Esophageal Doppler has also been used to guide intraoperative fluid management successfully while comparing different colloid regimens in thoracic surgery,[49] again showing the potential this method has for optimizing fluid management and hemodynamic status. Applying minimally invasive devices to monitor hemodynamic status allows a rational approach to perioperative fluid therapy and goal-directed fluid management has the potential to reduce and optimize overall fluid administration.[50]

There is currently difficulty in comparing the outcomes after surgery with regard to fluid administration in elderly patients. There is little consistency among studies, and many studies exclude patients that are high risk. However, there is a suggestion of improved outcomes in fluid restriction[43] in major abdominal and orthopedic operations. In a recent randomized study, restrictive intravenous fluid regimens in elderly patients with abdominal cancer showed better preservation of cellular immunity and a 50% decrease in pneumonia rate.[51] Further research regarding the use of GDFT and their effects on elderly patients undergoing pulmonary resection surgery is required.

The principles of fluid management that are suggested for pulmonary resection surgery for an average adult are[52]:

1. Total fluid balance in the first 24 hours postoperatively should not exceed 20 ml/kg.
2. Crystalloid administration should be limited to <2 L intraoperatively and <3 L in the first 24 hours postoperatively.
3. Colloids should only be used to replace an equivalent volume of blood loss if blood is not required.
4. Urine output >0.5 ml/kg/h is not necessary in the early postoperative period, unless patient is at risk of developing acute kidney injury.

Temperature Control

Thoracic surgery patients are especially at high risk for perioperative hypothermia. Along with aging, physiological function of both sympathetic and parasympathetic nervous systems gradually decreases. The effect of impaired autonomic activity may induce impaired thermoregulation in response to stress, causing elderly patients to be at high risk of hypothermia. During anesthesia the course of hypothermia is likely to be longer and more pronounced due to reduced muscle mass and a compromised ability to regain effective thermoregulatory control.[53] Perioperative hypothermia is associated with adverse outcomes that include postoperative delirium, increased perioperative blood loss, increased incidence of myocardial ischemia, poor wound healing, prolonged postoperative and hospital stay.[54]

Elderly patients are more difficult to rewarm once hypothermic, therefore measures to maintain temperature, and treatment, should be readily available perioperatively.

Positioning

The majority of thoracic procedures are performed in the lateral position. The anesthesiologist should take personal responsibility for the head, neck and airway during position change.

Because of limitations in mobility associated with aging, older patients are at high risk of preventable peripheral nerve injuries during prolonged surgery. Prevention of peripheral nerve injuries in the lateral position requires careful positioning. The most common injuries include the ulnar nerve when supine, the common peroneal nerve in lithotomy, the dependent radial nerve in the lateral position and the brachial plexus after prolonged periods of lateral neck flexion. Furthermore, elderly patients tend to have greatly reduced cervical spine mobility and increased degenerative changes of the spine. Care must be taken to accommodate pronounced thoracic kyphosis, neck flexion and additional support provided to prevent "free-hanging" of the head and neck.

Reduced skin depth, vascularity and reduced muscle mass predispose the older patient to tissue pressure necrosis, usually over bony protuberances, such as the heels, elbows and malleoli.

The Emerging Role of Minimally Invasive Surgical Techniques

Minimally invasive approaches are gradually replacing most open surgical procedures. Video-assisted thoracoscopic surgery (VATS) and robot-assisted thoracoscopic surgery have been described for every aspect of thoracic surgery.[55] The reported clinical benefits of VATS are perioperative decreases in blood loss, pain, inflammatory response, chest tube duration, improved postoperative pulmonary function and length of hospital stay.[56]

Particular operative strategies are also used to approach surgical resection in the elderly, including VATS to minimize chest wall trauma and by considering limited resections for the most elderly to minimize loss of lung tissue. VATS procedures in the elderly have been shown to have lower morbidity and lower rates of postoperative delirium, and result in earlier ambulation, a lower narcotic requirement and a faster recovery time[57,58] than standard thoracotomy procedures, making VATS the technique of choice in high-risk patients, such as the elderly and those with poor pulmonary function.

A recent study examined patients aged 65 years or older with stage I or II NSCLC who underwent thoracoscopic lobectomy, who were treated without tracheal intubation using epidural anesthesia, intrathoracic vagal blockade and sedation.[59] This study showed that thoracoscopic lobectomy without tracheal intubation under epidural anesthesia is a valid alternative for managing selected geriatric patients with NSCLC.

Randomized controlled trials are needed to evaluate VATS techniques for lobectomy in elderly patients. These trials should compare the outcomes, including long-term survival in elderly patients, with those standard open procedures.

Postoperative Management

The management of postoperative pain in the elderly patient undergoing thoracic surgical procedures represents a significant challenge to anesthesiologists. Choice of postoperative analgesic regimens may influence perioperative morbidity, particularly in this high-risk group of patients. A wide variety of modalities have been employed to control post-thoracotomy pain, but thoracic epidural analgesia (TEA) has long been considered the gold standard for patients undergoing open thoracic procedures.[60]

Placing a thoracic epidural catheter maybe more difficult in elderly patients. Appropriate positioning is difficult in the elderly patient due to kyphoscoliosis, arthritic joints and fixed flexion deformities. With advanced age, degenerative disc and joint disease causes distortion and compression of the epidural space. Older patients are more sensitive to the effects of epidurally administered local anesthetics (LA). Using the same volumes of LA, the concentration required to produce effective motor blockade decreases as patient age increases.[61]

Thoracic epidural administration of a fixed dose of a local anesthetic solution caused more extensive spread of analgesia, and faster onset of analgesia at the caudal segments[62] in elderly patients. Bradycardia and hypotension were also observed more in older patients with epidural analgesia.[63] Increased epidural compliance, decreased epidural resistance, increased residual epidural pressure and progressive sclerotic closure of the intervertebral foramina with advancing age may all contribute to enhanced epidural spread of local anesthetic solution in the elderly. It is therefore recommended to reduce epidural infusion rates in older patients.[64]

In post-thoracotomy patients, TEA has been shown to decrease splinting, reduce dynamic pain scores and improve mucociliary clearance, thereby improving postoperative respiratory mechanics[65] and decreasing postoperative respiratory complications.[66]

An additional advantage of TEA is to decrease cardiovascular complications in elderly patients by blunting the stress response and sympathetic outflow.[67] These authors also showed that age-related deterioration of diastolic function had no detrimental effect on the hemodynamic response to TEA in elderly patients. Additionally, TEA has been associated with a significant decrease in supraventricular arrhythmias, a complication in approximately 20–30% of post-thoracotomy patients.[68] TEA has also been associated with decreased length of intensive care unit (ICU) and hospital stay in high-risk patients.[69]

Postoperative Complications in Elderly Patients

Thoracic surgery involves stress on multiple organ systems that often uncovers clinically unrecognized vulnerability to stress. Complications are most often respiratory or cardiac. Risk factors for postoperative complications in elderly lung cancer patients include the existence of co-morbidities, mediastinal lymphadenectomy, pneumonectomy and prolonged surgery.[70] The most common reported complications in the elderly are arrhythmias (4–14%), prolonged air leak (7–11%) and pneumonia (6–10%).[71,72]

Another crucial aspect of postoperative geriatric care is comprehensive interprofessional discharge planning. Careful consideration of the appropriate setting for rehabilitation for individual patients is also very important, as many elderly patients will experience some cognitive or functional decline postoperatively and require assistance with one or more activities of daily living.

The average life expectancy of patients with untreated or palliated early stage NSCLC is 1.65 years.[73] Given that the average life expectancy of a person at 75 years of age exceeds 8 years, the life-limiting factor for patients with early stage lung cancer at age 75 years and older may not be their age, but instead, the cancer status.[74]

In the meantime lung cancer patients of any chronologic age should be evaluated on an individual basis in the context of a multidisciplinary approach in order to confer optimal treatment. Collectively, the data suggest that patients of age 80 or greater should not be disqualified from curative resection based on age alone.[75]

Critical for a successful outcome are careful preoperative assessment, identification of perioperative risk factors, choosing the proper operation and judicious postoperative care. Specialized multidisciplinary care provided by geriatric specialists, cardiologists, oncologists, surgeons, anesthesiologists, physical therapists and nutrition specialists should be included in decision-making.

From the data presented, anesthesiologists could directly exert a positive effect on elderly patient outcomes by facilitating restrictive intraoperative fluid management, administration of volatile anesthetics, use of protective ventilation modes and early extubation with the use of TEA.

References

1. Age invaders. *The Economist.* 2014. Available from: www.economist.com/news /briefing/21601248-generation-old-people-about-change-global-economy-they-will-not-all-do-so (Accessed July 12, 2017).

2. Vincent GK, Velkoff VA. *The Next Four Decades, The Older Population in the United States: 2010 to 2050, Current Population Reports, P25-1138.* Washington, DC, US Census Bureau, 2010.

3. Siegel R, Naishadham D, Jemal A. Cancer statistics, 2012. *CA Cancer J Clin.* 2012; 62:10–29.

4. Etzioni DA, Liu JH, Maggard MA, *et al.* The aging population and its impact on the surgery workforce. *Ann Surg.* 2003; 238:170–177.

5. Boffa DJ, Allen MS, Grab JD, *et al.* Data from The Society of Thoracic Surgeons General Thoracic Surgery database: the surgical management of primary lung tumors. *J Thorac Cardiovasc Surg.* 2008; 135:247–254.

6. Minino AM. Death in the United States, 2011. *NCHS Data Brief.* 2013; 115:1–8.

7. Janssens JP, Pache JC, Nicod LP. Physiological changes in respiratory function associated with ageing. *Eur Respir J.* 1999; 13:197–205.

8. Janssens JP. Aging of the respiratory system: impact on pulmonary function tests and adaptations to exertion. *Clin Chest Med.* 2005; 26:469–484.

9. Sprung J, Gajic O, Warner DO. Review article: age related alterations in respiratory function: anesthetic considerations. *Can J Anaesth.* 2006; 53(12):1244–1257.

10. Niewoenner D, Kleinerman J. Morphologic basis of pulmonary resistance in human lung and effects of aging. *J Appl Physiol.* 1974; 36:412–418.

11. Teramoto S, Ishii M. Aging, the aging lung, and senile ephysema are different. *Am J Respir Crit Care Med.* 2007; 175(2):197–198.

12. Zaugg M, Lucchinetti E. Respiratory function in the elderly. *Anesthesiol Clin N Am.* 2000; 18(1):47–58.

13. Svartengren M, Falk R, Philipson K. Long term clearence from small airways decreases with age. *Eur Respir J.* 2005; 26(4):609–615.

14. Sharma G, Goodwin J. Effect of aging on respiratory system physiology and immunology. *Clin Interven Aging.* 2006; 1(3):253–260.

15. Brown M, Hasser EM. Complexity of age-related change in skeletal muscle. *J Gerontol A Biol Sci Med Sci.* 1996; 51(2):B117–B123.

16. El Solh AA, Ramadan FH. Overview of respiratory failure in older adults. *J Intensive Care Med.* 2006; 21(6):345–351.

17. Taylor BJ, Johnson BD. The pulmonary circulation and exercise responses in the elderly. *Semin Respir Crit Care Med.* 2010; 31:528–538.

18. Humbert IA, Robbins J. Dysphagia in the elderly. *Phys Med Rehabil Clin North Am.* 2008; 19:853–866.

19. Paulsen F, Kimpel M, Lockemann U, *et al.* Effects of ageing on the insertion zones of the human vocal fold. *J Anat.* 2000; 196:41–54.

20. Lalley PM. The aging respiratory system: pulmonary structure, function and neural control. *Respir Physiol Neurobiol.* 2013; 187:199–210.

21. Crapo RO. *The Aging Lung: Pulmonary Disease in the Elderly Patient.* New York, Marcel Dekker, 1993: 1–21.

22. Cardús J, Burgos F, Diaz O, *et al.* Increase in pulmonary ventilation-perfusion inequality with age in healthy individuals. *Am J Respir Crit Care Med.* 1997; 156(2 Pt 1):648–653.

23. Sorbini LA, Grass V, Solinas E, *et al.* Arterial oxygen tension in relation to age in healthy subjects. *Respiration.* 1968; 25(1):3–13.

24. Connoly MJ, Crowley JJ, Charan NB, *et al.* Reduced subjective awareness of bronchoconstriction provoked by methacholine in elderly asthmatic and normal subjects as measured on a simple awareness scale. *Thorax.* 1992; 47: 410–413.

25. Sharma G, Goodwin J. Effect of aging on respiratory system physiology and immunology. *J Clin Interven Aging.* 2006; 1:253–260.

26. Panda A, Arjona A, Sapey E, *et al.* Humane innate immunosenescence: causes and consequences for immunity in old age. *Trends Immunol.* 2009; 30(7):325–333.

27. Lowery EM, Brubaker AL, Kuhlmann E, *et al.* The aging lung. *Clin Interv Aging.* 2013; 8:1489–1496.

28. Brunelli A, Kim AW, Berger KI, *et al.* Physiologic evaluation of the patient with lung cancer being considered for resectional surgery. *Chest* 2013; 143(5 Suppl):e166S–e190S.

29. Brunelli A, Charloux A, Bollinger CT, *et al.* ERS/ESTS clinical guidelines on fitness for radical therapy in lung cancer patients. *Eur Respir J.* 2009; 34(1):17–41.

30. Extermann M, Aapro M, Bernabei R, *et al.* Task Force on CGA of the International Society of Geriatric Oncology. Use of comprehensive geriatric assessment in older cancer patients: recommendations from the task force on CGA of the International Society of Geriatric Oncology (SIOG). *Crit Rev Oncol Hematol.* 2005; 55(3):241–252.

31. Schilling T, Kozian A, Kretzschmar M, *et al.* Effect of propofol and desflurane anesthesia on the alveolar inflammatory response to one-lung ventilation. *Br J Anesthesia.* 2007; 99:368–375.

32. Marik PE, Kaplan D. Aspiration pneumonia and dysphagia in the elderly. *Chest.* 2003; 124:328–336.

33. Cedborg AI, Sundman E, Boden K, *et al.* Pharyngeal function and breathing pattern during partial neuromuscular block in the elderly: effects on airway protection. *Anesthesiology.* 2014; 120:312–325.

34. Matteo RS, Ornstein E, Schwartz AE, *et al.* Pharmacokinetics and pharmacodynamics of rocuronium in elderly surgical patients. *Anesth Analg.* 1993; 77:1193–1197.

35. Cheng YD, Duan CJ, Zhang H, *et al.* Clinical controlled comparison between lobectomy and segmental resection for patients over 70 years of age with clinical stage I non-small cell lung cancer. *Eur J Surg Oncol.* 2012; 38:1149–1155.

36. Miller MR. Structural and physiological age-associated changes in aging lungs. *Semin Respir Crit Care Med.* 2010; 31:521–527.

37. Lohser J. Evidence-based management of one-lung ventilation. *Anesthesiol Clin.* 2008; 26(2):241–272.

38. Unzueta C, Tusman G, Suarez-Sipmann F, *et al.* Alveolar recruitment improves ventilation during thoracic surgery: a randomized controlled trial. *Br J Anaesth.* 2012; 108(3):517–524.

39. Downs JB, Robinson LA, Steighner ML, *et al.* Open lung ventilation optimizes pulmonary function during lung surgery. *J Surg Res.* 2014; 192:242–249.

40. Kozian A, Schilling T, Schutze H, *et al.* Ventilatory protective strategies during thoracic surgery: effects of alveolar recruitment maneuver and low-tidal volume ventilation on lung density distribution. *Anesthesiology.* 2011; 114:1025–1035.

41. Lin F, Pan L, Huang B, *et al.* Pressure-controlled versus volume-controlled ventilation during one-lung ventilation in elderly patients with poor pulmonary function. *Ann Thoracic Med.* 2014;9(4) 203–208.

42. Kozian A, Kretzschmar MA, Schilling T. Thoracic anesthesia in the elderly. *Curr Opin Anesthesiol.* 2015; 28:2–9.

43. Searl CP, Perrino A. Fluid management in thoracic surgery. *Anesthesiology Clin.* 2012; 30:641–655.

44. Arslantas MK, Kara HV, Tuncer BB, *et al.* Effect of the amount of intraoperative fluid administration on postoperative pulmonary complications following anatomic lung resections. *J Thorac Cardiovasc Surg.* 2015; 149:314–320.

45. Yao S, Mao T, Fang W, *et al.* Incidence and risk factors for acute lung injury after open thoracotomy for thoracic diseases. *J Thorac Dis.* 2013; 5(4):456–460.

46. Van der Heijden M, Verheij J, Amerongen GP, *et al.* Crystalloid or colloid fluid-loading and pulmonary permeability, edema and injury in septic and non-septic patients. *Crit Care Med.* 2009; 37:1275–1281.

47. Lee JH, Jeon Y, Bahk JH, *et al.* Pulse pressure variation as a predictor of fluid responsiveness during one-lung ventilation for lung surgery using thoracotomy: randomized controlled study. *Eur J Anaesthesiol.* 2011; 28:39–44.

48. Suehiro K, Okutani R. Influence of tidal volume for stroke volume variation to predict fluid responsiveness in patients undergoing one-lung ventilation. *J Anesth.* 2011; 25:777–780.

49. Abdallah MS, Assad OM. Randomised study comparing the effect of hydroxyethyl starch HES 130/0.4, HES 200/0.5 and modified fluid gelatin for perioperative volume replacement in thoracic surgery: guided by transoesophageal Doppler. *EJCTA.* 2010; 4:76–84.

50. Zhang J, Chen CQ, Lei XZ, *et al.* Goal directed fluid optimization based on stroke volume variation and cardiac index during one-lung ventilation in patients undergoing thoracoscopy lobectomy operations: a pilot study. *Clinics (Sao Paulo).* 2013; 68:1065–1070.

51. Gao T, Li N, Zhang JJ, *et al.* Restricted intravenous fluid regimen reduces the rate of postoperative complications and alters immunological activity of elderly patients operated for abdominal cancer: a randomized prospective clinical trail. *World J Surg.* 2012; 36:993–1002.

52. Chau EHL, Slinger P. Perioperative fluid management for pulmonary resection surgery and esophagectomy. *Semin Cardiothor and Vasc Anesth.* 2014; 18(1): 36–44.

53. National Confidential Enquiry into Patient Outcome and Death. Elective and emergency surgery in elderly: an age old problem. 2010. Available from: www .ncepod.org.uk/2010report3/downloads /EESE_fullreport.pdf (Accessed July 12, 2017).

54. National Institute for Health and Care Excellence. CG 65. Inadvertent perioperative hypothermia. 2008. Available from: www.nice.org.uk/ guidance/cg65 (Accessed July 12, 2017).

55. Lee P, Mathur PN, Colt H. Advances in thoracoscopy: 100 years since Jacobaeus. *Respiration.* 2010; 79(3):177–186.

56. Swanson SJ, Meyers BF, Gunnarson CL, *et al.* Video-assisted thoracoscopic lobectomy is less costly and morbid than open lobectomy: retrospective multi-institutional database analysis. *Ann Thorac Surg.* 2012; 93(4):1027–1032.

57. Jaklitsch MT, DeCamp MMJ, Liptay M, *et al.* Video-assisted thoracic surgery in the elderly. A review of 307 cases. *Chest.* 1996; 110:751–758.

58. Cattaneo SM, Park BJ, Wilton AS, *et al.* Use of video-assisted thoracic surgery for lobectomy in the elderly results in fewer complications. *Ann Thorac Surg.* 2008; 85:231–236.

59. Wu CY, Chen JS, Lin YS, *et al.* Feasibility and safety of nonintubated thoracoscopic lobectomy for geriatric lung cancer patients. *Ann Thorac Surg.* 2013; 95:405–411.

60. Joshi GP, Bonnet F, Shah R, *et al.* A systematic review of randomized trials evaluating regional techniques for postthoracotomy analgesia. *Anesth Analg.* 2008; 107:1026–1040.

61. Li Y, Zhu S, Bao F, *et al.* The effects of age on the median effective concentration of ropivacaine for motor blockade after epidural anesthesia with ropivacaine. *Anesth Analg.* 2006; 102:1847–1850.

62. Hirabayashi Y, Shimizu R. Effect of age on extradural dose requirement in thoracic extradural anesthesia. *Br J Anaesth*. 1993; 71:445–446.

63. Simon MJ, Veering BT, Stienstra R, *et al*. The effects of age on neural blockade and hemodynamic changes after epidural anesthesia with ropivacaine. *Anesth Analg*. 2002; 94:1325–1330.

64. Macintyre PE, Schug SA, Scott DA, *et al*. *Acute Pain Management: Scientific Evidence, 3rd edn*. Melbourne, ANZCA & FPM, 2010.

65. Warner DO, Warmer MA, Ritman EL. Human chest wall function during epidural anesthesia. *Anesthesiology*. 1996; 85:761–773.

66. Licker MJ, Widikker I, Robert J, *et al*. Operative mortality and respiratory complications after lung resection for cancer: impact of chronic obstructive pulmonary disease and time trends. *Ann Thorac Surg*. 2006; 81:1830–1837.

67. Wink J, Veering BT, Aarts L, *et al*. Effect of increasing age on the hemodynamic response to thoracic epidural anesthesia. *Eur J Anaesthesiol*. 2014; 31:597–605.

68. Oka T, Ozawa Y, Ohkubo Y. Thoracic epidural bupivacaine attenuates supraventricular tachyarrhythmias after pulmonary resection. *Anesth Analg*. 2001; 93:253–259.

69. Guay J. The benefits of adding epidural analgesia to general anesthesia: a metanalysis. *J Anesth*. 2006; 20:335–340.

70. Okami J, Higashiyama M, Asamura H, *et al*. Pulmonary resection in patients aged 80 years or over with clinical stage I NSCLC. Prognostic factors for overall survival and risk factors for postoperative complications. *J Thoracic Oncol*. 2009; 4:1247–1253.

71. Pei G, Zhou S, Han Y, *et al*. Risk factors for postoperative complications after lung resection for non-small cell lung cancer in elderly patients at a single institution in China. *J Thorac Dis*. 2014; 6(9):1230–1238.

72. Shiono S, Abiko M, Sato T. Postoperative complications in elderly patients after lung cancer surgery. *Interact Cardiovasc Thoracic Surg*. 2013; 16:819–823.

73. Woodward RM, Brown ML, Stewart ST, *et al*. The value of medical interventions for lung cancer in the elderly: results from SEER-CMHSF. *Cancer*. 2007; 110:2511–2518.

74. Mun M, Kohno T. Video assisted thoracic surgery for clinical stage I lung cancer in octogenerians. *Ann Thorac Surg*. 2008; 85:406–411.

75. Port JL, Mirza FM, Lee PC, *et al*. Lobectomy in octogenarians with non-small cell lung cancer: ramifications of increasing life expectancy and the benefits of minimally invasive surgery. *Ann Thorac Surg*. 2011; 92(6):1951–1957.

Geriatric Trauma: Principles and Anesthetic Considerations

Varun Rimmalapudi, Michael C. Lewis and
Carol Ann B. Diachun

Key Points

- The geriatric population has an increasing risk for traumatic injury as the number of elderly continues to increase.
- Geriatric patients are more likely to present in occult shock.
- Elderly patients have a decreased ability to compensate for the stress of trauma due to decreased organ function, decreased physiological reserve and increased incidence of co-morbidities.
- Early use of invasive hemodynamic monitoring will facilitate measurement of serial venous lactate and trends in vital signs to guide resuscitation therapies.
- Lower doses of induction agents, opioids and nondepolarizing neuromuscular blockers are needed due to trauma-induced hypovolemia and aging physiology.
- Epidural analgesia improves outcomes in thoracic trauma, particularly in the geriatric population.
- Postoperative delirium is a major complication and can be prevented by use of multimodal pain therapies to decrease sedative/opioid use and by use of clinical protocols targeting specific risk factors, like sleep deprivation, immobility and dehydration.

Introduction

Unintentional injuries are consistently in the top ten of mortality causes among people over 65 years, most due to falls (55%) and motor vehicle accidents (14%).[1,2] Falls are also the leading cause of nonfatal injuries (62% in 2013).[1,2] As the population lives longer, it is projected that geriatric patients will account for almost 39% of trauma admissions by 2050.[3]

Functional Reserve in the Elder

With age, there is a progressive decline in all organ function, resulting in diminishing capacity for adjustment.[4] As functional reserve declines with increasing age, the response of the older patient's organ system to injury is often inadequate, leading to decreased ability to effectively fight or prevent progression of systemic infection, inadequate organ function in the face of poor perfusion and increased chance of development of multi-organ dysfunction.[5] Compared to their younger counterparts, older trauma patients have an increase in mortality when adjusted for injury severity scale (ISS) and 150% increase in hospital complication rates.[6-9] The most common and clinically significant complications are cardiovascular events and pneumonia.[7]

There is significant interpatient variability in the rate of decline in functional reserve. Genetics, environmental factors, lifestyle choices and the presence of age-related diseases all play a role. Although patients over 65 are conventionally termed "geriatric," a functional definition may correlate better with outcomes rather than the standard age-based criteria.[10,11] Many aging adults are entering their sixth and seventh decades in better health and with better preinjury function than in previous generations.[12]

Increased Risk for Trauma

The incidence of trauma can be impacted by risk factors like drug and alcohol intoxication, and medical, environmental and behavioral factors. Several conditions place the geriatric population at risk for traumatic events and for worsened outcomes. Weakness or generalized deconditioning from chronic illness can lead to an increased rate of falls. Loss of visual acuity, unstable gait, slowed reaction times and cognitive impairment can all contribute to the increased incidence of traumatic events. Polypharmacy can greatly complicate management. Over 90% of geriatric patients use at least one drug per week, 40% take five or more drugs and 12–19% use 10 or more medications per week.[13,14] Drugs with anticholinergic effects have been associated with delirium and confusion in the perioperative period. Anticoagulant and antiplatelet agents significantly increase the morbidity associated with traumatic brain injury (TBI); with warfarin use resulting in a three- to tenfold increase.[15–17] Herbal remedies can also contribute to abnormalities of the coagulation system and hence a history of usage must be elicited wherever possible. Mixed outcomes are reported for preinjury beta-blocker therapy: improved outcomes in patients with burn injury and head trauma possibly due to reduced metabolism, but higher mortality in other studies possibly due to inhibition of the physiologic response to hypovolemic shock.[18–21] Co-morbid conditions that increase the risk of mortality significantly in the geriatric population include congestive heart failure, hepatic and renal insufficiency, and cancer.[22,23]

Prehospital Triage and Assessment

Pre-existing limitations in functional reserve necessitate the need for rapid transport of the elderly to a trauma center. Proper triage and treatment of the geriatric trauma patient can be life-saving. Decreases in postoperative infections, respiratory failure, length of stay and mortality have been demonstrated via establishment of trauma care networks and specific geriatric trauma care teams.[24,25] Unfortunately, elderly patients are consistently less frequently triaged to trauma centers due to lack of recognition of potential major injuries and underestimation of the severity of a traumatic event.[26,27] Both injury mechanism and vital signs can be unreliable while triaging elderly trauma patients. The American College of Surgeons and the Centers for Disease Control and Prevention currently recommend that emergency medical services transport trauma patients older than 55 years to a designated trauma center regardless of the severity of injury.[28,29]

Evaluation in the Trauma Center

Higher levels of vigilance are required while assessing elderly patients in the trauma center. Those who do not meet trauma activation criteria on initial evaluation often have occult injuries leading to higher morbidities.[30,31] Vital signs and physical examination can be falsely reassuring in this population, with a three-to fivefold increase in mortality in geriatric trauma patients with an SBP less than 90 mmHg.[6] The ATLS protocol should be followed, similar to younger patients, but with careful attention to the differences in physiology of geriatric patients.

Airway

Caution is advised for the use of nasopharyngeal airways in the unconscious or obtunded elderly patient. They have friable nasal mucosa and a higher likelihood of being on anti-platelet or anticoagulant medications, increasing the likelihood of nasal hemorrhage after nasal airway or nasogastric tube insertion. The oral cavity must be examined and poorly fitting or loose dental appliances must be removed. Edentulous patients may have oropharyngeal obstruction when positioned supine, complicating bag mask ventilation. Supplemental oxygen can benefit all elderly trauma patients by increasing apneic reserve in case a rapid sequence induction is needed.

When the decision is made to perform endotracheal intubation, the doses of induction medications may require adjustment in the elderly. Pharmacokinetics are altered due to trauma and to aging; decreases in total body water that decrease volumes of distribution, and reduced metabolism and excretion from declines in renal and hepatic function.[32-34] Bolus doses of barbiturates, benzodiazepines and opioids need to be reduced by as much as 25–50%.[35-37] Dosing of succinylcholine does not change significantly with aging. However, the doses of nondepolarizing neuromuscular blocking agents should be decreased.[38-40]

Laryngeal reflexes may diminish due to gradual deterioration of muscular structures and neurologic input, increasing the possibility of aspiration. Visualization of the vocal cords during intubation can be impaired due to bleeding from the more friable oropharynx and impaired cervical spine mobility from loss of the cervical lordotic curve, spondylosis, arthritis and spinal stenosis. Age-related osteoporosis increases the incidence of cervical spine injury during intubation in the elderly.[8]

Breathing

Maximum inspiratory and expiratory forces can be decreased by almost 50% due to the degenerative changes in the chest wall and respiratory musculature.[41] Elderly patients have a higher risk of respiratory failure, pneumonia and mechanical ventilation dependence due to a decrease in mucus production and a reduction in the ability to cough.[42,43] Osteoporosis increases the incidence of fractures of ribs, sternum, and first and second cervical vertebrae, which increases incidence of pulmonary contusions and poses severe limitations during pulmonary toilet and weaning from mechanical ventilation.[44] Epidural analgesia can provide superior pain control to other modalities and has been shown to improve pulmonary outcomes after thoracic trauma.[44,45] It must be considered early in patient management. The blunted response to hypoxia and hypercarbia may delay the onset of clinical signs of respiratory distress and hence arterial blood gases are valuable during respiratory assessment. Reduction in organ-dependent elimination of neuromuscular agents demands vigilance to prevent residual neuromuscular blockade and a resultant increase in pulmonary complications.

Circulation

The elderly trauma patient's response to hypovolemic shock is attenuated. Diminished catecholamine sensitivity, coronary atherosclerosis, myocyte fibrosis and conduction abnormalities can all play a role. Preinjury medications such as beta-blockers and calcium channel blockers can further hinder the tachycardic response to hypovolemia. Due to baseline hypertension, a "normal blood pressure" might actually indicate a state of hypoperfusion, increasing the chance of organ injury.[46] There is relative paucity of literature evaluating the endpoints of resuscitation in geriatric trauma patients. Prehospital shock index, trends in vital signs and venous lactate levels may provide better measures of perfusion and predictors of mortality.[47–49] Venous lactate over 4 mmol/l or a base deficit over 6 is associated with 40% mortality.[48] With the importance of frequent measurements combined with the higher incidence of cardiovascular co-morbidities, invasive hemodynamic monitoring may be useful in management of the elderly trauma patient.

Disability (Neurologic)

Total brain mass decreases by about 30% and cognition decline results in a drop in IQ by 1–2 standard deviations between the ages of 20 and 80.[50–52] The incidence of subclinical Alzheimer's disease, Parkinson disease, cerebrovascular disease and Lewy body dementia could be as high as 80% in individuals over the age of 60.[53] In addition, geriatric patients have a higher incidence of prior stroke. While the prevalence of cognitive dysfunction can be as high as 35% among geriatric patients, it is only recognized 6% of the time in the emergency room.[54] With delirium being the most common neurologic complication in the traumatized elder, every attempt has to be made to ascertain a baseline neurologic exam, especially level of cognition, prior to proceeding with any kind of intervention.

Exposure

Due to impaired thermoregulation in the elderly,[55] every attempt must be made to prevent hypothermia. Hypothermia predisposes to increased blood loss, increased risk of wound infection, impaired drug metabolism, increased myocardial ischemia and arrhythmias.[55–59] Active warming should be used.

Intraoperative Considerations and Resuscitation

Maintenance of hemodynamic stability in order to preserve the balance between myocardial oxygen supply and demand is crucial to minimize perioperative cardiovascular events. It is prudent to treat all traumatized elders similar to patients with known cardiac history in light of aging physiologic changes. Resuscitation must be determined based on adequacy of perfusion, which can be challenging due to pre-existing co-morbidities and medications that can alter the normal hemodynamic response to hypovolemia. Early invasive hemodynamic monitoring and serial lactate measurements can guide therapy. It is critical to make individualized assessments regarding the Starling curve of each patient during resuscitation. A reasonable approach would be to administer 500 ml crystalloid boluses while continually assessing patient response. The need for invasive central venous pressures, pulmonary artery pressures, cardiac output, mixed venous oxygen saturation and transesophageal echocardiography must be assessed on an individual basis, including co-morbidities, mechanism of trauma, physical examination findings and trends in the clinical picture.

Early PRBC transfusion has been shown to be an independent predictor of pulmonary complications, including ARDS and death in adult trauma patients.[60–62] The decision to transfuse must be based on evaluation of oxygen delivery–consumption balance, response to resuscitation, and cardiac, pulmonary and renal co-morbidities rather than standard cutoffs.

Postoperative Management

The most common postoperative complication in the geriatric population is postoperative delirium, with incidence varying from 15% to 50% based on the type of procedure performed.[63] The most important risk factors for postoperative delirium are dementia and advanced age.[64] Use of structured clinical protocols targeted at modifiable risk factors such as sleep deprivation, immobility, visual and hearing impairment, and dehydration are the only interventions shown to prevent delirium.[65,66] Prophylactic administration of haloperidol has lowered the severity and duration of episodes, but not the incidence of delirium.[67] Poor control of postoperative pain, usage of sedatives, narcotics and anticholinergics, and blood transfusions have been associated with postoperative delirium.[63,68,69] For the elderly trauma patient, it is vital to obtain a thorough preoperative history, including evaluation for cognitive dysfunction, to use a multimodal approach to pain control minimizing sedatives/opioids and to coordinate care with comprehensive geriatric care teams. Family members must be partners in the care of the patient. On a regular basis, the physician must have a frank discussion of rehabilitation expectations, disposition and outcomes, including mortality with the family.

Summary

Elderly patients represent one of the fastest-growing population segments and, due to an increasingly active lifestyle, are accounting for an increasing number of trauma admissions. They have worse outcomes compared to younger patients due to reduction in their functional reserve. Care of the traumatized elder requires a thorough understanding of the physiologic changes of aging. Falls account for over half of all unintentional injuries in the elderly. They are consistently undertriaged. Normal vital signs can indicate hypoperfusion. Early invasive hemodynamic monitoring can facilitate the use of serial arterial blood gases, venous lactates and trends in vital signs to guide therapy. Resuscitation must be individualized to the patient's Starling curve. The decision to transfuse must be based on careful evaluation of the patient's oxygen delivery–consumption balance, response to resuscitation, and cardiac, pulmonary and renal co-morbidities rather than standard cutoffs. Postoperative delirium is a major complication and can be prevented by the use of clinical protocols targeting specific risk factors. It is key to make the family a part of the care team and have realistic discussions regarding outcomes and rehabilitation. The benefits of medical or surgical intervention must always be balanced with prognosis, resource use and patient wishes.

References

1. CDC. National Vital Statistics Reports. 2013. Available from: www.cdc.gov/nchs/data/nvsr/nvsr62/nvsr62_06.pdf (Accessed July 13, 2017).

2. CDC. Ten leading causes of death and injury. 2015. Available from: www.cdc.gov/injury/wisqars/leadingcauses.html (Accessed July 13, 2017).

3. Pandya SR, Yelon JA, Sullivan TS, Risucci DA. Geriatric motor vehicle collision survival: the role of institutional trauma volume. *J Trauma*. 2011; 70(6):1326–1330.

4. Travis KW, Mihevc NT, Orkin FK, Zeitlin GL. Age and anesthetic practice: a regional perspective. *J Clin Anesth*. 1999; 11(3):175–186.

5. Frankenfield D, Cooney RN, Smith JS, Rowe WA. Age-related differences in the metabolic response to injury. *J Trauma.* 2000; 48(1):49–56; discussion 56–57.

6. Hashmi A, Ibrahim-Zada I, Rhee P, *et al.* Predictors of mortality in geriatric trauma patients: a systematic review and meta-analysis. *J Trauma Acute Care Surg.* 2014; 76(3):894–901.

7. Knudson MM, Lieberman J, Morris JA Jr., Cushing BM, Stubbs HA. Mortality factors in geriatric blunt trauma patients. *Arch Surg.* 1994; 129(4):448–453.

8. Shulman CI, Alouidor R, McKenney MG. Geriatric trauma. In: Feliciano DV, Matox KL, Moore EE, eds., *Trauma, 6th edn.* New York, McGraw-Hill Medical, 2008.

9. Caterino JM, Valasek T, Werman HA. Identification of an age cutoff for increased mortality in patients with elderly trauma. *Am J Emerg Med.* 2010; 28(2):151–158.

10. Joseph B, Pandit V, Zangbar B, *et al.* Superiority of frailty over age in predicting outcomes among geriatric trauma patients: a prospective analysis. *JAMA Surg.* 2014; 149(8): 766–772.

11. Ting B, Zurakowski D, Herder L, *et al.* Preinjury ambulatory status is associated with 1-year mortality following lateral compression Type I fractures in the geriatric population older than 80 years. *J Trauma Acute Care Surg.* 2014; 76(5):1306–1309.

12. Banks SE, Lewis MC. Trauma in the elderly: considerations for anesthetic management. *Anesthesiol Clin.* 2013; 31(1):127–139.

13. Qato DM, Alexander GC, Conti RM, *et al.* Use of prescription and over-the-counter medications and dietary supplements among older adults in the United States. *JAMA.* 2008; 300(24):2867–2878.

14. The Slone Survey. Patterns of medication use in the United States 2006. 2006. Available from: www.bu.edu/slone/files/2012/11/SloneSurveyReport2006.pdf (Accessed July 13, 2017).

15. Franko J, Kish KJ, O'Connell BG, Subramanian S, Yuschak JV. Advanced age and preinjury warfarin anticoagulation increase the risk of mortality after head trauma. *J Trauma.* 2006; 61(1):107–110.

16. Ivascu FA, Janczyk RJ, Junn FS, *et al.* Treatment of trauma patients with intracranial hemorrhage on preinjury warfarin. *J Trauma.* 2006; 61(2): 318–321.

17. Karni A, Holtzman R, Bass T, *et al.* Traumatic head injury in the anticoagulated elderly patient: a lethal combination. *Am Surg.* 2001; 67(11):1098–1100.

18. Neideen T, Lam M, Brasel KJ. Preinjury beta blockers are associated with increased mortality in geriatric trauma patients. *J Trauma.* 2008; 65(5):1016–1020.

19. Arbabi S, Campion EM, Hemmila MR, *et al.* Beta-blocker use is associated with improved outcomes in adult trauma patients. *J Trauma.* 2007; 62(1):56–61; discussion 61–62.

20. Arbabi S, Ahrns KS, Wahl WL, *et al.* Beta-blocker use is associated with improved outcomes in adult burn patients. *J Trauma.* 2004; 56(2):265–269; discussion 269–271.

21. Cotton BA, Snodgrass KB, Fleming SB, *et al.* Beta-blocker exposure is associated with improved survival after severe traumatic brain injury. *J Trauma.* 2007; 62(1):26–33; discussion 33–35.

22. Grossman MD, Miller D, Scaff DW, Arcona S. When is an elder old? Effect of preexisting conditions on mortality in geriatric trauma. *J Trauma.* 2002; 52(2):242–246.

23. Ferraris VA, Ferraris SP, Saha SP. The relationship between mortality and preexisting cardiac disease in 5,971 trauma patients. *J Trauma.* 2010; 69(3):645–652.

24. Ang D, Norwood S, Barquist E, *et al.* Geriatric outcomes for trauma patients in the state of Florida after the advent of a large trauma network. *J Trauma Acute Care Surg.* 2014; 77(1):155–160; discussion 160.

25. Mangram AJ, Mitchell CD, Shifflette VK, *et al.* Geriatric trauma service: a one-year experience. *J Trauma Acute Care Surg.* 2012; 72(1):119–122.

26. Chang DC, Bass RR, Cornwell EE, Mackenzie EJ. Undertriage of elderly trauma patients to state-designated trauma centers. *Arch Surg.* 2008; 143(8):776–781; discussion 782.

27. Phillips S, Rond PC III, Kelly SM, Swartz PD. The failure of triage criteria to identify geriatric patients with trauma: results from the Florida Trauma Triage Study. *J Trauma.* 1996; 40(2):278–283.

28. American College of Surgeons. Resources for optimal care of the injured patient 2014. 2015. Available from: www.facs .org/quality%20programs/trauma/vrc/ resources (Accessed July 13, 2015).

29. McCoy CE, Chakravarthy B, Lotfipour S. Guidelines for field triage of injured patients: in conjunction with the morbidity and mortality weekly report published by the Center for Disease Control and Prevention. *West J Emerg Med.* 2013; 14(1):69–76.

30. Demetriades D, Sava J, Alo K, *et al.* Old age as a criterion for trauma team activation. *J Trauma.* 2001; 51(4):754–756; discussion 756–757.

31. Lehmann R, Beekley A, Casey L, Salim A, Martin M. The impact of advanced age on trauma triage decisions and outcomes: a statewide analysis. *Am J Surg.* 2009; 197(5):571–574; discussion 574–575.

32. Muhlberg W, Platt D. Age-dependent changes of the kidneys: pharmacological implications. *Gerontology.* 1999; 45(5):243–253.

33. Buemi M, Nostro L, Aloisi C, *et al.* Kidney aging: from phenotype to genetics. *Rejuvenation Res.* 2005; 8(2): 101–109.

34. Peeters RP. Thyroid hormones and aging. *Hormones (Athens).* 2008; 7(1):28–35.

35. Chau DL, Walker V, Pai L, Cho LM. Opiates and elderly: use and side effects. *Clin Interv Aging.* 2008; 3(2): 273–278.

36. Linnebur SA, O'Connell MB, Wessell AM, *et al.* Pharmacy practice, research, education, and advocacy for older adults. *Pharmacotherapy.* 2005; 25(10): 1396–1430.

37. Rastogi R, Meek BD. Management of chronic pain in elderly, frail patients: finding a suitable, personalized method of control. *Clin Interv Aging.* 2013; 8:37–46.

38. Arain SR, Kern S, Ficke DJ, Ebert TJ. Variability of duration of action of neuromuscular-blocking drugs in elderly patients. *Acta Anaesthesiol Scand.* 2005; 49(3):312–315.

39. Sagir O, Yucesoy Noyan F, Koroglu A, Cicek M, Ilksen Toprak H. Comparison between the effects of rocuronium, vecuronium, and cisatracurium using train-of-four and clinical tests in elderly patients. *Anesth Pain Med.* 2013; 2(4):142–148.

40. Cope TM, Hunter JM. Selecting neuromuscular-blocking drugs for elderly patients. *Drugs Aging.* 2003; 20(2):125–140.

41. Narang AT, Sikka R. Resuscitation of the elderly. *Emerg Med Clin North Am.* 2006; 24(2):261–272, v.

42. Zaugg M, Lucchinetti E. Respiratory function in the elderly. *Anesthesiol Clin North Am.* 2000; 18(1):47–58, vi.

43. Chalfin DB. Outcome assessment in elderly patients with critical illness and respiratory failure. *Clin Chest Med.* 1993; 14(3):583–589.

44. Lomoschitz FM, Blackmore CC, Mirza SK, Mann FA. Cervical spine injuries in patients 65 years old and older: epidemiologic analysis regarding the effects of age and injury mechanism on distribution, type, and stability of injuries. *AJR Am J Roentgenol.* 2002; 178(3):573–577.

45. Wisner DH. A stepwise logistic regression analysis of factors affecting morbidity and mortality after thoracic trauma: effect of epidural analgesia. *J Trauma.* 1990; 30(7):799–804; discussion 804–805.

46. Heffernan DS, Thakkar RK, Monaghan SF, et al. Normal presenting vital signs are unreliable in geriatric blunt trauma victims. *J Trauma*. 2010; 69(4):813–820.

47. Salottolo KM, Mains CW, Offner PJ, Bourg PW, Bar-Or D. A retrospective analysis of geriatric trauma patients: venous lactate is a better predictor of mortality than traditional vital signs. *Scand J Trauma Resusc Emerg Med*. 2013; 21:7.

48. Callaway DW, Shapiro NI, Donnino MW, Baker C, Rosen CL. Serum lactate and base deficit as predictors of mortality in normotensive elderly blunt trauma patients. *J Trauma*. 2009; 66(4):1040–1044.

49. McNab A, Burns B, Bhullar I, Chesire D, Kerwin A. A prehospital shock index for trauma correlates with measures of hospital resource use and mortality. *Surgery*. 2012; 152(3):473–476.

50. Ramaiah R, Lam AM. Postoperative cognitive dysfunction in the elderly. *Anesthesiol Clin*. 2009; 27(3):485–496.

51. Meguro K, Shimada M, Yamaguchi S, et al. Cognitive function and frontal lobe atrophy in normal elderly adults: implications for dementia not as aging-related disorders and the reserve hypothesis. *Psychiatry Clin Neurosci*. 2001; 55(6):565–572.

52. Brody H. The aging brain. *Acta Neurol Scand Suppl*. 1992; 137:40–44.

53. Thal DR, Del Tredici K, Braak H. Neurodegeneration in normal brain aging and disease. *Sci Aging Knowledge Environ*. 2004; 2004(23):pe26.

54. Carpenter CR, DesPain B, Keeling TN, Shah M, Rothenberger M. The Six-Item Screener and AD8 for the detection of cognitive impairment in geriatric emergency department patients. *Ann Emerg Med*. 2011; 57(6):653–661.

55. Vaughan MS, Vaughan RW, Cork RC. Postoperative hypothermia in adults: relationship of age, anesthesia, and shivering to rewarming. *Anesth Analg*. 1981; 60(10):746–751.

56. Rajagopalan S, Mascha E, Na J, Sessler DI. The effects of mild perioperative hypothermia on blood loss and transfusion requirement. *Anesthesiology*. 2008; 108(1):71–77.

57. Sessler DI, Akca O. Nonpharmacological prevention of surgical wound infections. *Clin Infect Dis*. 2002; 35(11): 1397–1404.

58. Frank SM, Higgins MS, Breslow MJ, et al. The catecholamine, cortisol, and hemodynamic responses to mild perioperative hypothermia: a randomized clinical trial. *Anesthesiology*. 1995; 82(1):83–93.

59. Frank SM, Fleisher LA, Breslow MJ, et al. Perioperative maintenance of normothermia reduces the incidence of morbid cardiac events. A randomized clinical trial. *JAMA*. 1997; 277(14):1127–1134.

60. Chaiwat O, Lang JD, Vavilala MS, et al. Early packed red blood cell transfusion and acute respiratory distress syndrome after trauma. *Anesthesiology*. 2009; 110(2):351–360.

61. Croce MA, Tolley EA, Claridge JA, Fabian TC. Transfusions result in pulmonary morbidity and death after a moderate degree of injury. *J Trauma*. 2005; 59(1):19–23; discussion 23–24.

62. Claridge JA, Sawyer RG, Schulman AM, McLemore EC, Young JS. Blood transfusions correlate with infections in trauma patients in a dose-dependent manner. *Am Surg*. 2002; 68(7): 566–572.

63. Inouye SK. Delirium in older persons. *N Engl J Med*. 2006; 354(11):1157–1165.

64. Bitsch M, Foss N, Kristensen B, Kehlet H. Pathogenesis of and management strategies for postoperative delirium after hip fracture: a review. *Acta Orthop Scand*. 2004; 75(4):378–389.

65. Inouye SK, Bogardus ST Jr., Charpentier PA, et al. A multicomponent intervention to prevent delirium in hospitalized older patients. *N Engl J Med*. 1999; 340(9):669–676.

66. Monk TG, Weldon BC, Garvan CW, *et al.* Predictors of cognitive dysfunction after major noncardiac surgery. *Anesthesiology.* 2008; 108(1):18–30.

67. Bourne RS, Tahir TA, Borthwick M, Sampson EL. Drug treatment of delirium: past, present and future. *J Psychosom Res.* 2008; 65(3): 273–282.

68. Egbert AM. Postoperative pain management in the frail elderly. *Clin Geriatr Med.* 1996; 12(3):583–599.

69. Zhu SH, Ji MH, Gao DP, Li WY, Yang JJ. Association between perioperative blood transfusion and early postoperative cognitive dysfunction in aged patients following total hip replacement surgery. *Ups J Med Sci.* 2014; 119(3):262–267.

Major Surgery in the Elderly

James M. Hunter, Jr. and Thomas R. Vetter

Key Points

- Preoperative factors significantly associated with mortality include increasing age, worsening American Society of Anesthesiologists (ASA) physical status, a preoperative plasma albumin less than 30 g/l and undergoing nonscheduled surgery. Complications significantly associated with postoperative mortality include acute renal impairment, unplanned intensive care unit admission and systemic inflammation.
- Postoperative morbidity and mortality increase progressively with increasing age, as age is significantly associated with major wound, renal, cardiovascular and respiratory complications, as well as death at 30 days.
- Clinicians should carefully consider a patient's goals and wishes when assessing the need for surgical intervention at the end of life, to ensure that such interventions not only extend life, but also enhance the quality of life and reduce suffering.
- Enhanced Recovery After Surgery (ERAS) has been defined as a multifaceted perioperative care pathway designed to attenuate the stress response during all three phases of the perioperative period and the patient's journey through a surgical procedure, so as to facilitate the maintenance of bodily composition and organ function, and in doing so achieve early recovery.
- Key elements of ERAS include multimodal analgesia, maintenance of preoperative homeostasis by avoiding dehydration and promoting an anabolic state with preoperative oral liquids and carbohydrate loading, optimizing fluid therapy and avoiding volume overload, and utilizing anesthetic techniques that permit a more rapid return to normal cognitive function.
- A multimodal analgesic approach is recommended in order to provide adequate analgesia, reduce opioid consumption, reduce medication side effects and facilitate the achievement of ERAS milestones.

Introduction

If left unchecked, in the United States by 2023, there will be a projected 42% overall increase in cases of the seven primary chronic diseases of cancer, diabetes, hypertension, stroke, heart disease, pulmonary conditions, and mental disorders.[1] Therefore, by 2020, 157 million Americans are predicted to have one chronic disease, and 81 million will have multiple such chronic conditions. The reasons for this increased prevalence of chronic disease are multifactorial, but include the rising prevalence of obesity.[2] However, the future health care workforce in the United States is not similarly projected to include the appropriate mix of personnel capable of preventing and managing this substantial chronic disease burden.[2]

Conversely, the chronic disease burden from heart disease, hypertension, diabetes, obesity and arthritis is markedly less in Europe than in the United States.[2,3] This difference has been attributed to a generally healthier diet and lower poverty rates in Europe. This difference in chronic disease burden is also contributing to the marked health care spending gap between the United States and Europe.[2,3]

Furthermore, due to declining fertility, improved health care and greater longevity, the world's population is now aging at an unprecedented rate.[4] Specifically, in the United States, the population aged 65 years and older increased by 21% from 35.5 million in 2002 to 43.1 million in 2012. This number of older Americans is projected to more than double to 92 million in 2060.[5] This aging population in the United States has been accompanied by an increasing number of surgical procedures on elderly patients. Not surprisingly, many of these elderly surgical patients have major co-morbidity from chronic diseases.[6] Better strategies are emerging to prevent, or at least to properly manage, postoperative complications and thus to reduce the associated greater morbidity and mortality in elderly surgical patients.[7]

This chapter will initially review the epidemiology of major surgery in the elderly population. The chapter will then focus primarily on Enhanced Recovery After Surgery (ERAS) for major abdominal surgery, including its applicability in geriatric patients and some of its specific elements (prehabilitation, preoperative homeostasis, goal-directed fluid therapy, multimodal analgesia and anesthetic depth monitoring for facilitating more rapid recovery from anesthesia and reduction of the risk of delirium).

Epidemiology of Major Surgery in the Elderly

The relationship between the above international phenomenon of an aging population (the "Silver Tsunami"), perioperative care, and postoperative morbidity and mortality is complex.[7] The risk of complications and death following surgery in older patients has been extensively researched and well reviewed.[8] Among surgical patients 70 years and older, the overall 30-day mortality is approximately 6%; however, the mortality risk reportedly increases by 10% for every year after age 70.[7]

The prospective REASON study of 4158 noncardiac surgical patients 70 years or older, cared for in 23 hospitals in Australia and New Zealand, revealed that by postoperative day 30, 5% of patients had died, 20% had suffered major complications and 9.4% were admitted to an intensive care unit. Preoperative factors significantly associated with mortality included increasing age, worsening American Society of Anesthesiologists (ASA) physical status, a preoperative plasma albumin <3.0 g/dl and undergoing non-scheduled surgery. Complications significantly associated with postoperative mortality included acute renal impairment, unplanned intensive care unit admission and systemic inflammation.[9]

Based upon single institutional American College of Surgeons National Surgical Quality Improvement Program data from 2002 to 2005, among 7696 surgical patients, there was an overall 28% morbidity rate and 2.3% mortality rate. However, those patients older than 80 years of age had a morbidity rate of 51% and mortality rate of 7%. Postoperative morbidity and mortality increased progressively with increasing age, as age was significantly associated with major wound, renal, cardiovascular and respiratory complications, as well as death at 30 days.[6]

Cancer-related surveillance, treatment decision-making and surgery in the elderly present unique, multidimensional challenges. In the geriatric oncologic population, an impaired stress response, increased senescence and decreased immunity impact the risk/benefit ratio of cancer surgery.[10] This was borne out by a retrospective study of 8781 patients who underwent elective or emergent major thoracic, abdominal or pelvic resections for neoplasms in the 2005 to 2007 American College of Surgeons National Surgical Quality Improvement Program database. Increased age was also associated with higher operative mortality (4.83% for ages 75 years or older versus 1.09% for ages 40 to 55 years), a greater frequency of major complications and more prolonged hospital stays. However, the effect of age was comparable to the effects of other preoperative risk factors, supporting the use of individualized, risk-based surgical decision-making in older cancer patients.[11]

Notably, a retrospective cohort study of nearly 2 million elderly beneficiaries of fee-for-service Medicare in the United States, 65 years or older, who died in 2008, revealed that 31.9% underwent an inpatient surgical procedure during the year before their death, 18.3% underwent a procedure in their last month of life and 8.0% underwent a procedure during their last week of life. Importantly, the rate at which these older Americans underwent surgery varied substantially with age and by the region of the country, suggesting discretion in health care providers' decisions to intervene surgically at the end of life. These findings should prompt clinicians to carefully consider a patient's goals and wishes when assessing the need for surgical intervention at the end of life, to ensure that such interventions not only extend life, but also enhance the quality of life and reduce suffering.[12]

Enhanced Recovery After Surgery

Based on an increasing number of multinational, multicenter cohort studies, randomized studies and meta-analyses, the concept of a "fast-track" approach to surgery has evolved over the last three decades.[13-15] The application of multifaceted, evidence-based care within such a fast-track approach to surgery has been demonstrated to improve postoperative recovery and reduce morbidity.[14] The further integration of minimally invasive surgery techniques, pharmacological stress-reduction methods and effective multimodal, nonopioid analgesia can be expected to result in additional improvements in patient-centered outcomes.[14]

This multifaceted, evidence-based fast-track approach to surgery has subsequently been further substantiated and labeled as Enhanced Recovery After Surgery (ERAS) (Figure 14.1).[16,17] ERAS has been defined as a multifaceted perioperative care pathway designed to attenuate the stress response during all three phases of the perioperative period and the patient's journey through a surgical procedure, so as to facilitate the maintenance of bodily composition and organ function, and in doing so achieve early recovery.[16]

Repeated practice surveys from the United States, Europe, Australia and New Zealand have shown that adherence to an evidence-based perioperative care protocol like ERAS has been generally low.[18] The recent full scope of ERAS has thus transcended a simple protocol for perioperative care, with the creation of a novel multiprofessional, multidisciplinary medical society: the Enhanced Recovery After Surgery Society for Perioperative Care (www.erassociety.org). The ERAS Society is leading the development

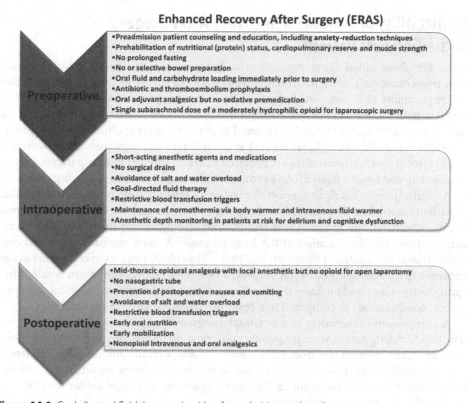

Enhanced Recovery After Surgery (ERAS)

Preoperative
- Preadmission patient counseling and education, including anxiety-reduction techniques
- Prehabilitation of nutritional (protein) status, cardiopulmonary reserve and muscle strength
- No prolonged fasting
- No or selective bowel preparation
- Oral fluid and carbohydrate loading immediately prior to surgery
- Antibiotic and thromboembolism prophylaxis
- Oral adjuvant analgesics but no sedative premedication
- Single subarachnoid dose of a moderately hydrophilic opioid for laparoscopic surgery

Intraoperative
- Short-acting anesthetic agents and medications
- No surgical drains
- Avoidance of salt and water overload
- Goal-directed fluid therapy
- Restrictive blood transfusion triggers
- Maintenance of normothermia via body warmer and intravenous fluid warmer
- Anesthetic depth monitoring in patients at risk for delirium and cognitive dysfunction

Postoperative
- Mid-thoracic epidural analgesia with local anesthetic but no opioid for open laparotomy
- No nasogastric tube
- Prevention of postoperative nausea and vomiting
- Avoidance of salt and water overload
- Restrictive blood transfusion triggers
- Early oral nutrition
- Early mobilization
- Nonopioid intravenous and oral analgesics

Figure 14.1 Goal-directed fluid therapy: algorithm for optimizing stroke volume.

of evidence-based guidelines that form the basis for implementing ERAS programs by translating its principles into practice.[17]

The subspecialty of colorectal surgery has been the earliest and most extensive adopter of ERAS principles and protocols.[19–23] ERAS has also been applied for a number of other major surgical procedures, including esophagectomy,[24,25] gastrectomy,[26,27] pancreatico-duodenectomy,[28,29] hepatectomy,[30,31] rectal/pelvic surgery[32] and radical cystectomy.[33,34] It has been applied to a lesser extent in gynecologic oncology surgery.[35,36]

The targets and strategies of ERAS thus appear supported by health care providers and their patients in the setting of major esophagogastric, hepatic, pancreatic and colorectal surgery. Nevertheless, controversies still exist about the relative importance of the individual components of ERAS.[37] Not surprisingly, strict adherence to ERAS protocols remains a challenge, and its benefits decrease with lower adherence. Maintaining optimal health care team adherence remains an ongoing challenge that requires repeated training and dedicated personnel.[38] Preliminary evidence suggests that a tailored implementation strategy based on the Knowledge to Action (KTA) cycle can be used to successfully disseminate and implement an ERAS program at multiple sites.[39] Additional supportive data are needed on the cost-effectiveness, long-term outcomes, health-related quality of life and other patient-centered outcomes with ERAS, and these issues thus remain important areas of future research.[18,40]

Applicability of Enhanced Recovery After Surgery to the Geriatric Patient

Given the above noted aging population and concomitant increasing number of surgical procedures on elderly patients,[6] there is understandable interest in the feasibility and applicability of a "fast-track" approach to major surgery, and specifically, ERAS, in geriatric patients. To date, only a handful of smaller-scale studies have examined this topic. Based upon a 2014 systematic review, ERAS can be safely applied in elderly patients in an effort to reduce complications and shorten length of hospital stay.[41] However, its authors noted that further studies are required to assess whether elderly patients are able to adhere to and benefit from ERAS protocols to the same extent as younger patients.[41]

An initial purely descriptive report of a fast-track rehabilitation program that enrolled 74 patients more than 70 years old, undergoing colonic surgery for benign or malignant disease, concluded the program was feasible and also decreased the number of overall complications and the duration of the hospital stay.[42] A more recent randomized controlled trial with 78 patients demonstrated that in the elderly patients over 65 years of age, undergoing laparoscopic colorectal surgery, a fast-track recovery program resulted in a significantly more rapid postoperative recovery, earlier discharge from hospital and fewer general complications as compared to a conventional postoperative protocol.[43]

A comparison of the safety of a fast-track program after laparoscopic colorectal surgery in 337 elderly versus younger patients observed no immediate postoperative differences in return of bowel function, advancement of diet, overall complications and length of postoperative stay. However, emergency department visits or readmission within a month after discharge were significantly more frequent in the patients older than 70 years (11.7%) than in the younger patients (4%).[44]

In another randomized controlled trial of 240 patients ≥70 years old with colorectal carcinoma undergoing open colorectal surgery, when compared to traditional perioperative management, a fast-track surgery approach significantly decreased the length of stay, facilitated the recovery of bowel function and reduced the occurrence of postoperative delirium and other complications.[45] Of note, the lower incidence of delirium may have been partly due to the reduced systemic inflammatory response mediated by and quantified with interleukin-6 (IL-6).[45]

Specific Elements of Enhanced Recovery After Surgery

Prehabilitation

"Prehabilitation" is an intervention to enhance functional capacity in anticipation of a forthcoming physiological stressor.[46] Prehabilitation aims to enhance functional capacity preoperatively for better toleration of surgery and to facilitate recovery.[47] Two burgeoning areas of interest in the geriatric surgical population are maximizing the opportunities for preoperative "prehabilitation" and concomitantly accurately predicting and then ideally reducing the need for prolonged postoperative, postdischarge institutional rehabilitation and convalescence.[48–51]

In colorectal cancer surgery patients, a prehabilitation program using exercise alone (walking and breathing exercises versus stationary cycling and strengthening), over a mean of 52 days preoperatively, had a limited impact and low adherence.[46] In another

trial of prehabilitation for colorectal surgery, patients whose physical function deterio-
rated preoperatively were at greater risk of complications requiring reoperation and/or
intensive care management.[52]

In contrast, an expanded, approximately 1-month trimodal prehabilitation program,
which added home-based, preoperative nutritional counseling, protein supplementa-
tion and relaxation exercises (anxiety reduction) to moderate aerobic and resistance
exercises, significantly improved functional recovery (walking capacity) at 4 weeks and
8 weeks postoperatively. However, postoperative complication rates and the hospital length
of stay were similar in the prehabilitation versus postoperative rehabilitation patients.[47,53]

Maintenance of Preoperative Homeostasis

The primary aim of ERAS is the reduction of the stress response to surgery,[16] thus accelerating the process of recovery. An important component of reducing the perioperative
stress response is optimizing the patient's condition at the time of presentation for surgery.

Traditional preparation of patients for gastrointestinal surgery included mechanical
bowel preparation, which was not only a source of discomfort, but also could result in the
patient presenting for surgery with a significant fluid deficit and electrolyte imbalances.[54]
More recently, it has been shown that forgoing mechanical bowel preparation does not
increase the risk of anastomotic or wound complications, may reduce the incidence of
postoperative ileus and improves the patient experience.[55-57] Routine use of mechanical
bowel preparation is not recommended within ERAS for open colorectal procedures,
though there may still be advantages to its use in laparoscopic procedures, as the reduction in bowel contents may improve surgical exposure.[55]

Modification of traditional recommendations for preoperative fasting has also been
found to be advantageous. Historically, patients were required to be *nil per os* (NPO)
after midnight the night prior to the procedure, regardless of whether the procedure
would be performed in the morning or later in the day. This resulted in patients presenting for surgery relatively dehydrated and in a metabolically "starved" state. Permitting
oral intake of clear liquids up to 2 hours prior to induction of anesthesia is now recognized to be safe.[58,59] It is associated with improved patient comfort, reduced anxiety
and decreased postoperative nausea and vomiting,[60] in addition to the obvious benefit
of allowing the patient to avoid dehydration caused by a prolonged period of no oral
intake. Fasting results in a reduction in insulin sensitivity, even in the absence of surgery
or trauma.[60] The combination of a fasting state and the effects of surgery results in a
greater stress response and reduction in insulin sensitivity than either fasting or surgery
alone.[60] The addition of carbohydrates (equivalent to 50 g of glucose) to preoperative
oral clear liquid intake can change the patient's metabolic state from a fasting (catabolic)
one, in which insulin levels are low and hepatic glycogen breakdown and gluconeogenesis are occurring, to a "fed" (anabolic) state, with increased insulin levels and a shift
to storage of energy as hepatic glycogen.[60] This practice reduces the stress response to
surgery, including a reduction in postoperative insulin resistance, reduced nitrogen loss
and preservation of muscle mass.[60] In the elderly population, who are already at risk for
dehydration, malnutrition and loss of muscle mass, the beneficial effects of these changes
to traditional NPO practices are apparent. They may also result in a decrease in intraoperative fluid requirements by eliminating, or at least mitigating, hypovolemia at the time
of presentation for surgery.

Goal-Directed Fluid Therapy

Optimal management of intravascular volume is an essential component of anesthetic management in patients undergoing major abdominal surgery. Too little intravascular volume results in tissue ischemia and may lead to multiple organ system failure.[61] Excessive fluid administration can lead to pulmonary edema, atrial fibrillation, and an increased risk of anastomotic breakdown and wound complications.[55,62,63] Administering the correct amount of replacement fluid is even more important in the elderly surgical patient than in younger patients, since the elderly are less able to compensate for hypovolemia or hypervolemia.[64] Despite its importance, determination of the optimal amount of fluid to administer to a given patient remains difficult.

It has been common practice to determine the intraoperative volume of intravenous fluids based on an estimate of pre-existing fluid deficits (e.g. those due to fasting and the use of mechanical bowel preparation), additional volume (5–7 ml/kg) administered to compensate for the venodilation produced by anesthesia and the fluid losses experienced intraoperatively, including blood loss and so-called "third space" losses (4–6 ml/kg/h for major abdominal surgery).[65] This approach typically results in an increase in weight of 3–6 kg postoperatively.[66] It has been observed that patients receiving larger quantities of fluid have worse outcomes,[66–69] calling into question these traditional methods of determining fluid requirements. In fact, the very existence of fasting-induced hypovolemia and of "third space" losses has been questioned.[70]

Goal-directed fluid therapy has some of its origins in the work of Shoemaker in the 1980s,[61,71,72] which demonstrated that patients who failed to achieve an increase in cardiac output and oxygen delivery in response to major surgery had higher mortality. Results of studies aimed at titration of fluids, blood products and inotropes to achieve the supra-normal levels of oxygen delivery seen in survivors were mixed, with no consistent mortality benefit.[73] However, the concept of titrating fluid therapy to specific hemodynamic endpoints remains logical. The optimal endpoint to be targeted (and, in particular, whether it is beneficial to use inotropes to reach those targets) remains unclear. Nevertheless, improvements in surgical morbidity and length of stay have been seen with standardized fluid resuscitation protocols, which utilize cardiac output monitoring to guide fluid administration,[73,74] at least in higher-risk procedures, including open procedures, prolonged procedures and those for which significant blood loss is expected.

Such goal-directed protocols most commonly take the approach of maximizing stroke volume: a fluid challenge is given and its effect on stroke volume is assessed using some means of monitoring cardiac output. If an increase in stroke volume of at least 10% is seen, additional fluid challenges are administered until there is no longer an increase in stroke volume. Once the maximal stroke volume has been determined, additional fluids are minimized unless stroke volume falls. Once maximal stroke volume has been attained, hypotension should be treated with vasopressors, provided there is no other evidence of hypoperfusion. Inotropic support should be reserved for situations where overt evidence of tissue hypoperfusion (such as lactic acidosis) persists after maximal stroke volume has been achieved with fluid resuscitation, and anemia has been corrected. While the optimal target for fluid administration remains unknown, and targeting maximal stroke volume may also result in some degree of volume overload,[70] this approach ensures that hypovolemia is avoided. It also provides an objective endpoint for limiting fluid administration, thus at least reducing the risk of fluid overload and redirecting the anesthesiologist's attention to other potential causes of hypotension.

Multimodal Analgesia

Effective analgesia is vital not only for humanitarian reasons and patient satisfaction, but also because poorly relieved postoperative pain contributes to the surgical stress response and impairs functional recovery.[75] Effective analgesia is important for both short-term and long-term postoperative outcomes, as inadequately controlled pain can lead to central nervous system sensitization (e.g. spinal cord wind-up) and chronic post-surgical pain that persists beyond the typical healing period of 1–2 months.[76–78] Such chronic postsurgical pain can have a sustained major adverse effect on a patient's health-related quality of life and activities of daily living.[78]

Elderly patients have age-related changes in their physiology, pharmacokinetics, pharmacodynamics and nociceptive processing, which can impact the effectiveness and safety of analgesic medications and modalities. The elderly may also experience other barriers (e.g. communication, social and cognitive issues) that may hamper effective postoperative pain treatment. The elderly are at increased risk of postoperative complications – especially in the presence of severe or uncontrolled pain.[78]

The efficacy of medications, but also their side effects are generally dose dependent.[79] Specifically, the historical ubiquitous and excessive use of opioids for postoperative analgesia has resulted in adverse effects like postoperative sedation, delirium, nausea and vomiting, urinary retention, ileus and respiratory depression, all of which can delay the return of functional status needed for discharge.[80]

A multimodal analgesic approach is thus recommended in order to provide adequate analgesia, reduce opioid consumption, reduce medication side effects and facilitate the achievement of ERAS milestones[80] – especially after major open or laparoscopic abdominal surgery.[75] Multimodal (or "balanced") analgesia is predicated on the use of more than one medication or pain treatment modality. Combining agents and modalities, with different mechanisms of action and receptor sites, can result in additive or synergistic analgesia and mitigate medication-related side effects, thereby achieving more effective and safer analgesia.[79,81]

As advocated by the PROcedure-SPECific Postoperative Pain ManagemenT (PROSPECT) Group (www.postoppain.org), a logical approach to such multimodal therapy for perioperative analgesia, especially in the elderly major surgery patient, is to tailor the regimen to the planned surgical procedure,[77,82,83] including for open versus laparoscopic abdominal surgery.[75]

A 2003 qualitative systematic review observed a beneficial association between epidural anesthesia and analgesia and multisystem physiology, the surgical stress response, immune function and cognition, as well as surgical complications and outcomes.[84] A 2014 systematic review and meta-analysis of 125 randomized controlled trials observed that the risk of death was decreased with epidural analgesia. Epidural analgesia also significantly decreased the risk of atrial fibrillation, supraventricular tachycardia, deep vein thrombosis, respiratory depression, atelectasis, pneumonia, ileus and postoperative nausea and vomiting, and also improved recovery of bowel function. Conversely, it significantly increased the risk of arterial hypotension, pruritus, urinary retention and motor blockade.[85]

Specifically, thoracic epidural analgesia has been demonstrated to provide significant pain control with improved gastrointestinal function after an open laparotomy procedure.[77] A thoracic epidural for 48 to 72 hours has thus been a mainstay for analgesia after open gastrointestinal surgery.[75] However, the data are less definitive for epidural analgesia for laparoscopic surgery, and many clinicians have migrated to other methods. One such alternative includes a single intrathecal dose of an opioid (e.g. hydromorphone), combined with perioperatively scheduled acetaminophen, a nonsteroidal anti-inflammatory drug, and a gabapentanoid.[75,77]

In a recent meta-analysis of 21 randomized controlled trials involving patients undergoing abdominal surgery, a perioperative intravenous lidocaine infusion was shown to be an effective adjuvant therapy by decreasing postoperative pain intensity, reducing opioid consumption, promoting return of gut function and reducing length of hospital stay, without significant systemic local anesthetic toxicity.[86] As a component of a multimodal analgesic regimen, the injection of liposomal bupivacaine into the surgical site is a new approach to extending the duration of postsurgical analgesia.[87]

Earlier Postoperative Recovery and Anesthetic Depth Monitoring

Earlier recovery of function after surgery requires prompt return of cognitive function to facilitate early oral intake and ambulation.[55] To this end, anesthetic plans should seek the return of normal cognitive function as soon as possible after surgery – including minimizing residual sedative effects of drugs used preoperatively, intraoperatively and postoperatively. This goal can be facilitated by avoiding long-acting sedatives, as recommended in the ERAS guidelines for colorectal surgery.[55] In many cases premedication is unnecessary, especially if anxiety can be mitigated by preoperative patient education and liberalizing preoperative oral fluids, including carbohydrates. For patients who require some degree of anxiolysis prior to general anesthesia, or to facilitate placement of a neuraxial block, a short-acting agent like midazolam, possibly in combination with fentanyl, is likely the best choice.

Concern has been raised that benzodiazepines are associated with an increased risk of postoperative cognitive dysfunction and delirium in the elderly.[88-90] Chronic benzodiazepine use, postoperative benzodiazepine use[91] and use of benzodiazepines for sedation in the intensive care unit[92,93] are associated with an increased risk of delirium. However, there are few data on whether the use of short-acting agents like midazolam in the immediate perioperative period (for anxiolysis or with regional anesthesia or monitored anesthesia care) increases the risk of postoperative delirium or cognitive dysfunction. Therefore, judicious use of short-acting benzodiazepines to alleviate anxiety or provide sedation seems justified.

While not a formal component of ERAS, the use of anesthetic depth monitoring can be considered a means to promote a fast-track approach to major surgery in the elderly patient – if its use can reduce the incidence of delayed emergence and postoperative delirium. While the efficacy of bispectral index (BIS) monitoring in reducing the risk of intraoperative awareness compared to end-tidal gas monitoring has not been demonstrated,[94,95] it may have a role in facilitating more rapid recovery from general anesthesia.[95] BIS monitoring thus may have a role in facilitating the goals of ERAS.[55] The use of BIS to guide intraoperative anesthetic dose has been reported to reduce total dose of anesthetic drugs and to decrease the time to awakening.[95-97] In addition, an association between low intraoperative BIS values and postoperative delirium has been reported, both in general anesthesia and in spinal anesthesia with sedation.[89,96,98] Additional research is needed before the routine use of BIS monitoring can be recommended, but its use may be prudent in those at highest risk for postoperative delirium.

Summary and Conclusions

The elderly are particularly at risk for postoperative morbidity and mortality, primarily due to the association of advanced age with greater co-morbidity and decreased physiologic reserve. Enhanced Recovery After Surgery (ERAS) programs hold the promise of decreasing complications and accelerating postoperative recovery by targeting reduction in the stress response to major surgery. However, implementation of these programs for major surgery remains inconsistent.[99] Key elements of this approach include multimodal analgesia, maintenance of preoperative homeostasis by avoiding dehydration and promoting an anabolic state with preoperative oral liquids and carbohydrate loading, optimizing fluid therapy and avoiding volume overload, and utilizing anesthetic techniques that permit a more rapid return to normal cognitive function. As pointed out by Henrik Kehlet, a seminal figure in the field, much work remains to be done to determine the optimal mix of interventions to achieve the goal of "pain- and risk-free operation."[99]

References

1. DeVol R, Bedroussian A. *An Unhealthy America: The Economic Burden of Chronic Disease*. Santa Monica, CA, Miliken Institute, 2007.

2. Bodenheimer T, Chen E, Bennett HD. Confronting the growing burden of chronic disease: can the U.S. health care workforce do the job? *Health Aff (Millwood)*. 2009; 28(1):64–74.

3. Thorpe KE, Howard DH, Galactionova K. Differences in disease prevalence as a source of the U.S.-European health care spending gap. *Health Aff (Millwood)*. 2007; 26(6):w678–w686.

4. Kinsella K, He W. *An Aging World: 2008, International Population Reports, P95/09-1*. Suitland, MD, US Census Bureau, 2009.

5. Administration on Aging. *A Profile of Older Americans: 2013*. Washington, DC, US Department of Health and Human Services, 2014.

6. Turrentine FE, Wang H, Simpson VB, Jones RS. Surgical risk factors, morbidity, and mortality in elderly patients. *J Am Coll Surg*. 2006; 203(6):865–877.

7. Story DA. Postoperative complications in elderly patients and their significance for long-term prognosis. *Curr Opin Anaesthesiol*. 2008; 21(3):375–379.

8. Story DA. Postoperative mortality and complications. *Best Pract Res Clin Anaesthesiol*. 2011; 25(3): 319–327.

9. Story DA, Leslie K, Myles PS, *et al.* Complications and mortality in older surgical patients in Australia and New Zealand (the REASON study): a multicentre, prospective, observational study. *Anaesthesia*. 2010; 65(10):1022–1030.

10. Kowdley GC, Merchant N, Richardson JP, *et al.* Cancer surgery in the elderly. *Sci World J*. 2012; 2012:9.

11. Al-Refaie WB, Parsons HM, Henderson WG, *et al.* Major cancer surgery in the elderly: results from the American College of Surgeons National Surgical Quality Improvement Program. *Ann Surg*. 2010; 251(2):311–318.

12. Kwok AC, Semel ME, Lipsitz SR, *et al.* The intensity and variation of surgical care at the end of life: a retrospective cohort study. *Lancet*. 2011; 378(9800):1408–1413.

13. Kehlet H, Wilmore DW. Multimodal strategies to improve surgical outcome. *Am J Surg*. 2002; 183(6):630–641.

14. Kehlet H, Wilmore DW. Evidence-based surgical care and the evolution of fast-track surgery. *Ann Surg*. 2008; 248(2):189–198.

15. Wilmore DW, Kehlet H. Management of patients in fast track surgery. *BMJ*. 2001; 322(7284):473–476.

16. Varadhan KK, Lobo DN, Ljungqvist O. Enhanced recovery after surgery: the future of improving surgical care. *Crit Care Clin*. 2010; 26(3):527–547, x.

17. Ljungqvist O. ERAS – Enhanced Recovery After Surgery: moving evidence-based perioperative care to practice. *JPEN J Parenter Enteral Nutr.* 2014; 38(5):559–566.

18. Segelman J, Nygren J. Evidence or eminence in abdominal surgery: recent improvements in perioperative care. *World J Gastroenterol.* 2014; 20(44):16615–16619.

19. Gustafsson UO, Scott MJ, Schwenk W, et al. Guidelines for perioperative care in elective colonic surgery: Enhanced Recovery After Surgery (ERAS(R)) Society recommendations. *Clin Nutr.* 2012; 31(6):783–800.

20. Fearon KC, Ljungqvist O, Von Meyenfeldt M, et al. Enhanced recovery after surgery: a consensus review of clinical care for patients undergoing colonic resection. *Clin Nutr.* 2005; 24(3):466–477.

21. Lassen K, Soop M, Nygren J, et al. Consensus review of optimal perioperative care in colorectal surgery: Enhanced Recovery After Surgery (ERAS) Group recommendations. *Arch Surg.* 2009; 144(10):961–969.

22. Gillissen F, Hoff C, Maessen JM, et al. Structured synchronous implementation of an enhanced recovery program in elective colonic surgery in 33 hospitals in The Netherlands. *World J Surg.* 2013; 37(5):1082–1093.

23. Miller TE, Thacker JK, White WD, et al. Reduced length of hospital stay in colorectal surgery after implementation of an enhanced recovery protocol. *Anesth Analg.* 2014; 118(5):1052–1061.

24. Findlay JM, Gillies RS, Millo J, et al. Enhanced recovery for esophagectomy: a systematic review and evidence-based guidelines. *Ann Surg.* 2014; 259(3):413–431.

25. Blom RL, van Heijl M, Bemelman WA, et al. Initial experiences of an enhanced recovery protocol in esophageal surgery. *World J Surg.* 2013; 37(10):2372–2378.

26. Lee J, Jeon H. The clinical indication and feasibility of the enhanced recovery protocol for curative gastric cancer surgery: analysis of 147 consecutive experiences. *Dig Surg.* 2014; 31(4-5):318–323.

27. Mortensen K, Nilsson M, Slim K, et al. Consensus guidelines for enhanced recovery after gastrectomy: Enhanced Recovery After Surgery (ERAS(R)) Society recommendations. *Br J Surg.* 2014; 101(10):1209–1229.

28. Lassen K, Coolsen MM, Slim K, et al. Guidelines for perioperative care for pancreaticoduodenectomy: Enhanced Recovery After Surgery (ERAS(R)) Society recommendations. *Clin Nutr.* 2012; 31(6):817–830.

29. Kagedan DJ, Ahmed M, Devitt KS, Wei AC. Enhanced recovery after pancreatic surgery: a systematic review of the evidence. *HPB (Oxford).* 2015; 17(1):11–16.

30. Page AJ, Ejaz A, Spolverato G et al. Enhanced recovery after surgery protocols for open hepatectomy–physiology, immunomodulation, and implementation. *J Gastrointest Surg.* 2015; 19(2):387–399.

31. Hughes MJ, McNally S, Wigmore SJ. Enhanced recovery following liver surgery:a systematic review and meta-analysis. *HPB (Oxford).* 2014; 16(8):699–706.

32. Nygren J, Thacker J, Carli F, et al. Guidelines for perioperative care in elective rectal/pelvic surgery: Enhanced Recovery After Surgery (ERAS(R)) Society recommendations. *Clin Nutr.* 2012; 31(6):801–816.

33. Cerantola Y, Valerio M, Persson B, et al. Guidelines for perioperative care after radical cystectomy for bladder cancer: Enhanced Recovery After Surgery (ERAS(R)) society recommendations. *Clin Nutr.* 2013; 32(6):879–887.

34. Mir MC, Zargar H, Bolton DM, Murphy DG, Lawrentschuk N. Enhanced Recovery After Surgery protocols for radical cystectomy surgery: review of current evidence and local protocols. *ANZ J Surg.* 2015; 85(7-8):514–520.

35. de Groot JJ, van Es LE, Maessen JM, et al. Diffusion of Enhanced Recovery principles in gynecologic oncology surgery: is active implementation still necessary? *Gynecol Oncol.* 2014; 134(3):570–575.

36. Nelson G, Kalogera E, Dowdy SC. Enhanced recovery pathways in gynecologic oncology. *Gynecol Oncol.* 2014; 135(3):586–594.

37. Hughes M, Coolsen MM, Aahlin EK, *et al.* Attitudes of patients and care providers to enhanced recovery after surgery programs after major abdominal surgery. *J Surg Res.* 2015; 193(1):102–110.

38. Bakker N, Cakir H, Doodeman HJ, Houdijk AP. Eight years of experience with Enhanced Recovery After Surgery in patients with colon cancer: impact of measures to improve adherence. *Surgery.* 2015; 157(6):1130–1136.

39. McLeod RS, Aarts MA, Chung F, *et al.* Development of an Enhanced Recovery After Surgery guideline and implementation strategy based on the knowledge-to-action cycle. *Ann Surg.* 2015; 262(6):1016–1025.

40. Stowers MD, Lemanu DP, Hill AG. Health economics in Enhanced Recovery After Surgery programs. *Can J Anaesth.* 2015; 62(2):219–230.

41. Bagnall NM, Malietzis G, Kennedy RH, *et al.* A systematic review of enhanced recovery care after colorectal surgery in elderly patients. *Colorectal Dis.* 2014; 16(12):947–956.

42. Scharfenberg M, Raue W, Junghans T, Schwenk W. "Fast-track" rehabilitation after colonic surgery in elderly patients – is it feasible? *Int J Colorectal Dis.* 2007; 22(12):1469–1474.

43. Wang Q, Suo J, Jiang J, *et al.* Effectiveness of fast-track rehabilitation vs conventional care in laparoscopic colorectal resection for elderly patients: a randomized trial. *Colorectal Dis.* 2012; 14(8):1009–1013.

44. Baek SJ, Kim SH, Kim SY, *et al.* The safety of a "fast-track" program after laparoscopic colorectal surgery is comparable in older patients as in younger patients. *Surg Endosc.* 2013; 27(4):1225–1232.

45. Jia Y, Jin G, Guo S, *et al.* Fast-track surgery decreases the incidence of postoperative delirium and other complications in elderly patients with colorectal carcinoma. *Langenbecks Arch Surg.* 2014; 399(1):77–84.

46. Carli F, Charlebois P, Stein B, *et al.* Randomized clinical trial of prehabilitation in colorectal surgery. *Br J Surg.* 2010; 97(8):1187–1197.

47. Li C, Carli F, Lee L, *et al.* Impact of a trimodal prehabilitation program on functional recovery after colorectal cancer surgery: a pilot study. *Surg Endosc.* 2013; 27(4):1072–1082.

48. Bouras AF. Hospital discharge of elderly patients after surgery: fast-track recovery versus the need for convalescence. *J Visc Surg.* 2014; 151(2):89–90.

49. Biffl WL, Biffl SE. Rehabilitation of the geriatric surgical patient: predicting needs and optimizing outcomes. *Surg Clin North Am.* 2015; 95(1):173–190.

50. Carli F, Brown R, Kennepohl S. Prehabilitation to enhance postoperative recovery for an octogenarian following robotic-assisted hysterectomy with endometrial cancer. *Can J Anaesth.* 2012; 59(8):779–784.

51. Cheema FN, Abraham NS, Berger DH, *et al.* Novel approaches to perioperative assessment and intervention may improve long-term outcomes after colorectal cancer resection in older adults. *Ann Surg.* 2011; 253(5):867–874.

52. Mayo NE, Feldman L, Scott S, *et al.* Impact of preoperative change in physical function on postoperative recovery: argument supporting prehabilitation for colorectal surgery. *Surgery.* 2011; 150(3): 505–514.

53. Gillis C, Li C, Lee L, *et al.* Prehabilitation versus rehabilitation: a randomized control trial in patients undergoing colorectal resection for cancer. *Anesthesiology.* 2014; 121(5):937–947.

54. Holte K, Nielsen KG, Madsen JL, Kehlet H. Physiologic effects of bowel preparation. *Dis Colon Rectum.* 2004; 47(8):1397–1402.

55. Gustafsson UO, Scott MJ, Schwenk W, *et al.* Guidelines for perioperative care in elective colonic surgery: Enhanced Recovery After Surgery (ERAS(R)) Society recommendations. *World J Surg.* 2013; 37(2):259–284.

56. Jung B, Lannerstad O, Pahlman L, *et al.* Preoperative mechanical preparation of the colon: the patient's experience. *BMC Surg.* 2007; 7:5.

57. Jung B, Pahlman L, Nystrom PO, Nilsson E; Mechanical Bowel Preparation Study G. Multicentre randomized clinical trial of mechanical bowel preparation in elective colonic resection. *Br J Surg.* 2007; 94(6):689–695.

58. Brady M, Kinn S, Stuart P. Preoperative fasting for adults to prevent perioperative complications. *Cochrane Database Syst Rev.* 2003(4):CD004423.

59. American Society of Anesthesiologists Committee. Practice guidelines for preoperative fasting and the use of pharmacologic agents to reduce the risk of pulmonary aspiration: application to healthy patients undergoing elective procedures: an updated report by the American Society of Anesthesiologists Committee on Standards and Practice Parameters. *Anesthesiology.* 2011; 114(3):495–511.

60. Nygren J. The metabolic effects of fasting and surgery. *Best Pract Res Clin Anaesthesiol.* 2006; 20(3):429–438.

61. Shoemaker WC, Appel PL, Kram HB. Tissue oxygen debt as a determinant of lethal and nonlethal postoperative organ failure. *Crit Care Med.* 1988; 16(11):1117–1120.

62. Holte K, Sharrock NE, Kehlet H. Pathophysiology and clinical implications of perioperative fluid excess. *Br J Anaesth.* 2002; 89(4):622–632.

63. Nicholau D. The postanesthesia care unit. In: Miller RD, ed., *Miller's Anesthesia, 7th edn.* Philadelphia, PA, Elsevier, 2010; 2708–2728.

64. Griffiths R, Beech F, Brown A, *et al.* Peri-operative care of the elderly 2014: Association of Anaesthetists of Great Britain and Ireland. *Anaesthesia.* 2014; 69 (Suppl 1):81–98.

65. Kaye AD, Riopelle JM. Intravascular fluid and electrolyte physiology. In: Miller RD, ed., *Miller's Anesthesia, 7th edn.* Philadelphia, PA, Elsevier, 2010; 1705–1735.

66. Brandstrup B, Tonnesen H, Beier-Holgersen R, *et al.* Effects of intravenous fluid restriction on postoperative complications: comparison of two perioperative fluid regimens: a randomized assessor-blinded multicenter trial. *Ann Surg.* 2003; 238(5):641–648.

67. Brandstrup B, Svendsen PE, Rasmussen M, *et al.* Which goal for fluid therapy during colorectal surgery is followed by the best outcome: near-maximal stroke volume or zero fluid balance? *Br J Anaesth.* 2012; 109(2):191–199.

68. Nisanevich V, Felsenstein I, Almogy G, *et al.* Effect of intraoperative fluid management on outcome after intraabdominal surgery. *Anesthesiology.* 2005; 103(1):25–32.

69. de Aguilar-Nascimento JE, Diniz BN, do Carmo AV, Silveira EA, Silva RM. Clinical benefits after the implementation of a protocol of restricted perioperative intravenous crystalloid fluids in major abdominal operations. *World J Surg.* 2009; 33(5):925–930.

70. Chappell D, Jacob M, Hofmann-Kiefer K, Conzen P, Rehm M. A rational approach to perioperative fluid management. *Anesthesiology.* 2008; 109(4):723–740.

71. Shoemaker WC. Oxygen consumption as an outcome predictor. *Intensive Care Med.* 1988; 15(1):64–66.

72. Shoemaker WC, Appel PL, Kram HB, Waxman K, Lee TS. Prospective trial of supranormal values of survivors as therapeutic goals in high-risk surgical patients. *Chest.* 1988; 94(6):1176–1186.

73. Grocott MP, Dushianthan A, Hamilton MA, *et al.* Perioperative increase in global blood flow to explicit defined goals and outcomes following surgery. *Cochrane Database Syst Rev.* 2012 (11):CD004082.

74. Corcoran T, Rhodes JE, Clarke S, Myles PS, Ho KM. Perioperative fluid management strategies in major surgery: a stratified meta-analysis. *Anesth Analg.* 2012; 114(3):640–651.

75. Fawcett WJ, Baldini G. Optimal analgesia during major open and laparoscopic abdominal surgery. *Anesthesiol Clin.* 2015; 33(1):65–78.

76. Vadivelu N, Mitra S, Narayan D. Recent advances in postoperative pain management. *Yale J Biol Med*. 2010; 83(1):11–25.

77. Gritsenko K, Khelemsky Y, Kaye AD, Vadivelu N, Urman RD. Multimodal therapy in perioperative analgesia. *Best Pract Res Clin Anaesthesiol*. 2014; 28(1):59–79.

78. Lovich-Sapola J, Smith CE, Brandt CP. Postoperative pain control. *Surg Clin North Am*. 2015; 95(2):301–318.

79. Buvanendran A, Kroin JS. Multimodal analgesia for controlling acute postoperative pain. *Curr Opin Anaesthesiol*. 2009; 22(5):588–593.

80. Tan M, Law LS, Gan TJ. Optimizing pain management to facilitate Enhanced Recovery After Surgery pathways. *Can J Anaesth*. 2015; 62(2):203–218.

81. White PF. Multimodal analgesia: its role in preventing postoperative pain. *Curr Opin Investig Drugs*. 2008; 9(1):76–82.

82. Joshi GP, Schug SA, Kehlet H. Procedure-specific pain management and outcome strategies. *Best Pract Res Clin Anaesthesiol*. 2014; 28(2):191–201.

83. Joshi GP, Kehlet H. Procedure-specific pain management: the road to improve postsurgical pain management? *Anesthesiology*. 2013; 118(4): 780–782.

84. Moraca RJ, Sheldon DG, Thirlby RC. The role of epidural anesthesia and analgesia in surgical practice. *Ann Surg*. 2003; 238(5):663–673.

85. Popping DM, Elia N, Van Aken HK, *et al*. Impact of epidural analgesia on mortality and morbidity after surgery: systematic review and meta-analysis of randomized controlled trials. *Ann Surg*. 2014; 259(6):1056–1067.

86. Sun Y, Li T, Wang N, Yun Y, Gan TJ. Perioperative systemic lidocaine for postoperative analgesia and recovery after abdominal surgery: a meta-analysis of randomized controlled trials. *Dis Colon Rectum*. 2012; 55(11): 1183–1194.

87. Golembiewski J, Dasta J. Evolving role of local anesthetics in managing postsurgical analgesia. *Clin Ther*. 2015; 37(6):1354–1371.

88. Trabold B, Metterlein T. Postoperative delirium: risk factors, prevention, and treatment. *J Cardiothorac Vasc Anesth*. 2014; 28(5):1352–1360.

89. Sieber FE, Zakriya KJ, Gottschalk A, *et al*. Sedation depth during spinal anesthesia and the development of postoperative delirium in elderly patients undergoing hip fracture repair. *Mayo Clin Proc*. 2010; 85(1):18–26.

90. Rasmussen LS, Steentoft A, Rasmussen H, Kristensen PA, Moller JT. Benzodiazepines and postoperative cognitive dysfunction in the elderly. ISPOCD Group. International Study of Postoperative Cognitive Dysfunction. *Br J Anaesth*. 1999; 83(4):585–589.

91. Marcantonio ER, Juarez G, Goldman L, *et al*. The relationship of postoperative delirium with psychoactive medications. *JAMA*. 1994; 272(19):1518–1522.

92. Pandharipande P, Shintani A, Peterson J, *et al*. Lorazepam is an independent risk factor for transitioning to delirium in intensive care unit patients. *Anesthesiology*. 2006; 104(1):21–26.

93. Pisani MA, Murphy TE, Araujo KL, *et al*. Benzodiazepine and opioid use and the duration of intensive care unit delirium in an older population. *Crit Care Med*. 2009; 37(1):177–183.

94. Avidan MS, Zhang L, Burnside BA, *et al*. Anesthesia awareness and the bispectral index. *N Engl J Med*. 2008; 358(11):1097–1108.

95. Punjasawadwong Y, Phongchiewboon A, Bunchungmongkol N. Bispectral index for improving anaesthetic delivery and postoperative recovery. *Cochrane Database Syst Rev*. 2014(6):CD003843.

96. Chan MT, Cheng BC, Lee TM, Gin T, Group CT. BIS-guided anesthesia decreases postoperative delirium and cognitive decline. *J Neurosurg Anesthesiol*. 2013; 25(1):33–42.

97. Wong J, Song D, Blanshard H, Grady D, Chung F. Titration of isoflurane using BIS index improves early recovery of elderly patients undergoing orthopedic surgeries. *Can J Anaesth*. 2002; 49(1):13–18.

98. Radtke FM, Franck M, Lendner J, *et al*. Monitoring depth of anaesthesia in a randomized trial decreases the rate of postoperative delirium but not postoperative cognitive dysfunction. *Br J Anaesth*. 2013; 110 (Suppl 1):i98–i105.

99. Kehlet H. Enhanced Recovery After Surgery (ERAS): good for now, but what about the future? *Can J Anaesth*. 2015; 62(2):99–104.

Chapter 15

Elective Orthopedic Surgery in the Geriatric Patient

Lisa Kunze and Elizabeth Fouts-Palmer

Key Points

- Geriatric patients account for a large proportion of orthopedic procedures; patients over 65 years old account for 30–36% of spine surgeries and 55–62% of joint arthroplasty procedures, while patients over 75 years old account for 9–14% of spine surgeries and 21–37% of joint arthroplasty procedures.
- The benefits demonstrated for neuraxial anesthesia, which are greater for elderly patients, include decreases in the incidence of surgical site infection, the need for blood transfusion, pulmonary complications and ICU admissions, shorter hospital stays and overall decreased short-term complications in patients.
- A multimodal, opioid-sparing approach to pain management may help reduce the incidence of chronic pain and complex regional pain syndrome (CRPS), as well as speeding recovery and limiting adverse side effects in the elderly population.
- Elderly patients have a greater risk of requiring transfusion; there is strong evidence that tranexamic acid administration in both total hip and total knee replacement procedures has shown significant reductions in blood loss and decreased transfusion requirements.
- The mechanism of bone implantation syndrome is complex, and likely due to embolic showering of marrow, bone and cement particles, which leads to acute pulmonary hypertension, right ventricular dysfunction and release of inflammatory cytokines. Management is largely supportive.
- The usual issues of positioning may be more challenging in the geriatric patient due to decreased range of movement in all joints, but specifically the neck, shoulders and hips, as well as increased fragility of the bones due to osteoporosis and osteopenia.

Introduction

Elective orthopedic surgical procedures, including total knee and hip arthroplasty, and spine surgery are among the most common surgical procedures in the United States, with over 5.6 million procedures done each year.[1] Patients over 65 years old account for 30–36% of spine surgeries and 55–62% of joint arthroplasty procedures, and those over 75 years old account for 9–14% of spine surgeries and 21–37% of joint arthroplasty procedures.[2] The number of these procedures is also predicted to escalate over the next 15 years. Primary and revision knee and hip arthroplasty is projected to increase 167–600% by 2030.[3] Today's anesthesiologist must optimize the perioperative management of these patients. Effective, efficient and evidence-based perioperative management of these patients is crucial in reducing complications and health care expenditures related to these procedures. This chapter discusses current strategies in anesthetic management, blood conservation, pain management and regional anesthesia for elective joint arthroplasty and spine surgery in the geriatric population.

Joint Replacement

Anesthetic Technique for Joint Replacement

There has been considerable controversy regarding the optimal anesthetic technique for hip and knee arthroplasty. Recently, several large, retrospective studies have demonstrated significant benefits of neuraxial anesthesia for joint replacement procedures.[4-7] The benefits demonstrated for neuraxial anesthesia include decreases in the incidence of surgical site infection, the need for blood transfusion, pulmonary complications and ICU admissions; shorter hospital stays and overall decreased short-term complications in patients. The benefits for neuraxial anesthesia were greater for patients in older age groups.[6] Patients with cardiopulmonary disease who are over 75 years old have a combined complication rate of 26% after total joint arthroplasty (TJA). This is compared to patients under 65 years old without cardiopulmonary disease who have a complication rate of 4.5%.[6] A recent comparison of general and spinal anesthesia in patients having total hip arthroplasty (THA) also noted that spinal anesthesia resulted in fewer unplanned, postoperative intubations, decreased risk of stroke, fewer cardiac arrests and decreased risk of blood transfusion.[7] There is no definitive data to support the use of neuraxial anesthesia to decrease the risk of perioperative delirium. However, a study including 220 patients over 70 years of age having TJA with spinal anesthesia and with opioid-sparing analgesia, followed patients for 12 days after surgery and found no cases of postoperative delirium.[8] It is not clear if it was the use of spinal anesthesia, opioid-sparing analgesia or the monitoring process that was responsible for these results.

The benefits of neuraxial anesthesia have been established predominantly based on retrospective data, which is more subject to bias than randomized controlled trials. However, taken in their entirety, the current evidence supports that neuraxial anesthesia confers significant medical benefits and decreases risks to patients undergoing elective total hip or knee arthroplasty.

Patients who are poor candidates for neuraxial anesthesia will require general anesthesia. Clear contraindications for neuraxial anesthesia include patients who have defects in blood coagulation and who have severe aortic stenosis or outflow tract obstruction. Patients who have had previous spinal reconstruction may be at increased risk of technical failure due to altered spinal anatomy. Spinal anesthesia may be acceptable in patients who have spinal cord stimulators after appropriate consultation and imaging,[9] but is contraindicated in patients with permanent indwelling epidural or intrathecal catheters. Relative contraindications to neuraxial anesthesia include psychological dysfunction that prohibits cooperation, severely altered anatomy of the spine and high surgical complexity. Additional consideration to type of anesthesia should be made in patients with BMI >40, known difficult airways or severe obstructive sleep apnea. These patients may be intolerant of sedation or have airways that are difficult to manage in the event that there is an intraoperative complication.

When general anesthesia is required, total intravenous anesthesia (TIVA) may be a good alternative to volatile anesthesia in the geriatric population. A small randomized, controlled trial in ASA I and II patients under 85 years old having TJA demonstrated that patients who had total intravenous anesthesia had less orthostatic hypotension and nausea than patients who had neuraxial anesthesia.[10] Patients had slightly reduced length of stay and less nausea with TIVA. In geriatric patients who require general anesthesia, it is critical to minimize the use of drugs that are known to cause delirium, to utilize opioid-sparing analgesia and to adhere to general principles for care of the geriatric patient, as described in other chapters of this book.

Multimodal Pain Management for Joint Replacement Surgery

The success of total joint replacement surgery is highly dependent on the ability of the patient to participate in physical therapy and rehabilitation during the immediate postoperative period. Factors that may preclude ability to participate in physical therapy include unstable hemodynamics, cognitive impairment, dizziness and inadequate analgesia. These factors may be directly related to management of anesthesia and analgesia. Therefore, a pain management plan that optimizes analgesia while minimizing adverse side effects is essential. Knee replacement surgery is also associated with the development of complex regional pain syndrome (CRPS)-like symptoms in up to 21% of patients 1 month postoperatively.[11] A multimodal, opioid-sparing approach to pain management may help reduce the incidence of chronic pain and CRPS, as well as speeding recovery and limiting adverse side effects in the elderly population.

Multimodal pain management strategies have been shown to be effective in shortening hospital stays, and improving pain control and range of movement after total knee replacements.[12] The key to pain management for these procedures appears to be combining regional pain management techniques with nonopiate pharmacologic strategies. Table 15.1 gives a brief summary of selected pharmacologic options.

Nonsteroidal anti-inflammatory agents (NSAIDs) are a mainstay for providing opioid-sparing analgesia plans. The detrimental effects on renal function, risk of cardiovascular

Table 15.1 Summary of selected pharmacologic options for multimodal pain management after total joint arthroplasty

	Dosing range	Comments
NSAIDs	Varies	Contraindicated in renal failure. Limited duration of use in THA. Relatively contraindicated in patients with cardiovascular disease
COX-2 inhibitors	Varies	Risk of myocardial infarction with long-term use
Gabapentin	50–300 mg (preop and TID days to weeks postop)	Reduce initial dose to limit sedation. Reduce dose in renal failure
Pregabalin	50–300 mg (preop and BID for days to weeks postop)	
Ketamine	Intraoperative bolus or infusion. Can continue infusion postop in patients with poor analgesia	Limited data regarding dosing in elderly patients
Acetaminophen	1000 mg TID–QID	Avoid in patients with cirrhosis or hepatic insufficiency

events, bleeding and bone fusion limit the use of these drugs for postoperative pain.[13,14] COX-2 inhibitors result in less platelet dysfunction, but have well-described cardiovascular risks with long-term use, and these drugs can affect bone healing.[13] Patients who are chronically anticoagulated or on potent antiplatelet agents may be at increased risk of bleeding if they are co-administered NSAIDS in the postoperative period. Surgeons often prohibit prolonged postoperative use of NSAIDS and COX-2 inhibitors in patients receiving a noncemented THA because these drugs may inhibit bone ingrowth into the prosthesis, which could lead to failure of the prosthesis.[14]

Gabapentin and pregabalin have been used in acute and chronic pain management, and can play a role in multimodal pain management after total joint replacement. Pregabalin has been shown to decrease the incidence of neuropathic pain after total knee arthroplasty (TKA),[15] as well as improving pain control after THR in combination with ketamine.[16] There is ongoing debate regarding the effectiveness of gabapentin after total joint arthroplasty. Several studies have shown decreased opiate use and improved function in the immediate postoperative period.[17,18] However, another study showed no change in opiate consumption.[19] These can be valuable drugs in a multimodal regimen, but given the risk for oversedation in elderly patients, pregabalin or gabapentin doses should start low and be given for as brief a course as possible.

Ketamine is also effective for pain management after total joint replacement. One randomized trial of a 0.5 mg/kg bolus followed by 2 mcg/kg/min infusion for 24 hours resulted in decreased opiate use and a decrease in chronic pain symptoms several months postoperatively.[20] Another randomized trial of a combination of ketamine and pregabalin also showed reduced opiate use, decreased pain with movement and decreased hyperalgesia,[16] emphasizing the importance of combining multiple agents into a multimodal regimen for maximal effects. Although the risk of hallucinations with ketamine might seem to be of concern in elderly patients at risk for delirium, there is some evidence that ketamine may actually decrease the incidence of postoperative delirium.[21] There are limited data available regarding the pharmacokinetics of ketamine in the elderly population so it is prudent to titrate doses cautiously.

Regional Techniques for Pain Management

Regional anesthesia techniques play an important role in multimodal analgesia following total joint replacement. Femoral nerve blocks have been used extensively for pain control after total knee replacement and provide excellent pain relief.[22] Both single-shot techniques and catheters have been used for analgesia.[23] The sensory innervation of the knee is complex and includes significant contributions from branches of the sciatic nerve as well. A sciatic or selective tibial nerve block may be considered for supplemental pain control, however the evidence demonstrates decreased pain only during the initial 3-12 hours after surgery.[24,25] The adductor canal block has also been used to decrease pain after TKA. This block provides good sensory blockade with a lower risk of motor blockade.[26] A recent randomized double-blinded controlled comparison of femoral and adductor canal blocks for analgesia for TKA showed significant improvement in quadriceps strength in patients receiving adductor canal blocks compared to those receiving femoral nerve blocks. The clinical significance remains unclear.[26]

The balance between providing adequate pain control using peripheral nerve blocks while avoiding excessive muscle weakness leading to falls or inadequate rehabilitation is a recurrent theme when considering peripheral nerve blocks for pain management after TKA. A large observational study failed to show any association between peripheral nerve blocks and inpatient falls after TKA.[27]

The use of peripheral nerve blocks for THA is not well established. A recent analysis reviewing the benefits of the use of lumbar plexus block, NSAIDS, intrathecal morphine and local anesthesia demonstrated that these techniques all provided some morphine-sparing effects, but there is no consensus as to which technique is superior.[28] Given the current knowledge, lumbar plexus blocks should be reserved for patients who have poor postoperative analgesia and intolerance to opioid and nonopioid therapies.

Many surgeons favor local infiltration of the wound in preference to peripheral nerve blocks. A recent review and meta-analysis concluded that local infiltration can be as effective for pain control as peripheral nerve blocks after TKA.[29,30] Unfortunately, results have been less promising for THA.[22,24] Use of liposomal bupivacaine, Exparel®, for peri-articular injection provided analgesia that was noninferior to the femoral nerve block.[31] A comparative study of Exparel® in TJA demonstrated significantly improved analgesia compared to periarticular injection of bupivacaine in both knee and hip arthroplasty, but there was high variability in VAS scores, depending on the surgeon.[32] Further research is required to fully elucidate the role of local anesthetics, including pain management for the arthroplasty patient.

Transfusion Practices in Total Joint Replacement

Historically, the transfusion rate for TJA patients was as high as 57%.[33] Transfusion with allogeneic blood increases the risk of respiratory or wound infection, which results in increased health care costs.[34] Patients who are older and have more co-morbidity have a greater risk of requiring transfusion.[35] Recent strategies for decreasing allogeneic transfusion include: (i) preoperative administration of erythropoietin, or intravenous iron, (ii) autologous donation, (iii) cell-salvage and (iv) administration of antifibrino-lytic agents.

Preoperative anemia occurs in approximately 20% of TJA patients. A recent review of erythropoietin use in patients with hemoglobin levels of 10–13 mg/dl demonstrated that it reduced the number of patients requiring transfusion, but was not cost effective.[36] Erythropoietin and intravenous iron therapy were found to be far less cost effective when compared to intraoperative tranexamic acid (TXA) or autologous donation.[37,38]

Intraoperative strategies for reducing allogeneic transfusion include cell-salvage, autologous donation and tranexamic acid. Use of spinal anesthesia may also reduce the need for transfusion, as described in the previous section. Cell-salvage has not demonstrated clear effectiveness in sparing transfusion in TJA.[36] In patients with hemoglobin levels greater than 13 mg/dl, cell-salvage did not decrease transfusion, but did increase cost. Cell-salvage is expensive in comparison to allogeneic transfusion,[39] so should be reserved for use in patients with anemia who are expected to have significant blood loss that will require transfusion. Cell-salvage may also be applicable in patients who refuse transfusion on a religious basis or who have a rare blood type.

Autologous donation is another useful technique for decreasing allogeneic transfu-sion in selected patients. Autologous blood transfusion is cost effective in patients with hemoglobin less than 12.5 mg/dl having TKA, but is not cost effective for use in all patients.[38,40] Autologous donation can increase the risk of transfusion, and is wasteful if the units go unused. Furthermore, patients who have baseline hemoglobin below 11 mg/dl are not candidates for autologous donation. The recommended strategy is for patients over 65 years old to donate one unit if their hemoglobin is 13-15 mg/dl and two units if their hemoglobin is 11–13 mg/dl. Patients under 65 years old should donate one unit if their hemoglobin in 11–13 mg/dl.[41] Unlike allogeneic transfusion, autologous transfusion does not increase the infection risk.[42] The clinician needs to consider cost, effectiveness, and risk of anemia and infection when choosing this blood conservation strategy.

Tranexamic acid administration is probably the safest, least expensive and easiest method for reducing transfusion of allogeneic blood in TJA. It is available in both oral and intravenous formulations and has also been used in topical applications.[43] Meta-analyses of randomized trials of TXA administration in both total hip and total knee replacement procedures have shown significant reductions in blood loss and decreased transfusion requirements.[44,45] Although it might seem counterintuitive to give antifibrinolytic agents during procedures known for their high risk of clotting complications, some evidence suggests that TXA administration may actually be associated with a lower risk of thromboembolic complications.[46] A variety of dosing regimens have been reported, with bolus doses ranging from 10–20 mg/kg, sometimes followed by redosing at 3–6 hour intervals or followed by an infusion for several hours after the initial dose. The standard practice at our institution is to give a 10 mg/kg bolus over 15 minutes prior to incision for most patients undergoing total hip or total knee arthroplasty. Contraindications to TXA administration include a history of thromboembolic events, the need for chronic anticoagulation and acquired color blindness.

In addition to individualized blood conservation planning, restrictive transfusion practices should be utilized. The current evidence does not support transfusion to patients with hemoglobin greater than 8 mg/dl.[47] Studies in elderly, hypertensive rats indicate that acute anemia causes perioperative cognitive dysfunction.[48] POCD is of great concern to patients and their families. Further research is required to elucidate the balance between the detrimental effects of anemia and the risks of transfusion, specifically in the geriatric patient.

Venous Thromboembolic Events in TJA

TJA patients are at high risk for postoperative thromboembolic events (VTEs). The American Academy of Orthopedic Surgeons has issued guidelines recommending prophylactic anticoagulation for all patients after total joint replacement.[49] Low-molecular-weight heparin is a commonly used agent, but there has been interest in the use of newer oral anticoagulants such as dabigatran and rivaroxaban for DVT prophylaxis after total joint arthroplasty.[50] Risks of bleeding and falls are increased with advancing age, so there is increasing support for use of aspirin for VTE prophylaxis in patients over 80 years old.[51] The use of neuraxial anesthesia and peripheral nerve catheters and injections should be coordinated with administration of VTE prophylaxis using the ASRA 2014 guidelines.[52]

Bone Cement Syndrome

Current practice in hip arthroplasty minimizes the use of cemented femoral components.[53] However, in patients with poor bone quality or with narrow femoral canals, cemented components are required. Unfortunately, these issues occur with greater frequency in older patients. When cement is applied to the intramedullary part of the bone it poses a risk of an intraoperative reaction, termed "bone cement implantation syndrome." This syndrome manifests as hypoxia, hypotension and altered mental status. The mechanism of this reaction is complex, and likely due to embolic showering of marrow, bone and cement particles, which leads to acute pulmonary hypertension, right ventricular dysfunction and release of inflammatory cytokines. Management of bone cement implantation syndrome is largely supportive. Patients with significant cardiopulmonary co-morbidities who develop bone cement implantation syndrome may benefit from advanced hemodynamic monitoring and postoperative ICU care.[54]

Spine Procedures

Spine procedures are among the top five common surgical procedures in patients between 65 and 80 years old. Disease processes of the spine that are commonly encountered include complications of osteoporosis, fractures resulting from falls, cervical myelopathy due to spondylosis and lumbar stenosis resulting from degeneration of intervertebral discs and facet joints.[55] US data from 2011 showed over 140,000 spine surgeries performed in adults age 65–74, and nearly 70,000 such procedures in patients over 75 years.[1,2] These numbers are expected to increase with the upward shift in the population age. Multiple co-morbidities can contribute to short- and long-term complication rates as high as 62% in patients having multilevel spinal deformity surgery.[56] The complication rate was 10-fold higher in patients over 70 years with hypertension alone. However, lumbar and cervical laminectomies provide good results without greatly increased complications in patients over 70 years old compared with more conservative measures such as nerve blocks or neurotomy.[57,58]

The geriatric spine patient will benefit from comprehensive, multidisciplinary perioperative evaluation and planning.[55] Appropriate preoperative optimization of medical issues is crucial. These patients may be on potent antiplatelet therapy and chronic anticoagulation, which will require input from cardiology or hematology in the perioperative period. Primary intraoperative challenges in spine reconstruction of the geriatric patient include positioning, pain management and blood conservation strategies. The usual issues of prone positioning may be more challenging in the geriatric patient due to decreased range of movement in all joints, but specifically the neck, shoulders and hips, as well as increased fragility of the bones due to osteoporosis and osteopenia. Great care needs to be taken to avoid skeletal injury and compression of the peripheral nerves. Pain management should follow a multimodal, opioid-sparing paradigm.[55,59] Blood management strategies elucidated for the TJA patients are also applicable to the spine patient. Neuro-monitoring is an anesthetic technique commonly requested by surgeons for certain spinal reconstruction procedures. This technique requires total intravenous anesthesia with avoidance of neuromuscular blockade. The hemodynamic effects of the propofol, dexmedetomidine, ketamine and remifentanil required to provide an immobile patient may be more pronounced in the geriatric patient, and sedation may be more enduring in the postoperative period. BIS monitoring is advocated to minimize the hemodynamic effects, but may not be as useful in the geriatric patient.[60] The effect of the total intravenous anesthesia required for neuro-monitoring on postoperative delirium is controversial.[61] Recent research comparing total intravenous anesthesia to inhaled anesthetic agents showed equivocal effects on delirium in the postoperative period.[62]

Minimally Invasive Spine Procedures

Elderly patients may present with spine pathology related to the process of aging. Spinal compression fractures are one of the most common complications of osteoporosis, and although they are often managed conservatively, these patients may require surgical treatment such as kyphoplasty or vertebroplasty to reduce pain and disability. Both procedures involve percutaneous insertion of filling cannulas into the vertebral bodies and injection of cement for stabilization. In kyphoplasty, the vertebral body is first reamed and expanded with a balloon to correct the deformity, whereas in vertebroplasty the cement is simply injected for stabilization. Performance of these procedures has been controversial since 2009 publications indicated that these procedures provided no reduction in pain, but ongoing research suggests that these procedures are cost effective compared to non-operative management of compression fractures.[63]

The anesthetic management of these percutaneous spine procedures can be challenging. The procedures are performed in the prone position, and monitored anesthesia care is often the preferred option, especially for vertebroplasty. Pain can often be well controlled with local anesthetics, including intraosseous lidocaine. Lower doses of sedatives may be required to provide adequate patient comfort. Procedures involving multiple levels and kyphoplasty procedures may be more painful and require general anesthesia.[64]

A rare but potentially severe complication of minimally invasive spine surgery is embolization of fat, air or bone marrow during reaming or injection of cement, similar to the bone cement implantation syndrome described above. This may present with right heart failure and circulatory collapse, and there have been reports of intraoperative death with multiple pulmonary emboli visualized on transesophageal echocardiogram.[65] There have also been reports of intravascular spread of cement, sometimes presenting years later.[66] Given the potential severity of these complications, it is imperative that the anesthesia provider ensure adequate monitoring, IV access and that resources for resuscitation are available, particularly when these procedures are performed in remote settings with a prone patient and an unsecured airway.

Summary

Today's anesthesiologist can expect to see rising numbers of elderly patients presenting for reconstructive orthopedic procedures, and it is imperative that the most effective, evidence-based approaches are utilized for the perioperative management of these patients. In the preceding sections, we have summarized current options for anesthetic management, postoperative pain control strategies, blood management and VTE prophylaxis in elderly patients undergoing joint arthroplasty and reconstructive spine procedures in the geriatric population. We encourage the reader to remain alert for new information on this fascinating and highly clinically relevant topic.

There is a paucity of data in the literature regarding the effects of aging on spinal somatosensory and motor-evoked potentials, and it remains unclear whether anesthetic techniques require modification to allow for adequate neuro-monitoring in geriatric patients.

References

1. Centers for Disease Control and Prevention *National Hospital Discharge Survey: 2010, with Special Feature on Death and Dying.* Hyattsville, MD, National Center for Health Statistics, 2011.

2. Centers for Disease Control and Prevention. Health research and quality: cost of hospital discharges with common hospital operating room procedures in nonfederal community hospitals, by age and selected principle procedure: United States 2000-2010. 2012. Available from: www.cdc.gov/hchs/hus/contents2012 .htm#115 (Accessed July 14, 2017).

3. Kurtz S, Ong K, Lau E, Mowat F, Halpern M. Projections of primary and revision hip and knee arthroplasty in the United States from 2005 to 2030. *J Bone Jt.* 2007; 89:780–785.

4. Pugely AJ, Martin CT, Gao Y, Mendoza-Lattes S, Callaghan JJ. Differences in short-term complications between spinal and general anesthesia for primary total knee arthroplasty. *J Bone Joint Surg Am.* 2013; 95:193–199.

5. Memtsoudis SG, Sun X, Chiu Y-L, *et al.* Perioperative comparative effectiveness of anesthetic technique in orthopedic patients. *Anesthesiology.* 2013; 118:1046–1058.

6. Memtsoudis SG, Rasul R, Suzuki S, *et al.* Does the impact of the type of anesthesia on outcomes differ by patient age and comorbidity burden? *Reg Anesth Pain Med.* 2014; 39:112–119.

7. Basques BA, Toy JO, Bohl DD, Golinvaus NS, Grauer JN. General compared with spinal anesthesia for total hip arthroplasty. *J Bone Joint Surg Am.* 2015; 97:455–461.

8. Krenk L, Rasmussen LS, Hansen TB, *et al.* Delirium after fast-track hip and knee arthroplasty. *Br J Anaesth.* 2012; 108:607–611.

9. Patel S, Das S, Stedman RB. Urgent cesarean section in a patient with a spinal cord stimulator: implications for surgery and anesthesia. *Ochsner J.* 2014; 14:131–134.

10. Harsten A, Kehlet H, Ljung P, Toksvig-Larsen S. Total intravenous anaesthesia vs. spinal anaesthesia for total hip arthroplasty: a randomized, controlled trial. *Acta Anaesth Scand.* 2015; 59:298–309.

11. Harden RN, Bruehl S, Stanos S, *et al.* Prospective examination of pain-related and psychological predictors of CRPS-like phenomena following total knee arthroplasty: a preliminary study. *Pain.* 2003; 106:393–400.

12. Hebl JR, Dilger JA, Byer DE, *et al.* A pre-emptive multimodal pathway featuring peripheral nerve block improves perioperative outcomes after major orthopedic surgery. *Reg Anesth Pain Med.* 2008; 33:510–517.

13. Kurmis AP, Kurmis TP, O'Brien JX, Dalen T. The effect of nonsteroidal anti-inflammatory drug administration on acute phase fracture-healing: a reivew. *J Bone Joint Surg Am.* 2012; 94:815–823.

14. Trelle S, Reichenbach S, Wandel S, *et al.* Cardiovascular safety of non-steroidal anti-inflammatory drugs: network meta-analysis. *BMJ.* 2011; 342:c7086.

15. Buvanendran A, Kroin JS, Della Valle CJ, *et al.* Perioperative oral pregabalin reduces chronic pain after total knee arthroplasty: a prospective, randomized, controlled trial. *Anesth Analg.* 2010; 110:199–207.

16. Martinez V, Cymerman A, Ben Ammar S, *et al.* The analgesic efficiency of combined pregabalin and ketamine for total hip arthroplasty: a randomised, double-blind, controlled study. *Anaesthesia.* 2014; 69:46–52.

17. Clarke H, Pereira S, Kennedy D, *et al.* Gabapentin decreases morphine consumption and improves functional recovery following total knee arthroplasty. *Pain Res Manag.* 2009; 14:217–222.

18. Clarke H, Katz J, McCartney C, *et al.* Perioperative gabapentin reduces 24 hour opioid consumption and improves in-hospital rehabilitation but not postdischarge outcomes after total knee arthroplasty with peripheral nerve block. *Br J Anaesth.* 2014; 113(5):855–864.

19. Paul J, Nantha-Aree M, Buckley N, *et al.* Gabapentin did not reduce morphine consumption, pain, opioid-related side

effects in total knee arthroplasty. *Can J Anaesth*. 2013; 60(5):423–431.

20. Remérand F, Le Tendre C, Baud A, *et al.* The early and delayed analgesic effects of ketamine after total hip arthroplasty: a prospective, randomized, controlled, double-blind study. *Anesth Analg*. 2009; 109:1963–1971.

21. Mu JL, Lee A, Joynt GM. Pharmacologic agents for the prevention and treatment of delirium in patients undergoing cardiac surgery. *Crit Care Med*. 2015; 43(1):194–204.

22. Chan EY, Fransen M, Parker DA, Assam PN, Chua N. Femoral nerve blocks for acute postoperative pain after knee replacement surgery. *Cochrane Database Syst Rev*. 2014(5):CD009941.

23. Machi AT, Sztain JF, Kormylo NJ *et al.* Discharge readiness after tricompartment knee arthroplasty: adductor canal versus femoral continuous nerve blocks-a dual-center randomized trial. *Anesthesiology*. 2015; 123:444–456.

24. Abdallah FW, Brull R. Is sciatic nerve block advantageous when combined with femoral nerve block for postoperative analgesia following total knee arthroplasty? A systematic review. *Reg Anesth Pain Med*. 2011; 36(5):493–498.

25. Nagafuchi M, Sato T, Sakuma T, *et al.* Femoral nerve block-sciatic nerve block vs. femoral nerve block-local infiltration analgesia for total knee arthroplasty: a randomized controlled trial. *BMC Anesthesiol*. 2015; 15:182–188.

26. Grevstad U, Mathiesen O, Valentiner LS, *et al.* Effect of adductor canal block versus femoral nerve block on quadriceps strength, mobilization, and pain after total knee arthroplasty. *Reg Anesth Pain Med*. 2015; 40(1):3–10.

27. Memtsoudis S, Danniger T, Rasul R, *et al.* Inpatient falls after total knee arthroplasty. *Anesthesiology*. 2014; 120:551–563.

28. Peder A, Karlsen H, Geisler A, *et al.* Postoperative pain treatment after total hip arthroplasty: a systematic review. *Pain*. 2015; 156:8–30.

29. Fan L, Zhu C, Zan P, *et al.* The comparison of local infiltration analgesia with peripheral nerve block following TKA: a systematic review with meta-analysis. *J Arthroplasty*. 2015; 30(9):1664–1671.

30. Andersen LØ, Kehlet H. Analgesic efficacy of local infiltration analgesia in hip and knee arthroplasty: a systematic review. *Br J Anaesth*. 2014; 113 (3):360–374.

31. Surdam JW, Licini DJ, Baynes NT, Arce BR. The use of Exparel (liposomal bupivacaine) to manage postoperative pain in unilateral total knee arthroplasty patients. *J Arthrop*. 2015; 30:325–329.

32. Barrington JW, Oluseun O, Lovald S, Liposomal bupivacaine: a comparative study of more than 1000 total joint arthroplasty cases. *Orthop Clin N Am*. 2015; 46:469–477.

33. Bierbaum BE, Callaghan JJ, Galante JO, *et al.* An analysis of blood management in patients having a total hip or knee arthroplasty. *J Bone Joint Surg*. 1999; 81-A:1–10.

34. Friedman R, Homering M, Holberg G, Berkowitz SD. Allogeneic blood transfusions and postoperative infections after total hip or knee arthroplasty. *J Bon Joint Surg Am*. 2014; 96:272–278.

35. Danninger T, Rasul R, Poeran J, *et al.* Blood transfusion in total hip and knee arthroplasty: an analysis of outcomes. *Sci World J*. 2014:1–10.

36. So-Osman C, Nelissen RG, Koopman-van Gemert AW, *et al.* Patient blood management in elective total hip and knee replacement surgery: Part 1. *Anesthesiology*. 2014; 120:839–851.

37. Phan DL, Ani F, Schwarzkopf R. Cost analysis of tranexamic acid in anemic total joint arthroplasty patients. *J Arthroplasty*. 2016; 31(3):579–582.

38. Green WS, Toy P, Bozic KJ. Cost minimization analysis of perioperative erythropoietin vs autologous and allogeneic blood donation in total joint arthroplasty. *J Arthoplasty*. 2010; 25:93–96.

39. So-Osman C, Nelissen RG, Koopman-van Gemert AW, *et al.* Patient blood

management in elective total hip and knee replacement surgery: Part 2. *Anesthesiology*. 2014; 120:852–860.

40. Kim S, Bou Monsef J, King EA, Sculco TP, Boettner F. Nonanemic patients do not benefit from autologous blood donation before total knee replacement. *HSSJ*. 2011; 7:141–144.

41. Bong MR, Patel V, Chang E, *et al.* Risks associated with blood transfusion after total knee arthroplasty. *J Arthroplasty*. 2014; 19:281–287.

42. Friedman R, Homering M, Holberg G, Berkowitz SD. Allogeneic blood transfusions and postoperative infections after total hip or knee arthroplasty. *J Bone Joint Surg Am*. 2014; 96:272–278.

43. Gilbody J, Dhotar HS, Perruccio AV, Davey JR. Topical tranexamic acid reduces transfusion rates in total hip and knee arthroplasty. *J Arthoplasty*. 2014; 29:681–684.

44. Alshryda S, Sarda P, Sukeik M, *et al.* Tranexamic acid in total knee replacement: a systematic review and meta-analysis. *J Bone Joint Surg Br*. 2011; 93(12):1577–1585.

45. Oremus K, Sostaric S, Trkulja V, Haspl M. Influence of tranexamic acid on postoperative autologous blood retransfusion in primary total knee and hip arthroplasty: a randomized, controlled trial. *Transfusion*. 2014; 54:31–41.

46. Poeran J, Rasul R, Suzuki S, *et al.* Tranexamic acid use and postoperative outcomes in patients undergoing total hip or knee arthroplasty in the United States: retrospective analysis of effectiveness and safety. *BMJ*. 2014; 349:g4829.

47. Ponnusamy KE, Kim TJ, Khanjua HS. Perioperative blood transfusions in orthopaedic surgery. *J Bone Joint Surg Am* 2014; 96:1836–1844.

48. Li M, Bertout JA, Ratcliff SJ, *et al.* Acute anemia elicits cognitive dysfunction and evidence of cerebral cellular hypoxia in older rats with systemic hypertension. *Anesthesiology*. 2010; 113:845–858.

49. Jacobs JJ, Mont MA, Bozic KJ, *et al.* American Academy of Orthopaedic

Surgeons clinical practice guideline on preventing venous thromboembolic disease in patients undergoing elective hip and knee arthroplasty. *J Bone Jt Surg*. 2012; 94:746–747.

50. Galanis T, Merli GJ. New oral anticoagulants: prevention of VTE in phase III studies in total joint replacement surgery and the hospitalized medically-ill patients. *J Thromb Thrombol*. 2013; 36(2):141–148.

51. Raphael IJ, Tischler EH, Huang R, *et al.* Aspirin: an alternative for pulmonary embolism prophylaxis after arthroplasty? *Clin Orthop Relat Res*. 2014; 472:482–488.

52. Horlocker TT, Wedel DJ, Rowlingson JC, *et al.* Regional anesthesia in the patient receiving antithrombotic or thrombolytic therapy: American Society of Regional Anesthesia and Pain Medicine evidence-based guidelines (third edition). *Reg Anesth Pain Med*; 35:64–101.

53. Khanuja HS, Vakil JJ, Goddard MS, Mont MA. Cementless femoral fixation in total hip arthroplasty. *J Bone Joint Surg Am*. 2011; 93:500–509.

54. Donaldson A, Thomson H, Harper N, Kenny N. Bone cement implantation syndrome. *Br J Anaesth*. 2009; 102(1):12–22.

55. Brallier JW, Diener S. The elderly spine surgery patient: pre- and intraoperative management of drug therapy. *Drugs Aging*. 2015; 32:601–609.

56. Acosta FL, McClendon J, O'Shaughnessy BA, *et al.* Morbidity and mortality after spinal deformity surgery in patients 75 years and older: complication and predictive factors. *J Neurosurg Spine*. 2011; 15:667–674.

57. O'Lynnger TM, Zuckerman SL, Morone PJ, Vasquez Castellonos RA, Cheng JS. Trends for spine surgery for the elderly: implication for access to healthcare in North America. *Neurosurgery*. 2015; 77:S136–S141.

58. McGirt MJ, Parker SL, Hilibrand A, *et al.* Lumbar surgery in the elderly provides significant health benefits in the US health care system: patient-reported outcomes in

4370 patients from the N2QOD registry. *Neurosurgery*. 2015; 77:S125–S135.

59. Puvanesarajah V, Liauw JA, Lina IA, *et al.* Analgesic therapy for major spine surgery. *Neruosurg Rev*. 2015; 38: 407–419.

60. Chan MT. BIS-guided anesthesia decreases postoperative delirium and cognitive decline. *J Neurosurg Anesthesiol*. 2013; 25:33–42.

61. Radke F. Monitoring depth of anesthesia decreases the rate of postoperative delirium but not postoperative cognitive dysfunction. *Br J Anaesth*. 2013; 110(Suppl 1):i98–i105.

62. Deiner S, Lin HM, Bodansky D, Silverstein J, Sano M. Do stress markers and anesthetic technique predict delirium in the elderly? *Dement Geriatr Cogn Disord*. 2014; 38:366–374.

63. Goldstein CL, Chutkan NB, Choma TJ, Orr RD. Management of the elderly with vertebral compression fractures. *Neurosurgery* 2015; 77:S33–S45.

64. Luginbühl M. Percutaneous vertebroplasty, kyphoplasty and lordoplasty: implications for the anesthesiologist. *Curr Opin Anaesthesiol*. 2008; 21:504–513.

65. Chen H-L, Wong C-S, Ho S-T, *et al.* A lethal pulmonary embolism during percutaneous vertebroplasty. *Anesth Analg*. 2002; 95(4):1060–1062.

66. Lim KJ, Yoon SZ, Jeon YS, *et al.* An intraatrial thrombus and pulmonary thromboembolism as a late complication of percutaneous vertebroplasty. *Anesth Analg*. 2007; 104(4):924–926.

Chapter 16

Regional and Neuraxial Anesthesia in the Geriatric Population

Shachi C. Patel and Anasuya Vasudevan

Key Points

- In the elderly a sympathectomy from neuraxial technique causes an exaggerated drop in blood pressure with poor ability to adjust stroke volume due to ventricular stiffening.
- Elderly patients are more sensitive to effects of local anesthetics due to age-related changes such as increased volume of distribution, decreased plasma proteins and unpredictable duration of local anesthetic effects.
- Old age is an independent risk factor for developing positioning-related nerve injuries.
- There has not been shown to be a demonstrable difference between regional anesthesia and general anesthesia with regards to cardiovascular outcomes.
- There is convincing evidence to support the use of neuraxial anesthesia in thoracic surgery to reduce the incidence of pulmonary complications.
- When compared with systemic opioid analgesia after general anesthesia, the use of thoracic epidural analgesia with a local anesthetic-based regimen is associated with significantly earlier return of gastrointestinal function after abdominal surgery.

Introduction

According to the CDC data for the United States, the fastest growing population includes the elderly aged 65 and older, comprising approximately 43 million people in the United States. By 2050 that number is expected to double and reach 89 million.[1] Furthermore, this population comprises 13 million hospital admissions.[1] With this steadily rising elderly population, the number of geriatric patients presenting for anesthetic care during surgery is growing. Though there has been no evidence of decreased morbidity or mortality with regional anesthesia, with the advent of new regional techniques, anesthesia providers and surgeons appear to favor regional anesthesia techniques in elderly patients presenting for surgical care. In this chapter we discuss age-related physiologic changes, the risks and benefits of regional versus general anesthetic technique, as well as important considerations for age-related changes in anatomy, pharmacodynamics, pharmacokinetics and local anesthetic metabolism pertaining to regional and neuraxial techniques.

Effect of Geriatric Physiology on Regional Anesthesia

Cardiovascular Changes

The aging heart has significant hemodynamic consequences on regional and neuraxial anesthesia (Table 16.1).

Systemic Vascular Resistance

Age-related vascular changes are the most systemic changes observed in the elderly. The Framingham Heart Study presented the effects of aging on vascular changes. Of note, there was nearly linear increase in systolic blood pressure from age 30 to 84 years.[2] In particular, elderly patients have been shown to have a 50–75% increase in arterial stiffness and a 25% increase in systemic vascular resistance.[2]

Cardiac Function

The aging heart alters cardiac responsiveness to β-adrenergic stimuli, thus catecholamine or exercise-induced increases in contractility and heart rate are blunted in elderly patients.[3,4] Significant deposition of collagen and fatty infiltration into the conduction fibers of an aging heart promotes arrhythmias and conduction abnormalities.[4]

The elderly heart undergoes ventricular hypertrophy propagated by age-related vascular stiffening, limiting the heart's ability to adjust its stroke volume, as well as impairing passive early diastolic filling, despite preservation of its systolic function.[4] Due to these functional limitations, the aging heart can compensate for high metabolic demands by increasing preload volume, indirectly increasing stroke volume and therefore cardiac output.[3]

Effect of Neuraxial Anesthesia on the Cardiovascular System

Clinically, these changes have dramatic consequences when elderly patients undergo regional and neuraxial techniques as part of their anesthetic care. For example, the decreased elasticity of myocardial and vascular structures promote left ventricular hypertrophy and hypertension in elderly patients. Thus, in the elderly a sympathectomy from neuraxial technique causes an exaggerated drop in blood pressure with poor ability to adjust stroke volume due to ventricular stiffening. In addition, age-related fibrosis of the cardiac conduction system makes elderly patients more prone to arrhythmias, especially when attempting to use medications such as ephedrine to help resuscitate hypotension after sympathectomy or with accidental vascular injection of epinephrine with regional techniques. Lastly, a decreased catecholamine response to peripheral β-adrenergic receptors causes elderly patients to have a poor ability to respond to hypovolemia and hypotension by increasing heart rate. As described above, they are therefore preload dependent to maintain stroke volume. Additionally, providing a large rapid volume of fluid to compensate makes them prone to pulmonary edema, unlike young patients who benefit from fluid boluses prior to neuraxial placement.

Pulmonary Changes

Age-related pulmonary changes can cause significant respiratory effects with regional and neuraxial anesthesia.

The thoracic cavity of the elderly, like the myocardium, becomes stiffer, causing changes in lung compliance and mechanics. As we age, the chest wall compliance decreases due

Table 16.1 Cardiovascular physiologic changes impacting regional and neuraxial anesthesia

Physiologic changes	Clinical consequences
• Decreased elasticity of myocardial and vascular structures • Fibrosis of conduction system • Decreased catecholamine response	• Left ventricular hypertrophy and hypertension • Sympathectomy from neuraxial technique causes exaggerated drop in blood pressure • Stiff left ventricle with poor ability to adjust stroke volume • More prone to arrhythmias • Poor ability to respond to hypovolemia and hypotension by increasing heart rate • Preload dependent to maintain metabolic need for higher stroke volume • Large and rapid volume of fluid places elderly patients at risk for pulmonary edema

to thoracic wall stiffening, causing increased work of breathing and reduced maximal minute ventilation.[5] Additionally, aging structural changes in the lung parenchyma cause a gradual reduction in lung elastic recoil, causing an increase in closing capacity.[5] This closing capacity will exceed the functional residual capacity by age 65, promoting atelectasis.[4] In the supine position, closing capacity may reach functional residual capacity (FRC) by 44 years of age.[4] Furthermore, the decreases in chest wall compliance with a reduction of inward elastic lung recoil cause age-related changes to pulmonary mechanics. Particularly, residual volume and functional residual capacity both increase with age – 5–10% and 1–3% per decade, respectively – whereas the forced expiratory volume in 1 second is reduced approximately 6–8% per decade.[4]

Effect of Pulmonary Changes on Regional Anesthesia

The physiological changes of the aging lung have important consequences when elderly patients undergo regional and neuraxial techniques as part of their anesthetic care. Lung compliance is decreased, and closing capacity surpasses functional residual capacity making patients prone to atelectasis and poor oxygenation. In the perioperative period, regional techniques confer the benefit of less pain-limited inspiration, especially for thoracic and abdominal procedures, preventing less hypoxic events. However, with the use of neuraxial techniques, particularly in the thoracic region, there is a risk of blocking the use of accessory respiratory muscles making patients feel weak and short of breath. Furthermore, if blockade is high enough it can cause a "high spinal," risking the need for general anesthesia (Table 16.2).

Neurologic Changes

The aging of the central and peripheral nervous system has significant neurophysiologic consequences with regional and neuraxial anesthesia. The elderly brain experiences a loss of cortical gray matter as it ages, causing age-related cerebral atrophy.[6] This loss of cortical gray matter in the central nervous system is due more to loss of neural volume, as opposed to overall neural loss.[4,6] Cerebral autoregulation involving cerebral metabolic rate and blood flow remain intact.[4] Furthermore, in addition to the age-related loss of neural density, there are also biochemical changes, including decreased concentration of neurotransmitters.[6] Of note, the spinal cord of the elderly is also associated with neuronal loss, causing age-related demyelization and shrinkage of nerve fibers attributing to

Table 16.2 Pulmonary physiologic changes impacting regional and neuraxial anesthesia

Physiologic changes	Clinical consequences
• Decreased chest wall compliance • Increased residual volume and functional residual capacity • FEV, reduced • Closing capacity increased greater than functional residual capacity	• Increased work of breathing and reduced maximal minute ventilation • Prone to atelectasis and poor oxygenation • Regional techniques confer the benefit of less pain-limited inspiration • Risk of high spinal requiring general anesthesia with use of thoracic epidurals

spinal cord atrophy.[6] In addition, the anatomy of the spinal canal changes with aging, as it becomes narrower due to age-related osteoporotic changes to the bony spine.

Effect of Neurological Changes on Regional Anesthesia

Clinically, these changes have important consequences when elderly patients undergo regional and neuraxial techniques as part of their anesthetic care. The anatomical narrowing of the spinal canal promotes increased cephalad spread of subarachnoid and epidural local anesthetics and opioids. The decreased central nervous system neuron density, as well as decreased concentration of central neurotransmitters permits a decreased minimum alveolar concentration (MAC) of anesthetic due to increased sensitivity to anesthetics. Furthermore, increased demyelination of neurons promotes neuropathy and decreased conduction velocity, which leads to increased risk of falls, longer duration of regional blocks and the need for lower concentration of drugs due to the increased sensitivity to local anesthetics in the elderly population (Table 16.3).

Effect of Age-Related Pharmacologic Changes on Regional Anesthesia

Age-related changes to the liver and renal system cause significant pharmacodynamics and pharmacokinetic consequences on regional and neuraxial anesthesia. With an aging kidney, elderly patients are prone to renal insufficiency. There is a progressive decline in renal blood flow and loss of renal parenchyma.[4] In patients 80 years and older, nephrons become sclerotic, reducing the functional capacity of the already reduced nephron number.[4] As a consequence, these age-related processes result in a progressive decline in glomerular filtration rate.[4] In addition to the changes in the kidney's filtration function, there are also age-related changes in the kidney's ability to maintain fluid homeostasis. This is complicated by alterations in thirst mechanisms and ADH release that frequently result in dehydration.[4] As a result, the elderly kidney is prone to the deleterious effects of low cardiac output, hypotension, hypovolemia and hemorrhage. Clinically, the use of anesthetics, surgical stress, pain, sympathetic stimulation and renal vasoconstrictive drugs may all compound subclinical renal insufficiency.[4]

Effect of Hepatic and Renal Changes on Regional Anesthesia

Hepatic changes in the elderly impact the dosing and metabolism of many anesthetic drugs used perioperatively. Of note, there is a decrease in plasma proteins and albumin from chronic illness and poor nutrition causing systemic changes in hepatic drug

Table 16.3 Neurologic physiologic changes impacting regional and neuraxial anesthesia

Physiologic changes	Clinical consequences
• Narrowing of central spinal canal • Decreased neuron density and concentration of neurotransmitters • Increased demyelination of neurons promoting neuropathy and decreased conduction velocity	• Increased cephalad spread of subarachnoid and epidural LA/opioids • Decreased MAC • Increased risk of falls, longer regional block and the need for lower concentration of drugs due to increased sensitivity

metabolism.[4] The age-related changes in plasma proteins can cause decreased drug protein binding and increased free drug fraction.[4] Clinically, these age-related changes have a potential to increase the pharmacologic effect of drugs used perioperatively.[4] With aging there is decrease in lean body mass and total body water, and an increased proportion of body fat.[4] As a consequence, there is systemic alterations in the volume of distribution and redistribution of drugs, which ultimately alter the rates of clearance and elimination of many drugs.[4] Ultimately, alterations in cardiac output, renal, or hepatic clearance may change drug plasma concentrations and their duration of action.

Due to these extensive age-related renal and hepatic changes, there is an impact on absorption, distribution and clearance of local anesthetic metabolism in the elderly undergoing regional and neuraxial techniques. Elderly patients are more sensitive to effects of local anesthetics due to these age-related changes. As mentioned previously, there is age-related loss of neural density and decreased concentration of neurotransmitters, which provide increased sensitivity to epidural and spinal absorption of local anesthetics.[7] These anatomical changes at the level of neurons in the spinal cord as well as anatomical changes in the spinal canal predispose elderly patients to a higher level of sensory blockade following both spinal and epidural anesthesia. Furthermore, the age-related changes in lean body mass, total body water and total body fat increase the volume of distribution of local anesthetics. Consequently, elderly patients have varied peak drug concentrations after local anesthetic boluses and infusions, as well as varied duration of local anesthetic effects.[7] Furthermore, increased half-life of local anesthetics and decreased clearance of local anesthetics with age promote a prolonged blockade.[7] According to Tsui et al., caution should be taken when administering repeated doses or continuous infusions of local anesthetics because the clearance of local anesthetics is reduced in elderly patients.[7] Clinically, this translates to small doses, increased sensitivity, prolonged blockade and less frequent redosing when using local anesthetics in the elderly.

Physiological Changes in the Musculoskeletal System in the Elderly

With aging, the incidence of arthritis, degenerative joint disease (DJD) and reduction in mobility becomes inevitable. Advancement in DJD gradually leads to significant restrictions and limitations in range of motion. Elderly patients may have reduced range of motion in the cervical spine, reduced flexibility of the spine, kyphoscoliotic changes and reduction in the range of motion of the major joints. Arthritic changes to the vertebral column may cause significant disc degeneration, loss of height of vertebral bodies, calcification of the spinal ligaments and narrowing of intervertebral spaces.

Impact of Musculoskeletal Changes on Regional Anesthesia

The calcification and limitations in range of movements can offer considerable challenges with neuraxial anesthesia. The narrowing and calcification of intervertebral spaces can be severe enough that the neuraxial procedure may need to be abandoned. Elderly patients with spinal stenosis and history of receiving anticoagulation therapy are at increased risk of developing epidural hematomas. Old age is an independent risk factor for developing positioning-related nerve injuries. Limitations with cervical spine range of motion can be challenging for managing the airway. Similarly reduced range of motion of other joints can reduce the success of peripheral nerve blocks. Even under ultrasound guidance, positioning the probe and acquiring satisfactory windows to perform nerve blocks may be challenging.

Risk Versus Benefit of Regional Anesthesia Versus General Anesthesia in the Geriatric Population

There is debate on whether regional and neuraxial anesthesia or general anesthesia provide better surgical outcomes in the geriatric population. In this section, we create an outline of organ-based outcome measurements seen in regional and neuraxial techniques versus general anesthesia to outline the controversy surrounding this topic in the elderly population

Many anesthesiologists prefer regional anesthesia in the elderly because theoretically it can provide a stable cardiovascular profile and superior pain relief with avoidance of large quantities of opioids. This confers the advantages of reducing postoperative respiratory complications by avoiding general anesthesia, as well as medications causing respiratory depression. However, literature on this subject has shown no overall difference in outcome and mortality between regional and general anesthesia in the elderly.[8]

Cardiovascular System

Numerous studies have been conducted to evaluate for improved hemodynamic outcomes in regional versus general anesthesia following surgery in the elderly population. O'Hara et al. conducted a retrospective cohort study in hip fracture patients undergoing surgical repair to evaluate the effect of type of anesthesia on postoperative morbidity and mortality. The primary outcome was defined as death within 30 days of the operation and secondary cardiac outcome included postoperative myocardial infarction, postoperative congestive heart failure and 7-day mortality after anesthesia.[9] Like many similar studies, there was no demonstrable evidence that regional anesthesia was associated with better cardiovascular outcomes over general anesthesia in elderly patients. However, when deciding on an anesthetic plan in the clinical setting, it is important to consider that regional anesthesia techniques offer minimal sedation, a pain-free anesthetic approach and may be cost effective by minimizing drug-related complications and side effects.

Respiratory System

Respiratory outcomes have been measured in patients undergoing regional versus general anesthesia following surgery in the elderly population. The pulmonary system is one of the few organ systems that has convincing data on the overall benefits of neuraxial anesthesia over general anesthesia. Elderly patients undergoing abdominal and thoracic surgery under general anesthesia are prone to respiratory morbidity due to associated use of systemic opioids for postoperative pain control, in conjunction with atelectasis, and attenuation of respiratory effort due to pain, or splinting. Ballantyne *et al.* performed a meta-analysis of randomized controlled trials and found a decrease in the incidence of atelectasis in postoperative patients receiving epidural opioids versus systemic opioids for postoperative pain control.[10] Furthermore, compared with systemic opioids, postoperative epidural analgesia with local anesthetics significantly decreased the incidence of pulmonary morbidity.[10,11] Of note, compared with systemic opioids, epidural opioids decreased the incidence of atelectasis, but did not significantly diminish the incidence of pulmonary complications.[10,11] It is therefore important to consider use of neuraxial techniques in elderly patients as they exhibit a better respiratory profile due to protection from pain-related respiratory compromise and postsurgical atelectasis that can prevent postoperative hypoxemic events.

Neurological and Cognitive Recovery Profiles

It is perceived by many that the incidence of long-term postoperative cognitive decline would be far less in patients undergoing regional or neuraxial anesthesia in comparison to elderly patients undergoing general anesthesia. This is particularly because regional and neuraxial anesthesia can be done with minimal sedation and potentially prevents postoperative delirium due to superior analgesia from these techniques. However, Wu *et al.* have demonstrated that there is no difference found in long-term postoperative cognitive decline or dysfunction between general anesthesia and neuraxial techniques.[12] They reviewed 24 trials of patients 60 and older who underwent a wide range of neuropsychometric tests to evaluate cognitive function. All but 1 of the 24 trials did not demonstrate a benefit from neuraxial anesthesia in decreasing the incidence of postoperative cognitive dysfunction.[12]

Coagulation Systems

General anesthesia is associated with a hypercoagulable state. Wu *et al.* suggest that the possible mechanisms include potentiation by the surgical stress response, endothelial damage with tissue factor activation and synergism with inflammation.[11] Several studies have shown that the use of regional anesthesia is associated with a significant decrease in procoagulation-related events in orthopedic and vascular surgery patients, in whom hypercoagulation can be problematic. Of note, numerous randomized trials have shown that regional anesthesia decreases the incidence of DVT after orthopedic surgeries.[13–15]

Gastrointestinal System

It is well known that abdominal surgery is associated with increased incidence of postoperative ileus, causing delayed gastric function and prolonged hospitalization. Wu *et al.* suggest that the causes of increased incidence of postoperative gastrointestinal dysfunction include an increased sympathetic efferent outflow from pain or stress response, postoperative use of opioids for analgesia and spinal reflex inhibition of gastrointestinal motility.[11] Furthermore, use of perioperative opioids is associated with slowing of the gastrointestinal tract. When compared with systemic opioid analgesia after general anesthesia, the use of thoracic epidural analgesia with a local anesthetic-based regimen is associated with significantly earlier return of gastrointestinal function after abdominal surgery.[12] It is important to note while there is evidence that epidural local anesthetic is associated with earlier return of gastrointestinal motility after abdominal surgery, there are unclear data on whether neuraxial opioids confer a benefit in earlier return of GI function compared to systemic opioids.

Conclusion

Appropriate selection of elderly patients for neuraxial and regional anesthesia offers at least short-term benefits. Evidence to date suggests regional anesthesia provides better perioperative analgesia, reduced perioperative opioid requirement and a reduction in pulmonary and embolic complications. Some elderly patients, especially those with unstable cardiac disease, may benefit from general anesthesia as the hemodynamic changes can be better controlled. Even in this high-risk population, regional anesthesia should be considered as an adjunct to general anesthesia. When there are no contraindications to regional anesthesia, the benefits from regional anesthesia make it a desirable choice in this patient population.

References

1. Gill J, Moore M. The state of aging and health in America 2013. 2013. www.cdc.gov/aging/pdf/state-aging-health-in-america-2013.pdf (Accessed July 17, 2017).

2. Franklin SS, Gustin W IV, Wong ND, et al. Hemodynamic patterns of age-related changes in blood pressure: the Framingham Heart Study. *Circulation*. 1997; 96(1):308–315.

3. Ferarri A, Radaelli A, Centola M. Invited review: aging and the cardiovascular system. *Circulation*. 2003; 95(6):2591–2597.

4. Cook D, Rooke A. Priorities in perioperative geriatrics. *Anesth Analg*. 2003; 95(6):2591–2597.

5. Sprung J, Gajic O, Warner D. Review article: age-related alterations in respiratory function – anesthetic considerations. *Anesth Analg*. 2006; 95(6):2591–2597.

6. Sieber FE. Changes which occur in the central nervous system with aging. In: *Geriatric Anesthesia*. New York, McGraw-Hill, Medical Pub. Division, 2015.

7. Tsui BC, Wagner A, Finucane B. Regional anaesthesia in the elderly. *Drugs Aging*. 2004; 21(14):895–910.

8. Roy RC. Choosing general versus regional anesthesia for the elderly. *Anesthesiol Clin North Am*. 2000; 18(1):91–104.

9. O'Hara DA, Duff A, Berlin JA, et al. The effect of anesthetic technique on postoperative outcomes in hip fracture repair. *Anesthesiology*. 2000; 92(4):947–957.

10. Ballantyne JC, Carr DB, deFerranti S, et al. The comparative effects of postoperative analgesic therapies on pulmonary outcome: cumulative meta-analyses of randomized, controlled trials. *Anesth Analg*. 1998; 86:598–612.

11. Wu CL, Fleisher LA. Outcomes research in regional anesthesia and analgesia. *Anesth Analg*. 2000; 91:1232–1242.

12. Wu CL, Hsu W, Richman JM, Raja SN. Postoperative cognitive function as an outcome of regional anesthesia and analgesia. *Reg Anesth Pain Med*. 2004; 29(3):257–268.

13. Modig J, Borg T, Karlstrom G, et al. Thromboembolism after total hip replacement: role of epidural and general anesthesia. *Anesth Analg*. 1983; 62:174–180.

14. McKenie PJ, Wishart HY, Gray I, Smith G. Effects of anaesthetic technique on deep vein thrombosis: a comparison of subarachnoid and general anaesthesia. *Br J Anaesth*. 1985; 57:853–857.

15. Jorgensen LN, Rasmussen LS, Nielsen PT, et al. Antithrombotic efficacy of continuous extradural analgesia after knee replacement. *Br J Anaesth*. 1991; 66:8–12.

Anesthesia for Urologic and Gynecologic Surgery in the Elderly

Kristine E. W. Breyer

Key Points

- Elderly patients are commonly seen in medical practice for urologic and gynecologic pathologies.
- Obturator nerve and lateral femoral cutaneous nerve injury risk with lithotomy positioning.
- Robotic surgery is common and attention must be paid to proper positioning.
- Robotic surgery with steep Trendelenburg causes physiologic changes that may be less well tolerated in an elderly population with multiple co-morbidities.
- Transurethral resection (TUR) syndrome is an iatrogenic fluid overload with hypotonic hyponatremia and patients at risk are those undergoing TUR prostatectomy, TUR bladder and tumour resections, cystoscopy and also hysteroscopy procedures.
- Regional or local anesthesia may confer unique advantages for TUR procedures and hysteroscopy by allowing for better neurologic monitoring and possibly less fluid absorption.

Introduction

Urologic and gynecologic surgeries are common in the geriatric population. Most often these types of surgical procedures are performed for urinary obstruction, urinary incontinence and cancer. The majority of these procedures are amenable to regional or general anesthesia techniques. This chapter will outline some of the most common urologic and gynecologic procedures in the geriatric population, specific procedural complications and the pros and cons of different anesthetic techniques.

Elderly patients make up a significant portion of office visits to urologists and gynecologists. Approximately half of all urology office visits are with patients aged 65 years and older and greater than 60% of all urologic surgical procedures are performed on this same age group.[1] For male patients the most common indications for urologic surgery in the elderly include benign prostatic hypertrophy (BPH), urinary incontinence, nephrolithiasis and cancer. Elderly female patients are most commonly seen for urinary incontinence, pelvic organ prolapse and abnormal uterine bleeding. Age is an independent risk factor for incontinence, BPH and cancer.

In men, BPH can cause bladder outlet obstruction, which can lead to urinary retention, bladder stones, nephrolithiasis, recurrent urinary tract infections (UTI) and renal insufficiency. Surgery for BPH has declined significantly over the past several decades due to improvements in pharmacotherapy. Surgical candidates have moderate to severe symptoms, have failed medical therapy or have complications from BPH.[2] Surgical options include transurethral resection or vaporization, open prostatectomy and transurethral incision. Transurethral resection of the prostate (TURP) is the most common operation for BPH.

Urinary incontinence is a significant problem for males and for females in this age group with an estimated incidence between 10% and 28% for male patients and upwards of 60% for females. Urinary incontinence contributes to depression, decreased social interactions and decreased overall quality-of-life scores. Studies indicate that urinary incontinence may be an independent risk factor for nursing home admission.[3] Postoperative mortality for incontinence surgery has been shown to correlate more with co-morbidities than advanced age itself. Surgical procedures for urinary incontinence can often be performed under regional (spinal) anesthesia.

Geriatric female patients are commonly seen by physicians for pelvic organ prolapse (POP). POP often co-exists and contributes to urinary incontinence and severe POP can also cause hydronephrosis. Prevalence of POP is as high as 40% for females, according to a 2014 study by the Women's Health Initiative.[4] POP is the most common reason for hysterectomy in patients greater than 55 years old.

Prostate cancer is the second most frequently diagnosed cancer in males and the sixth leading cause of death. Current American Urology Association (AUA) guidelines recommend screening for prostate cancer in patients with a greater than 10-year life expectancy, regardless of age.[5] It is not uncommon for elderly males to undergo prostatectomy. Other common urologic oncologic surgical procedures include cystectomies and nephrectomies.

On the other hand the American Congress of Obstetricians and Gynecologists, along with the US Preventive Services Task Force, do not recommend routine cervical cancer screening for women greater than 65 years old unless that patient is at higher risk than the general population.[6] However, the peak incidence of endometrial cancer is in the 70–80-year-old cohort and represents the third most prevalent type of female cancer. Overall, cancer is the second most common reason for hysterectomy in the elderly.

Lithotomy Positioning

Lithotomy is a common patient position for many urologic and gynecologic surgeries. Lithotomy classically involves flexion of the hips and knees with abduction of the legs to approximately 30–45 degrees.[7] Lithotomy has been associated with nerve injuries. In 2000, a prospective study of 991 patients revealed an overall nerve injury incidence of 1.5%. The obturator nerve was most frequently injured, followed closely by the lateral femoral cutaneous nerve, as well as sciatic and peroneal nerves. Neuropathy was present within 4 hours of the surgical end time. Symptoms were mostly parasthesias and pain, no motor weakness was found in any injury, and for 14/15 of the patients the symptoms resolved within 4 months of surgery. Length of surgery greater than 2 hours was the only risk factor found in this study.[8] An older retrospective review of almost 200,000 patients indicated that the lateral femoral cutaneous nerve was the most common motor neuropathy from lithotomy.[7] General attention to padding and correct positioning in lithotomy is important. Legs should be raised and lowered simultaneously in order to prevent spine torsion. In the elderly population osteoarthritis and prosthetic joints are common and it is essential to ask the patient about specific positioning limitations prior to anesthesia. Some have advocated placing the patient in the surgical lithotomy position prior to induction of anesthesia to ensure patient comfort.

Robotic Surgery

Robotic surgery came into use around 1999 and has quickly become an increasingly utilized modality for both urologic and gynecologic surgical procedures. From 2003 to 2007 the use of minimally invasive prostatectomies rose from 9% to 43% for prostate cancer and from 2007 to 2010 the use of robotic hysterectomies for benign pathology increased from 0.5% to 9.5%.[9,10] Most commonly the robot is used for prostatectomies; however, it is now also being used for cystectomies, nephrectomies and radial hysterectomies. The procedural advantages of robotic surgery include increased laparoscopic instrument range of motion and accuracy. Patient benefits of robotic prostatectomy include shorter hospital length of stays and lower surgical complications. For open versus robotic prostatectomies no significant difference has been found for cancer control or overall quality of life.[9,11] Robotic hysterectomies offer the benefit of significantly shorter hospital length of stays, but without a difference in surgical complications or blood transfusions.[10]

Robotic surgery does introduce some positioning and physiologic challenges for the anesthesiologist. Robotic surgery is laparoscopic and is generally performed with the patient in steep Trendelenburg (30–45°), the patients arms are usually both tucked into the sides and the patient may also be in lithotomy. The robot itself is docked near the patient, therefore direct access to the patient is limited. Positioning the patient in such steep Trendelenburg mandates that the patient is very well secured to the bed to avoid slipping and injury. Many institutions use a combination of a nonslip mattress (such as a bean bag and foam) on the bed and gel shoulder braces. Chest straps (usually placed in an X-fashion) over the chest can be used to further anchor the patient. Tucked arms should be placed in an anatomically neutral position with thumbs up. It is common to place the patient in steep Trendelenburg prior to the start of surgery in order to test the positioning stability. The test should include an assessment of both the patient's mobility or stability in the position, as well as physiologic tolerance. It is important to look for slipping or stretching at the shoulders and neck in order to prevent brachial plexus injury. Once surgery has begun and the robot is docked it is difficult to access the patient, particularly the upper extremities. Therefore it is essential that all monitors are in place before surgery starts, including any additional intravenous lines or invasive lines that could potentially be required during the case. In an emergent situation it is possible to access the patient's arms; however, the robot will need to be undocked first. The endotracheal tube should be well secured to avoid migration. A small metal tray or additional padding can be positioned above the patient's face in order to afford protection from laparoscopic equipment.[12–14]

Robotic surgery is also challenging from a physiologic standpoint. Most of the physiologic perturbations result from laparoscopic insufflation. Systemic vascular resistance (SVR) is increased with the pneumoperitoneum via both mechanical and neurohormonal factors.[7] A recent study investigated the hemodynamic consequences of laparoscopic insufflation and steep Trendelenburg position in 16 American Society of Anesthesiologists (ASA) class I and II patients undergoing robotic radical prostatectomy. The authors used both pulmonary artery catheters and transesophageal echocardiography in their analysis. Mean arterial blood pressure increased with abdominal insufflation, but did not change further with Trendelenburg. Both central venous pressure (CVP) and pulmonary capillary wedge pressure increased significantly with the steep Trendelenburg position. In fact, wedge pressures of greater than 18 mmHg were found in most patients. Similarly, systolic pulmonary arterial blood pressures greater than 35 mmHg were found in over 75% of the studied patients. Cardiac output did not change, but cardiac stroke work indices increased by nearly 65%. All values normalized following return to normal supine position and removal of abdominal insufflation.[15] There were no hemodynamic complications from the surgical procedure in this study, but these were all relatively healthy patients. Patients with known pulmonary hypertension or heart failure may have difficulty tolerating this procedure.

Respiratory mechanics also change with laparoscopic surgery and steep Trendelenburg. Functional residual capacity (FRC) is decreased with both laparoscopy and also with Trendelenburg. Respiratory compliance can decrease as much as 50% with resultant peak airway pressures and plateaus rising approximately 25–45% upon abdominal insufflation and then increasing more with the addition of steep Trendelenburg. This can make intraoperative mechanical ventilation difficult in healthy patients and particularly in any patient with underlying lung disease.[12–15]

Carbon dioxide is the most commonly used laparoscopic gas. A steady increase in arterial carbon dioxide for the first 15–30 minutes of laparoscopy is normal, after this initial rise the level should begin to plateau. Further increases in arterial carbon dioxide warrant investigation into optimization of mechanical ventilation and also for accidental extraperitoneal insufflation causing subcutaneous emphysema. Risk factors for subcutaneous emphysema include older patients and longer surgery times (greater than 3 hours). Suspicion should be raised with end-tidal carbon dioxide levels exceeding 50 mmHg. Treatment includes prolonging ventilation at the end of the procedure in order to normalize arterial blood gases as much as possible. Gas embolism is another known complication from laparoscopy. This occurs most frequently at the start of the surgical procedure, but can also occur in radial prostatectomies during dissection off the prostatic venous plexus. Pneumothorax and pneumomediastinum are also rare but reported complications.[7,12,15]

Other complications from robotic laparoscopic surgeries include laryngeal edema and optic neuropathy. Consider checking for airway leaks at the start and at the end of the surgical procedure, prior to extubation. Although there are very few reported incidences of ischemic optic neuropathy from robotic surgeries there have been several recent studies investigating changes in ocular pressure during these procedures. This may be particularly applicable to the elderly patient population with higher prevalence of glaucoma. Intraocular pressures (IOP) rose significantly with both abdominal insufflation and also with Trendelenburg, and combined, these two more than doubled IOP in healthy eyes. In patients with glaucoma these numbers may be further exaggerated. Importantly, in healthy eyes the IOP returned to baseline immediately postoperatively. There are no studies to date on glaucoma and robotic surgery; however, this is something to take into consideration for those affected patients.[13,16–18]

Transurethral Resection Syndrome

Excessive fluid absorption can lead to fluid overload and dilutional hyponatremia during transurethral resections, cystoscopy, hysteroscopy and some percutaneous lithotripsy procedures. This syndrome was described in the 1950s with TURP procedures and is called transurethral resection (TUR) syndrome. The principle behind these types of procedures involves distending the operative cavity with fluid in order to improve visualization and facilitate the surgical procedure. The overall incidence of TUR syndrome is 1–8%.[19]

TUR syndrome is an iatrogenic fluid overload with hypotonic hyponatremia, defined as a serum sodium level less than or equal to 120 meq/l, along with at least two clinical signs or symptoms.[7] Signs and symptoms include chest tightness, agitation, confusion, headaches, slowed pupillary light reflexes and shortness of breath. Initially systemic blood pressure may go up, but this can be masked in the setting of significant surgical bleeding. At serum sodium levels less than 120 meq/l symptoms include restlessness, confusion and also signs of pulmonary edema and heart failure. At serum sodium levels less than 115 meq/l symptoms include nausea and somnolence and signs include widened QRS, ST segment changes and ectopy. At serum sodium levels less than 100–110 meq/l patients can have seizures, become comatose and are at risk for respiratory and cardiac arrest.[19,20]

The type of distending fluid utilized varies depending upon the use of monopolar or bipolar cautery. Early TUR procedures were done with monopolar electrocautery and this limits the type of distending media. Monopolar cautery contains an active electrode that releases electricity to the targeted tissue. This energy must then go back via a return circuit, which is usually in the form of a topically placed pad on the patient. Bipolar cautery, on the other hand, self-contains both the active and return circuits together in the same resectoscope. Therefore, energy travels a much shorter distance with bipolar electrocautery than with monopolar. Because energy travels a much longer distance with monopolar cautery the distending fluid must be nonconductive, whereas this is not the case for bipolar resections.[21] Prior to the use of bipolar resectoscopes, fluid for TUR procedures included sterile water and glycine solutions, all of which are nonconductive and also hypotonic. If a bipolar resectoscope is being used, normal saline can be used as the distending fluid. Although normal saline can still cause fluid overload, it does not cause some of the other problems seen in this syndrome and outlined below.[21,22]

Glycine and Cytal are the most common distending solutions used today for monopolar TURPs. Water was historically used, but carries a high risk of hemolysis. Glycine is an inhibitory neurotransmitter and, in addition to causing a dilutional hyponatremia, glycine also exerts direct effects. Normal serum glycine levels are approximately 13–17 mg/l, higher serum glycine levels can directly cause decreased respiratory rate, nausea, decreased urine production, central nervous system (CNS) changes and seizures. Glycine is converted to ammonia and elevated ammonia levels can also cause CNS alterations by inhibiting dopamine and norepinephrine release.[7,20] Cytal is a combination of sorbitol and mannitol. Mannitol may contribute to circulatory overload.

Average fluid absorption is approximately 1 l per hour (or 10–30 ml/minute). The more fluid that is absorbed puts the patient at a higher risk for TUR syndrome. Recommendations for prevention include limiting resecting time to less than 1 hour, limiting the height of the fluid column to less than 60 cm above the site of resection and monitoring the fluid absorption intraoperatively. One method for assessing volume absorbed is to continually calculate the fluid instilled and subtract the fluid returned back out. Of course this volumetric method is flawed in that fluid can be lost and significant bleeding can confound the calculation.[22] Specific risk factors for TUR syndrome are age greater than 80 years, prostate gland size greater than 45 g (for TURP), resection time greater than 90 minutes and capsular perforation (for TURP).[20]

Symptoms of TUR syndrome can begin as early as 15 minutes into the procedure. In awake patients, complaints such as chest tightness and shortness of breath or sudden agitation should prompt investigation into possible TUR syndrome. Reducing the height of the irrigating fluid and shortening procedure length should be considered. Treatment involves supportive care, fluid restriction, loop diuretics and in severe cases, sodium therapy.[7,20,22]

Type of Anesthesia

Many urologic and gynecologic surgeries lend themselves to anesthesia by either regional (RA) or general (GA) techniques. There is more research assessing type of anesthesia for hip fractures than for urologic and gynecologic surgeries. A 2004 Cochrane review of regional anesthesia versus general anesthesia for hip fractures found a small decrease in mortality for patients undergoing regional anesthesia, but with borderline significance. There was significantly less postoperative delirium in the regional anesthesia group (9.4% versus 19.2%).[23] A review of anesthesia for noncardiac surgery revealed a small decrease, but an insignificant difference in postoperative delirium for patients receiving RA. This difference did not persist at 3 months postoperatively.[24] More recent studies evaluating for postoperative cognitive dysfunction (POCD) following genito-urinary surgeries found that POCD correlated more with nonelective surgery, intraoperative hypotension, personal history of delirium and impaired preoperative IADLs, and did not correlate with general versus regional anesthesia nor with open versus endoscopic surgical techniques.[25-27]

Regional or local anesthesia may confer unique advantages for TUR procedures and hysteroscopy. One benefit of regional anesthesia for TUR procedures is the ability to assess the patient for signs and symptoms of TUR syndrome, many signs and symptoms are otherwise masked under general anesthesia. Recent data for hysteroscopy patients suggest that patients receiving local anesthesia, versus either general or epidural anesthesia, have significantly less fluid absorption. This may be partly explained by less vasodilation with local anesthesia.[28,29]

Summary

Urologic and gynecologic surgeries in the geriatric population are common. Most often these types of surgical procedures are performed for urinary obstruction, urinary incontinence and cancer. Many urologic and gynecologic procedures are amenable to either regional anesthesia techniques or general anesthesia techniques. Recent studies evaluating for postoperative cognitive dysfunction (POCD) following genito-urinary surgeries found that POCD correlated more with nonelective surgery, intraoperative hypotension, personal history of delirium and impaired preoperative IADLs, and did not correlate with general versus regional anesthesia nor with open versus endoscopic surgical techniques. Regional or local anesthesia may confer unique advantages for transurethral resection (TUR) procedures and hysteroscopy, as these patients are at risk for TUR syndrome. Higher incidences of osteoarthritis and also prosthetic joints in the elderly population make it essential to ask the patient about specific positioning problems prior to anesthesia, particularly with regard to lithotomy positioning. Robotic surgery also introduces positioning and also physiologic challenges to the anesthesiologist. Robotic surgery came into use around 1999 and has quickly become an increasingly utilized modality for both urologic and gynecologic surgical procedures. Most commonly the robot is used for prostatectomies; however, it is now also being used for cystectomies, nephrectomies and radical hysterectomies.

Acknowledgments

I would like to thank Dr. Benjamin Breyer, MD (associate professor) and Dr. Anne Suskind, MD (assistant professor) both in the Department of Urology at the University of California, San Francisco, for their contribution to this chapter.

References

1. Drach GW, Griebling TL. Geriatric urology. *J Am Geriatr Soc.* 2003; 51(7 Suppl):S355–S358.

2. McVary KT, Roehrborn CG, Avins AL, *et al.* Update on AUA guideline on the management of benign prostatic hyperplasia. *J Urol.* 2011; 185(5):1793–1803.

3. Coward RT, Horne C, Peek CW. Predicting nursing home admissions among incontinent older adults: a comparison of residential differences across six years. *Gerontologist.* 1995; 35(6):732–743.

4. Wu JM, Matthews CA, Conover MM, Pate V, Jonsson Funk M. Lifetime risk of stress urinary incontinence or pelvic organ prolapse surgery. *Obstetr Gynecol.* 2014; 123(6):1201–1206.

5. Carter HB, Albertsen PC, Barry MJ, *et al.* Early detection of prostate cancer: AUA Guideline. *J Urol.* 2013; 190(2):419–426.

6. Moyer VA. Screening for cervical cancer: U.S. Preventive Services Task Force recommendation statement. *Ann Intern Med.* 2012; 156(12):880–891, W312.

7. Miller RD. *Miller's Anesthesia, 7th edn.* New York, Churchill Livingstone Elsevier, 2010.

8. Warner MA, Warner DO, Harper CM, Schroeder DR, Maxson PM. Lower extremity neuropathies associated with lithotomy positions. *Anesthesiology.* 2000; 93(4):938–942.

9. Hu JC, Gu X, Lipsitz SR, *et al.* Comparative effectiveness of minimally invasive vs open radical prostatectomy. *JAMA.* 2009; 302(14):1557–1564.

10. Wright JD, Ananth CV, Lewin SN, *et al.* Robotically assisted vs laparoscopic hysterectomy among women with benign gynecologic disease. *JAMA.* 2013; 309(7):689–698.

11. Alemozaffar M, Sanda M, Yecies D, *et al.* Benchmarks for operative outcomes of robotic and open radical prostatectomy: results from the Health Professionals Follow-up Study. *Eur Urol.* 2015; 67(3):432–438.

12. Gainsburg DM. Anesthetic concerns for robotic-assisted laparoscopic radical prostatectomy. *Minerva Anestesiol.* 2012; 78(5):596–604.

13. Hsu RL, Kaye AD, Urman RD. Anesthetic challenges in robotic-assisted urologic surgery. *Rev Urol.* 2013; 15(4):178–184.

14. Kalmar AF, De Wolf AM, Hendrickx JFA. Anesthetic considerations for robotic surgery in the steep Trendelenburg position. *Adv Anesth.* 2012; 30:75–96.

15. Lestar M, Gunnarsson L, Lagerstrand L, Wiklund P, Odeberg-Wernerman S. Hemodynamic perturbations during robot-assisted laparoscopic

radical prostatectomy in 45 degrees Trendelenburg position. *Anesth Analg.* 2011; 113(5):1069–1075.

16. Mondzelewski TJ, Schmitz JW, Christman MS, *et al.* Intraocular pressure during robotic-assisted laparoscopic procedures utilizing steep Trendelenburg positioning. *J Glaucoma.* 2015; 24(6):399–404.

17. Taketani Y, Mayama C, Suzuki N, *et al.* Transient but significant visual field defects after robot-assisted laparoscopic radical prostatectomy in deep Trendelenburg position. *PloS One.* 2015; 10(4):e0123361.

18. Awad H, Santilli S, Ohr M, *et al.* The effects of steep Trendelenburg positioning on intraocular pressure during robotic radical prostatectomy. *Anesth Analg.* 2009; 109(2):473–478.

19. Vijayan S. TURP syndrome. *Trends Anaesth Crit Care.* 2011; 1:46–50.

20. Gainsburg DM. *Geriatric Anesthestiology, 2nd edn.* Berlin, Springer Science+Business Media, LLC, 2008.

21. Issa MM. Technological advances in transurethral resection of the prostate: bipolar versus monopolar TURP. *J Endourol.* 2008; 22(8):1587–1595.

22. Issa MM, Young MR, Bullock AR, Bouet R, Petros JA. Dilutional hyponatremia of TURP syndrome: a historical event in the 21st century. *Urology.* 2004; 64(2):298–301.

23. Parker MJ, Handoll HH, Griffiths R. Anaesthesia for hip fracture surgery in adults. *Cochrane Database Syst Rev.* 2004 (4):CD000521.

24. Newman S, Stygall J, Hirani S, Shaefi S, Maze M. Postoperative cognitive dysfunction after noncardiac surgery: a systematic review. *Anesthesiology.* 2007; 106(3):572–590.

25. McRae PJ, Peel NM, Walker PJ, de Looze JW, Mudge AM. Geriatric syndromes in individuals admitted to vascular and urology surgical units. *J Am Geriatr Soc.* 2014; 62(6):1105–1109.

26. Tognoni P, Simonato A, Robutti N, *et al.* Preoperative risk factors for postoperative delirium (POD) after urological surgery in the elderly. *Arch Gerontol Geriatr.* 2011; 52(3):e166–e169.

27. Tai S, Xu L, Zhang L, Fan S, Liang C. Preoperative risk factors of postoperative delirium after transurethral prostatectomy for benign prostatic hyperplasia. *Int J Clin Exp Med.* 2015; 8(3):4569–4574.

28. Bergeron ME, Ouellet P, Bujold E, *et al.* The impact of anesthesia on glycine absorption in operative hysteroscopy: a randomized controlled trial. *Anesth Analg.* 2011; 113(4):723–728.

29. Goldenberg M, Cohen SB, Etchin A, Mashiach S, Seidman DS. A randomized prospective comparative study of general versus epidural anesthesia for transcervical hysteroscopic endometrial resection. *Am J Obstet Gynecol.* 2001; 184(3):273–276.

Chapter 18

Cataract Surgery in the Elderly

George A. Dumas and Gwendolyn L. Boyd

Key Points

- Routine preoperative testing prior to cataract surgery is unnecessary.
- To perform a retrobulbar block a small volume of local anesthesia is injected inside the cone formed by the eye muscles. This block achieves rapid anesthesia and akinesia of the eye.
- Orbital complications of a nerve block include globe perforation, globe rupture, optic nerve damage, extraocular muscle injury, retrobulbar hemorrhage, conjunctival hemorrhage, corneal abrasion and chemosis.
- Central nervous system spread of local anesthesia from unintentional arterial injection via reverse flow from the ophthalmic artery to the anterior cerebral or internal carotid artery can result in seizures and even death.
- Accidental globe perforation and rupture is a devastating complication of needle blocks. Risk factors associated include: recession of the eye, limited operator experience and increased optical axial length, e.g. from myopia, staphyloma and previous scleral buckle surgery.
- Topical anesthesia advantages include simplicity, rare systemic complications, minimal pain with application and rapid recovery postoperatively.

Introduction

Cataract extraction with intraocular lens insertion is the most commonly performed operation in the geriatric population. Patients present with multiple co-morbidities that may affect the anesthetic technique chosen for this procedure. In this chapter, we will review the preoperative assessment of these patients, intraoperative regional, topical and general anesthetic options, sedation issues, postoperative pain concerns and finally the unique benefits of successful cataract surgery in this population. Consideration of visual function improvement with associated cognitive and quality-of-life benefits underlies the importance of this procedure to our patients.

Surgical Technique

A cataract is an opacity of the crystalline lens of the eye. Vision is obstructed by cataracts, particularly when centrally located in the posterior aspect of the lens.

Typically the lens is removed by ultrasonic vibrations known as the phacoemulsification technique. A small incision is made, the lens is then fragmented and removed via aspiration and irrigation. An artificial intraocular lens is positioned in the capsular bag. The small incision size, minimal postoperative pain, less astigmatism, refractive stabilization and fast patient recovery make this technique particularly attractive.[1]

Extracapsular cataract extraction involves removal of the lens and leaves the posterior capsule intact. This technique may be required for extremely hard cataracts or when phacoemulsion cannot be used.

Intracapsular cataract extraction involves removal of the lens and the lens capsule. Retinal detachment and macular edema are common complications with this rarely used technique.[2]

Preoperative Assessment

Elimination of unnecessary and wasteful preoperative testing in the elderly cataract patient is wise. A large clinical trial found that preoperative testing (ECG, electrolytes, urea nitrogen, creatinine and glucose) did not affect outcomes for cataract surgery.[3] Abnormalities found from routine testing in this study were rarely acted upon.[3] Ignoring these abnormalities may also leave the provider at greater liability than if the results were never obtained.

According to the American College of Cardiology and the American Heart Association guidelines on perioperative cardiovascular evaluation and management of patients undergoing noncardiac surgery, ophthalmic surgery is categorized as a very low-risk procedure. In general patients should proceed to the operating room without further cardiac testing unless they present with an acute coronary syndrome or the estimated perioperative risk of major adverse cardiac event (MACE) based on combined clinical/surgical risk is elevated and they have poor functional capacity, and further testing will impact patient care.[4] Another study found that preoperative consultations for Medicare patients undergoing cataract surgery do not affect outcome and vary by nonmedical factors.[5] Costs associated with patients who had routine preoperative medical testing were shown to be 2.55 times higher.[6]

On the day of surgery the elderly patient's medications should be verified with the patient and caregiver, if applicable. Intraoperative floppy iris syndrome may occur in patients taking α-1 receptor antagonists such as tamsulosin (Flomax®) for benign prostatic hypertrophy.[7] Unfortunately, this effect appears irreversible and discontinuing tamulosin prior to cataract surgery does not decrease the risk of this complication. Cognitive and physical factors that may affect cooperation during local anesthesia should be identified preoperatively, such as a hearing aid. Patient positioning may be challenging – especially in patients with significant kyphosis or neck arthritis.

In general coordination of care of the geriatric patient with primary care, the surgeon and anesthesiologist can lead to a reduction of unnecessary consultations and testing.[8]

Antithrombotic Therapy

Older cataract patients are frequently on antithrombotic therapies. Management of these medicines involves weighing the risk of thrombotic complications against the risk of hemorrhagic complications. Discontinuation of anticoagulant or antiplatelet therapy substantially increases the risk of thromboembolic events, particularly in patients with prosthetic heart valves, atrial fibrillation or recent coronary stents.[9,10] Cataract surgery is an avascular procedure and considered to be at very low risk for bleeding complications.

Regional needle blocks during use of routine anticoagulant and antiplatelet medications in general are found to be safe, provided that therapy levels were in the usual therapeutic window.[9] Most cataract surgeries are in fact performed under topical anesthesia or topical and intracameral anesthesia. In general, provided the surgeon is agreeable, it is recommended that antiplatelet and anticoagulant treatment are continued for surgery, including retinal surgery under retrobulbar block.[11] However, insufficient data exist regarding the safety of needle and cannula blocks for patients taking the newer anticoagulant drugs (dabigatran, rivaroxaban, apixaban) and newer antiplatelet medications (prasugrel, ticagrelor).[10] Considering reduced clearance of these newer medications in the elderly, special consideration and management may be warranted before needle or cannula block. This may involve consultation with the patient's cardiologist regarding the risk of discontinuation of any anticoagulant medications.

Anesthetic Techniques

In cataract surgery, the need for total akinesia or immobility of the eye is greatly reduced when using the phacoemulsion technique, as the ultrasound probe mechanically immobilizes the eye. In contrast, for extracapsular extraction of the cataract, the surgeon and patient will likely benefit from greater akinesia of the eye, possibly requiring a retrobulbar block. Irrespective of the technique, avoidance of patient movement, general restlessness, anxiety and discomfort are important to perform the surgery successfully. Coughing may impair the surgical field and raise intraocular pressure, and can be particularly problematic. Some patients may experience visual sensations, including seeing lights, colors and surgical instruments under topical or regional anesthesia. Because some of these patients may find these sensations disturbing, preoperative explanation about the possibility of such visual sensations is beneficial.[12] Rarely, general anesthesia may be the only viable option in certain patients due to psychological, medical or surgical issues. Patient factors, surgeon preferences and anesthesia provider skill set will all factor into determining the best anesthetic technique.

Needle Blocks

Retrobulbar block is an intraconal block. Anesthesia is achieved by injecting a small volume of local anesthesia inside the cone formed by the eye muscles (Figure 18.1). This block achieves rapid anesthesia and akinesia of the eye.

Peribulbar block is an extraconal block. Anesthesia is achieved by injecting a larger volume of anesthesia outside of the cone formed by the eye muscles (Figure 18.2). The anesthesia is placed further from key nerves and requires higher volumes for diffusion. The onset of anesthesia and akinesia is typically longer for the peribulbar approach.

Needle block complications can be divided into systemic and orbital complications. Orbital complications may include globe perforation, globe rupture, optic nerve damage, extraocular muscle injury, retrobulbar hemorrhage, conjunctival hemorrhage, corneal abrasion and chemosis. Systemic complications can include brainstem anesthesia from injection under the dural sheath in the optic nerve or directly through the optic foramen.[13] Central nervous system spread of local anesthesia from unintentional arterial injection via reverse flow from the ophthalmic artery to the anterior cerebral or internal carotid artery can result in seizures.[14]

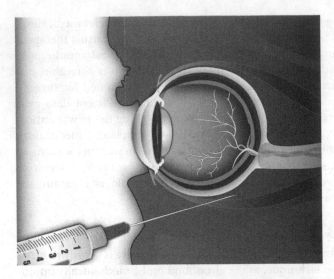

Figure 18.1 Intraconal block or retrobulbar injections within the cone formed by the extraocular muscles of the eye.
(From Kumar, Dodds, and Gayer, *Ophthalmic Anesthesia*; used with permission Oxford University Press.)

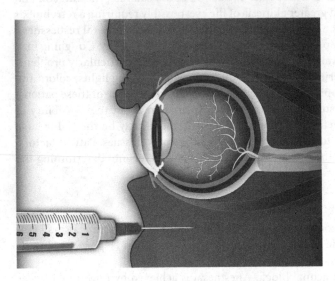

Figure 18.2 Extraconal block or peribulbar injections outside the cone formed by the extraocular muscles.
(From Kumar, Dodds, and Gayer, *Ophthalmic Anesthesia*; used with permission Oxford University Press.)

Accidental globe perforation and rupture can be a devastating complication of needle blocks. Some of the risk factors associated with accidental globe perforation with the needle include: recession of the eye, limited operator experience and increased optical axial length.[15] Ultrasound measurement of axial length can make this determination. Myopia, staphyloma and previous scleral buckle surgery are associated with increased anterior–posterior distance and thus higher risk of globe perforation.[16]

Retrobulbar hematoma results from damage to the arterial or venous vessels inside the orbit. Arterial bleeds are rapid and may present with worsening proptosis. Retinal perfusion becomes compromised and surgical consultation for urgent decompression via lateral canthotomy is warranted. Venous bleeding may be less severe and will likely resolve with pressure and time.[17] Arterial fragility in diabetic and hypertensive elderly patients is a greater risk factor than clotting problems for retrobulbar hematoma.[10]

Sub-Tenon's Block

Sub-Tenon's block can be achieved by placing either a needle or a blunt cannula into the episcleral space below Tenon's capsule. Typically a blunt cannula is used for an improved safety profile. Local anesthesia is injected through the cannula and diffuses around and into the muscle cone.[13] Excellent sensory anesthesia is obtained, while more variable amounts of akinesia are obtained depending on the volume and characteristics of the local anesthetic agent used.[18,19]

The primary benefit of the sub-Tenon's cannula block is safety. Blind placement of the needle into the orbit is avoided. Minor complications include loss of anesthetic volume during injection, pain during injection, chemosis and subconjunctival hemorrhage.[17] Major complications may still occur, despite the improved safety profile over needle-based techniques.[20] Any major needle block complication may occur after sub-Tenon's block, but the incidence should be lower.[21]

Topical Anesthesia

Topical anesthesia offers several advantages, including simplicity, noninvasiveness, extremely rare systemic complications, minimal pain with application and rapid recovery postoperatively. The risks of retrobulbar hemorrhage and optic nerve injury that are associated with regional blocks are eliminated with topical anesthesia.[22] Local anesthetic drops and gels provide surface analgesia. Anesthetic gels provide higher concentrations in the anterior chamber compared to equivalent doses of anesthetic drops and may provide improved analgesia.[23]

Disadvantages of topical anesthesia include eye movement, possible incomplete analgesia, visual awareness, corneal damage and unanticipated patient movement. Intracameral injection of local anesthetics is one way to improve analgesia.[24] This involves injecting local anesthetic into the anterior chamber of the eye. However, this may have toxic effects on corneal endothelium.[25] Compensating for inadequate topical anesthesia with overly aggressive sedation may lead to patient disinhibition and movement leading to poor outcomes.[26] A comparison of local anesthetic techniques is shown in Table 18.1.

Table 18.1 Comparison of anesthetic blocks and topical anesthesia for cataract surgery

Technique	Safety/complication risk	Globe akinesia	Eyelid akinesia	Sensory block
Topical	Extremely safe	None	None	Adequate, may need supplementation
Retrobulbar block	Highest risk	Excellent	May require facial nerve block	Excellent
Peribulbar block	High risk	Good	Good	Excellent
Sub-Tenon's block	Moderate risk	Variable	Good	Excellent

Monitored Sedation

Although not mandatory, sedation is often given with local anesthesia for cataract surgery. Anxiety over discomfort during the procedure is often present in these patients. This anxiety is not only troubling for the patient, but can make the procedure more difficult for the surgeon as well. The catecholamine release precipitated by anxiety may be detrimental to this elderly patient population. Hypertension, angina, history of myocardial infarction or a condition treated by coronary artery bypass, and arrhythmia have been shown to be prevalent in patients scheduled for cataract surgery.[3] These co-morbidities may be exacerbated with tachycardia and hypertension. Also, anxiety, pain and fear during cataract surgery have been shown to produce lower patient satisfaction scores.[27]

Sedation has been implicated as a risk factor for adverse intraoperative medical events in cataract surgery. A large study found that adjuvant agents used to alleviate pain and anxiety during cataract surgery were associated with such events.[28] Treatment for brady-arrhythmias and hypertension were the most common of these events. Furthermore, as the number of agents administered increased, so did the prevalence of these adverse events.[28] Providers must always be prepared to manage airway complications, particularly upper airway obstruction, which is common in patients with obstructive sleep apnea. Oversedation may result in an uncooperative and disoriented patient. In demented or older patients, the loss of cooperation occurs at even smaller doses of sedation. This may result in unwanted patient movements resulting in challenging surgical conditions. It should also be noted that over 20% of closed claims for monitored anesthesia care cases occurred during ophthalmic surgery.[29] Unwanted patient movement and eye block accounted for the majority of these events.[29] Preoperative counseling, intraoperative communication and appropriate reassurance during the procedure are additional strategies to help alleviate patient fear and anxiety.

Anxiety, pain and discomfort during cataract surgery may be managed with a variety of different agents. Local anesthesia injections and suboptimal local anesthesia during the procedure are common causes of this discomfort. Ideally, the agents chosen to reduce these symptoms will have a rapid onset, rapid offset, be free of significant physiologic alterations and be void of residual effects postoperatively. Patients should be able to respond to commands during cataract extraction. Medications with anticholinergic properties, such as diphenhydramine, are best avoided in the elderly.[30] Confusion and delirium may result, as the elderly are more sensitive to the central effects of anticholinergics.[30] Meperidine and benzodiazepines are also best avoided as these agents are known to increase the risk of delirium.[31] Medications in these three classes: anticholinergics, sedative-hypnotics and meperidine have been shown to more than double the risk of postoperative delirium. It is recommended by the American Geriatrics Society guidelines on postoperative delirium in older adults to avoid these medications if possible.[31] If required, judicious titration should be utilized.

Midazolam, due to its rapid, short-acting properties, can be given if the patient has a history of alcohol abuse or benzodiazepine dependence. It is known to produce anxiolysis, amnesia, hypnosis and sedation. As its effects are increased in the elderly, care must be exhibited when choosing and titrating this agent. Adequate time, from 5 to 10 minutes, must be allowed for the effect to be evaluated.[32] Propofol is a sedative-hypnotic notable for its rapid onset, rapid offset and lack of residual effect. Respiratory depression and hypotension are potential side effects. Also, abrupt changes in consciousness produced by propofol can result in patient movement. In a study of elderly same-day cataract patients, propofol was deemed to be useful via patient-controlled administration (PCA).[33] Narcotic analgesics to consider include fentanyl, alfentanil and remifentanil. Intravenous fentanyl is commonly used with doses of 25–50 mcg providing analgesia with minimal sedation when given alone. Fentanyl has been shown to provide patient comfort and improve patient satisfaction during cataract surgery under topical anesthesia when given via PCA.[32,34] Respiratory depression and nausea are known side effects. Dexmedetomidine is an α-2 receptor agonist with sedative, analgesic and anxiolytic properties. Side effects include bradycardia and hypotension. It also has minimal effects on respiration, but may be associated with patient movement during stimulation. Although successfully used in cataract surgery,[35] more widespread use is limited by cost.

General Anesthesia

General anesthesia may be the best or only option for some patients. This is likely due to medical, psychological or surgical factors. Mental issues, Parkinson disease or pain issues are examples of patient factors that may not allow them to lie still for surgery. As mentioned before, oversedation can cause problems that a general anesthetic with airway control will prevent. Elderly patients will also need additional time for adequate pre-oxygenation compared to their younger counterparts.[36] Allowing sufficient time for the induction agent to work is important to prevent unnecessary overdosing. Although the elderly are known to have reduced esophageal sphincter tone and reduced gastrointestinal mobility, a supraglottic airway device such as the laryngeal mask airway (LMA) is our usual choice for airway control. The LMA provides smooth emergence conditions, and residual muscle paralysis is not a concern.

Postoperative Pain

Typically, there is no pain or only mild postoperative pain after cataract surgery.[37] Severe pain should be concerning for a complication like infection or inflammation. However, severe pain postoperatively may not be associated with surgical complication and counseling and pain management may be needed.[37] Surgical trauma and topical drops, which can contain preservatives like benzalkonium chloride, may also cause postoperative pain. Eye patching, acetaminophen, topical NSAIDs and preservative-free topical steroids may be beneficial in minimizing this pain.[37] If there are not any contraindications, NSAIDs and COX-2 inhibitors can also be used for mild to moderate pain. Topical anesthetic drops postoperatively can provide short-term pain relief, but should be utilized judiciously. Opiates are very rarely needed. Postoperative pain control, preferably with non-opiates, is important, as pain contributes to delirium in older patients.[31]

Benefits for the Elderly

Increased mortality is associated with cataracts and visual impairment.[38,39] One study not only supported previous studies that associated visual impairment with mortality, but also showed that successful cataract surgery resulted in a 40% reduction in long-term mortality risk for older persons with cataracts.[40] Visual improvement leads to improved physical and psychological well-being. This likely contributes to a longer life span.[40] Cataract surgery is considered an "essential surgery" in the Disease Control Priorities, i.e. it is a procedure that provides great value and is cost effective where there are limited resources.[41] It has been shown that good clinical outcomes are attainable in cataract surgery in very elderly patients despite multiple systemic and ocular co-morbidities.[42] Improved visual function, as well as vision and health-related quality of life have also been shown to be improved after cataract surgery. Additional gains in vision and health-related quality of life are well documented after second eye cataract surgery.[43]

Cognitive impairment and cognitive decline have been associated with vision loss. Early cataract extraction may slow this decline or even improve cognition.[44,45] Depression is also associated with cataracts in the elderly.[46] Vision-related quality of life, cognitive impairment and depressive mental status are related.[47] Cognitive impairment related to depression has been called depressive pseudodementia.[48] If poor vision is the cause of depression and pseudodementia, then cataract surgery may lead to improvements in all of these areas.[47] Improved blue-light transmission after cataract surgery may also benefit cognition and improve sleep in the elderly.[49,50]

Fall risk has been linked to cataracts in the elderly.[51,52] Binocular vision is important in preventing falls and other motor functions. It is likely important to have expedited second eye cataract surgery, if required, to optimize binocular vision and help prevent falls.[53]

References

1. Watson A, Sunderraj P. Comparison of small-incision phacoemulsification with standard extracapsular cataract surgery: postoperative astigmatism and visual recovery. *Eye.* 1992; 6:626–629.

2. Harper RA, Shock JP. Lens. In: Riordan-Eva P, Cunningham ET Jr., eds., *Vaughan & Asbury's General Ophthalmology, 18th edn.* New York, McGraw-Hill, 2011; Chapter 8.

3. Schein OD, Katz J, Bass EB, *et al.* Study of medical testing for cataract surgery: the value of routine preoperative medical testing before cataract surgery. *N Engl J Med.* 2000; 342(3):168–175.

4. Fleisher LA, Fleischmann KE, Auerbach AD, *et al.* 2014 ACC/AHA guideline on perioperative cardiovascular evaluation and management of patients undergoing noncardiac surgery: a report of the American College of Cardiology/American Heart Association Task Force on Practice Guidelines. *J Am Coll Cardiol.* 2014; 64:e77–e137.

5. Thilen SR, Treggiari MM, Lange JM, *et al.* Preoperative consultations for medicare patients undergoing cataract surgery. *JAMA Intern Med.* 2014; 174(3):380–388.

6. Keay L, Lindsley K, Tielsch J, *et al.* Routine preoperative medical testing for cataract surgery. *Cochrane Database Syst Rev.* 2012(3):CD007293.

7. Chang DF, Campbell JR. Intraoperative floppy iris syndrome associated with tamsulosin. *J Cataract Refract Surg.* 2005; 31(4):664–673.

8. Dexter F, Wachtel RE. Strategies for net cost reductions with the expanded role and expertise of anesthesiologists in the Perioperative Surgical Home. *Anesth Analg.* 2014; 118(5):1062–1071.

9. Katz J, Feldman MA, Bass EB, *et al.* Risks and benefits of anticoagulant and antiplatelet medication use before cataract surgery. *Ophthalmology.* 2003; 110(9):1784–1788.

10. Bonhomme F, Hafezi F, Boehlen F, Habre W. Management of antithrombotic therapies in patients scheduled for eye surgery. *Eur J Anaesthesiol.* 2013; 30(8):449–454.

11. Mason JM, Gupta SR, Compton CJ, *et al.* Comparison of hemorrhagic complications of warfarin and clopidogrel bisulfate in 25-gauge vitrectomy versus a control group. *Ophthalmology.* 2011; 118(3):543–547.

12. Haripriya A, Tan CS, Venkatesh R, *et al.* Effect of preoperative counseling on patient fear from visual sensations during phacoemulsification under topical anesthesia. *J Cataract Refract Surg.* 2011; 37:814–818.

13. Kumar C, Dowd T. Ophthalmic regional anaesthesia. *Curr Opin Anaesthesiol.* 2008; 21:632–637.

14. Aldrete JA, Romo-Salas F, Arora S, *et al.* Reverse arterial blood flow as a pathway for central nervous system toxic responses following injection of local anesthetics. *Anesth Analg.* 1978; 57:428–433.

15. Duker JS, Belmony JB, Benson WE, *et al.* Inadvertent globe perforation during retrobulbar and peribulbar anesthesia: patient characteristics, surgical management, and visual outcome. *Ophthalmology.* 1991; 98:519–526.

16. Gayer S, Kumar CM. Ophthalmic regional anesthesia techniques. *Minerva Anesthesiol.* 2008; 74(1-2):23–33.

17. Kumar CM, Dowd TC. Complications of opthalmic regional blocks: their treatment and prevention. *Ophthalmologica.* 2006; 220:73–82.

18. Verghese I, Sivaraj R, Lai YK. The effectiveness of sub-Tenon's infiltration of local anaesthesia for cataract surgery. *Aust N Z J Ophthalmol.* 1996; 24:117–120.

19. Guise P. Sub-Tenon's anesthesia: a prospective study of 6000 blocks. *Anesthesiology.* 2003; 98:964–968.

20. El-Hindy N, Johnston RL, Jaycock P, *et al.*; UK EPR User Group. The Cataract National Dataset electronic multicenter audit of 55,567 operations: anaesthetic techniques and complications. *Eye.* 2009; 23:50–55.

21. Ruschen H, Bremmer FD, Carr C. Complications after sub-Tenon's eye block. *Anesth Analg* 2003; 96:273–277.

22. Kershner RM. Topical anesthesia for small incision self-sealing cataract surgery: a prospective evaluation of the first 100 patients. *J Cataract Refract Surg.* 1993; 19:290–292.

23. Bardocci A, Lofoco G, Perdicaro S, *et al.* Lidocaine 2% gel versus lidocaine 4% unpreserved drops for topical anesthesia in cataract surgery: a randomized controlled trial. *Ophthalmology.* 2003; 110:144–149.

24. Karp CL, Cox TA, Wagoner MD, *et al.* Intracameral anesthesia: a report by the American Academy of Ophthalmology. *Ophthalmology.* 2001; 108:1704–1710.

25. Eggeling P, Pleyer U, Hartman C, Rieck PW. Corneal endothelial toxicity of different lidocaine concentrations. *J Cataract Refract Surg.* 2000; 26:1403–1408.

26. Gayer S. Key components of risk associated with ophthalmic anesthesia. *Anesthesiology.* 2006; 105:859.

27. Fung D, Cohen MM, Stewart S, Davies A. What determines patient satisfaction with cataract care under topical local anesthesia and monitored sedation in a community hospital setting? *Anesth Analg.* 2005; 100:1644–1650.

28. Katz J, Feldman MA, Bass EB, *et al.* Adverse intraoperative medical events and their association with anesthesia management strategies in cataract surgery. *Ophthalmology.* 2001; 108:1721–1726.

29. Bhananker SM, Posner KL, Cheney FW, *et al.* Injury and liability associated with monitored anesthesia care: a closed claims analysis. *Anesthesiology.* 2006; 104:228–234.

30. Barnett SR. Polypharmacy and perioperative medications in the elderly. *Anesthesiol Clin.* 2009; 27(3):377–389.

31. Inouye SK, Robinson T, Blaum C, *et al.*; The American Geriatrics Society Expert Panel on Postoperative Delirium in Older Adults. Postoperative delirium in older adults: best practice statement from the American Geriatrics Society. *J Am Coll Surg.* 2015; 220(2):136–148.

32. Greenhalgh DL, Kumar CM. Sedation during ophthalmic surgery. *Eur J Anaesthesiol.* 2008; 25:701–707.

33. Janzen PR, Christys A, Vucevic M. Patient-controlled sedation using propofol in elderly patients in day-case cataract surgery. *Br J Anaesth.* 1999; 82:635–636.

34. Aydin ON, Ku F, Ozkan SB, Gusoy F. Patient-controlled anaesthesia and sedation with fentanyl in phacoemulsification under topical anesthesia. *J Cataract Refract Surg.* 2002; 28:1968–1972.

35. Woo JH, Au Eong KG, Kumar CM. Conscious sedation during ophthalmic surgery under local anesthesia. *Minerva Anesthesiol.* 2009; 75:211–219.

36. Kang H, Park HJ, Baek SK, *et al.* Effects of preoxygenation with the three minutes tidal volume breathing technique in the elderly. *Korean J Anesthesiol.* 2010; 58(4):369–373.

37. Porela-Tiihonen S, Kaarniranta K, Kokki H. Postoperative pain after cataract surgery. *J Cataract Refract Surg.* 2013; 39(5):789–798.

38. McCarty CA, Nanjan MB, Taylor HR. Vision impairment predicts 5 year mortality. *Br J Ophthalmol.* 2001; 85:322–326.

39. Wang JJ, Mitchell P, Simpson JM, *et al.* Visual impairment, age related cataract, and mortality. *Arch Ophthalmol.* 2001; 119:1186–1190.

40. Fong CS, Mitchell P, Rochtchina E, *et al.* Correction of visual impairment by cataract surgery and improved survival in older persons: The Blue Mountain Eye Study cohort. *Ophthalmology.* 2013; 120(9):1720–1727.

41. Prajna NV, Ravilla TD, Srinivasan S. Cataract Surgery. In: Jamison DT, Nugent R, Gelband H, Horton S, Jha P, Laxminarayan R, eds., *Disease Control Priorities: Essential Surgery, 3rd edn.* Washington, DC, World Bank, 2015; Chapter 11, 197–212.

42. Lai FH, Lok JYC, Chow PPC, Young AL. Clinical outcomes of cataract surgery in very elderly adults. *J Am Geriatr Soc.* 2014; 62(1):165–170.

43. Desai P, Reidy A, Minassian DC, *et al.* Gains from cataract surgery: visual function and quality of life. *Br J Ophthalmol.* 1996; 80:868–873.

44. Rosen PN. Cognitive impairment and cataract surgery. *J Cataract Refract Surg.* 2004; 30:2459–2460.

45. Tamura H, Tsukamoto H, Mukai S, *et al.* Improvement in cognitive impairment after cataract surgery in elderly patients. *J Cataract Refract Surg.* 2004; 30:598–602.

46. Rovner BW, Ganguli M. Depression and disability associated with impaired vision: the MoVIES project. *J Am Geriatr Soc.* 1998; 46:617–619.

47. Ishii K, Kabata T, Oshika T. The impact of cataract surgery on cognitive impairment and depressive mental status in elderly patients. *Am J Ophthalmol.* 2008; 146(3):404–409.

48. Fischer P. The spectrum of depressive pseudo-dementia. *J Neural Transm Suppl.* 1996; 47:193–203.

49. Asplund R, Lindblad BE. Sleep and sleepiness 1 and 9 months after cataract surgery. *Arch Gerontol Geriatr.* 2004; 38(1):69–75.

50. Schmoll C, Tendo C, Aspinall P, Dhillon B. Reaction time as a measure of enhanced blue-light mediated cognitive function following cataract surgery. *Br J Ophthalmol.* 2011; 95:1656–1659.

51. Ivers RQ, Cumming RG, Mitchell P, Attebo K. Visual impairment and falls in older adults: the Blue Mountains Eye Study. *J Am Geriatr Soc.* 1998; 46:58–64.

52. Harwood RH, Foss AJE, Osborn F, *et al.* Falls and health status in elderly women following first eye cataract surgery: a randomized controlled trial. *Br J Ophthalmol.* 2005; 89:53–59.

53. Meuleners LB, Fraser ML, Ng J, Morlet N. The impact of first- and second-eye cataract surgery on injurious falls that require hospitalisation: a whole-population study. *Age Ageing.* 2014; 43:341–346.

Chapter

19

Critical Care of the Elderly Patient

Abirami Kumaresan and Shahzad Shaefi

Key Points

- Older adults account for 50% or more of ICU admissions and the increasing age of this population predisposes them to increased morbidity and mortality. Morbidity and mortality after ICU admission is directly related to prior health status, preadmission functional impairment and age.
- Frailty has been shown to be associated with longer durations of both ICU and in-hospital stay, and with less likelihood of independence upon discharge. Frail patients also have a higher risk of a major adverse events during their hospital stay compared with their less frail or nonfrail counterparts.
- Multidisciplinary team involvement including early involvement of palliative care teams, physical therapists and the patient's geriatrician or primary care physician may help the intensivist arrive at an informed decision about triage, impact on survival and quality of life after discharge.
- The decision to admit to the ICU should be based on objective criteria, without a strict age cutoff. Physicians should avoid providing futile care to any one group of patients, regardless of age, as this may lead to delays and divert care from another group or patient that may benefit.
- Geriatric trauma patients have higher rates of admission after injury, longer length of stay, and higher morbidity and mortality, even with less severe injury, than their younger counter parts.
- There is evidence that critical illness may have an impact, in a dose-dependent fashion, on the incidence and severity of cognitive dysfunction.

Introduction

This chapter addresses the care of the elderly surgical patient admitted to the intensive care unit (ICU), including risk assessment and appropriate triage, as well as common complications and outcomes following admission. The objective of this chapter is to assist perioperative physicians in the management of critically ill geriatric surgical patients.

A Brief History of Critical Care Medicine

Long before the first ICU came into existence, health care providers realized the need for specialized care of the critically ill. During the Crimean War, Florence Nightingale insisted that wounded soldiers be cared for in special areas of the medical treatment tent, especially after surgery. She is frequently credited with the first recorded attempt at critical care medicine. She recognized the need for more intense treatment of very ill patients. In 1927 Dr. Walter Dandy, of Johns Hopkins University, established a special area within the main hospital for patients to recover following surgery. Finally, the polio epidemic in the 1950s increased the demand for mechanical ventilation and specialty intensive care nursing; thus the modern day ICU was born.

By the early 1960s, institutions such as the University of California Los Angeles and the University of Pittsburg were among the first to have designated units for critically ill patients. These units resembled the modern day ICU with early models of invasive monitoring systems and multidisciplinary teams. By the late 1980s the American Board of Medical Specialties approved certification for practice of critical care medicine for the field of anesthesiology; now critical care specialists come from many backgrounds, including medicine, surgery, emergency medicine, and obstetrics and gynecology.

Today there are over 60,000 ICU beds in the US alone, and as a country, the US cares for over 5 million critically ill patients per year. This chapter will address the growing portion of the patient population defined as older adults (age >65) to the very old (>85 years of age) who are receiving an increasingly larger percentage of ICU care.

Demographics

Older adults, defined as those aged 65 and greater, are the fastest growing segment of the world's population. According to the 2010 US census data, 45 million Americans are older than 65 years of age. It is estimated that by 2050 this number will increase to almost 84 million or 20% of the total population.

As the population ages there is a parallel increase in demand for intensive care services for the critically ill elderly patients. The increase in demand is reflected in the dramatic increase in the number of ICU beds, now estimated to be more than 67,000 nationally. As this demographic group approaches end of life, costs increase – with the majority of Medicare cost accruing in the last 2 months of life.[1] Currently, the cost of ICU care is almost 1% of the Gross National Product,[2] and elderly patients account for between 42% and 52% of ICU admissions and 60% of all ICU days.[3] It is important for both the intensivist and the non-ICU physician to be cognizant of the increase in the demand for ICU resources in order to help allocate appropriate resources to patients, providing the most benefit and limiting potential harm.

Where do ICU Patients Come From?

A non-ICU team member, such as the primary care physician or admitting team, generally performs the initial evaluation of the very ill patient. This initial evaluation often forms the cornerstone of the patient's history, including baseline health status and management of chronic conditions, as well as the patient's wishes for invasive treatments and advanced care. Once this evaluation reveals critical illness or the potential for rapid deterioration, the patient is generally evaluated by someone from the ICU team, and the patient is either admitted to the ICU or further managed by the primary team.

Patients can be admitted to the ICU from anywhere in the hospital; one study examining Medicare data estimated 43.8% of ICU admissions were "postprocedural" while 33.4% were under the category of "general medical." The most common diagnostic procedural codes for the ICU Medicare population (>65 years) included total hip replacement, hip and femur fracture, cardiac catheterization and bypass grafting. Common medical admissions include congestive heart failure, pneumonia, stroke, myocardial infarction, COPD and infection or sepsis. Not infrequently, older patients have both medical and surgical issues prompting ICU admission.

Assessment of Health Status and Risk of Hospitalization

Morbidity and mortality after ICU admission is directly related to prior health status, preadmission functional impairment and age. Thus a full understanding of the elderly patient's preadmission health status is vital when admitting a patient to the ICU. There are several tools available to help physicians assess and risk stratify their patients. These tools can help predict which patients will have the greatest benefit from ICU admission and those who are at greatest risk for mortality or posthospital impairment.

It is well known that greater age is associated with increased chronic illness and functional impairment.[4] However, age alone fails to take into consideration the heterogeneity of patients in older age groups. This has direct relevance for the ICU, as differences in "reserve" and "resilience," both cognitively and physiologically, have a large impact on the course and outcomes during and after an ICU admission. Patients with reduced reserve are more susceptible to infection, have higher rates of co-morbidity and decreased functional status when compared to younger and healthier patient populations. Identifying risk factors and using them to predict ICU course and postdischarge outcomes of old and very old patients continues to remain a challenge for providers.

ICU and Frailty

Although the definition varies, the concept of "frailty" has been used in medicine to facilitate outcome prediction and assess pre-existing risk. The combinations of signs and symptoms defining frail elderly patients have a significant impact on mortality, depletion of medical resources and caregiver stress. Fried *et al.*[5] defined frailty as three or more of the following: decreased grip strength on the dominant side, self-reported exhaustion, slow walking speed, unintentional weight loss and low physical activity. Sternberg *et al.*[6] performed a systematic review of over 4000 abstracts geared at identifying the operational definition of frailty, tools for identification of frailty and screening for the severity of frailty. They identified several high-quality assessments, a few of which are highlighted below (Table 19.1).

Frailty has been demonstrated to predict falls, dependence, hospitalizations and mortality for elderly in the community, independent of co-morbidities and disability. The incidence of frailty and disability increases with age, independent of co-morbidities.[5] Frailty is thus useful in assessing a patient's preadmission health status and in risk-stratifying patients who face possible admission to the ICU.[7] Frailty has been shown to be associated with longer durations of both ICU and in-hospital stays and with less likelihood of independence upon discharge. Frail patients also have a higher risk of a major adverse event during their hospital stay compared with their less frail or nonfrail counterparts. One year after discharge, frail patients had a higher rate of hospital readmission. The evaluation of frailty may help to identify patients that would benefit from the multidisciplinary coordination of ICU care, rehabilitation and follow-up care to improve mortality, functional independence and quality of life. Examples of possible areas of intervention include minimization of unnecessary sedation, early and frequent screening for delirium, nutritional support and early mobilization.[8]

Table 19.1 Various definitions of frailty

Ávila-Funes	Fried criteria+ 1. Cognitive impairment
Rothman	Fried criteria+ 1. Cognitive impairment 2. Depressive symptoms
Ensrud	Weight loss 1. Time to get up five times from a chair 2. Decreased energy level 3. Score: 0 = robust; 1 = prefrail; 2+ = frail
Rockwood	1. Modified MMSE 2. Cumulative Illness Rating Scale 3. History of falls 4. Delirium 5. Cognitive impairment or dementia 6. Functional status 7. Urinary incontinence 8. ADL 9. Cognitive impairment, no dementia 10. Mobility Score: 1 (very fit) to 7 (severely frail)
Puts	1. Static: BMI, peak expiratory flow, MMSE, vision, hearing, incontinence, mastery, depression, low physical activity 2. Dynamic: weight loss, decline in peak flow, decline in cognition, loss of vision or hearing, new incontinence, decline in "mastery," activity
Fried	1. Weight loss 2. Grip strength 3. Exhaustion 4. Walking time 5. Physical activity Frail = ≥3 criteria Prefrail = 1 or 2 criteria

The six highest scoring articles that attempted to define, identify and score severity of frailty based on systematic review from Sternberg SA, Schwartz AW, Karunananthan S, Bergman H, Mark Clarfield A. The Identification of Frailty: A Systematic Literature Review. *J Am Geriatr Soc.* 2011;59(11):2129–2138.

Co-Morbidities

Co-morbidity can be defined based on the number of conditions in a given individual and the impact of those conditions on overall health. It is agreed upon that co-morbidities and pre-existing disability have known consequences on outcomes after acute institutionalization. Co-morbidities are associated with increased health care cost, more complex care plans and poorer outcomes.[9] Measures such as co-morbidity can be used as predictors of postdischarge mortality and may help to risk stratify patients and allocate resources.[10] Co-morbid conditions such as degenerative brain disease, cerebrovascular disease, congestive heart failure, chronic obstructive pulmonary disease, diabetes and malnutrition are associated with a greater institutional dependency in the elderly.

Table 19.2 Charlson Comorbidity Index: weighted scores and associated conditions

1	Myocardial infarct, congestive heart failure, peripheral vascular disease, dementia, cerebrovascular disease, chronic lung disease, connective tissue disease, ulcer, chronic liver disease, diabetes
2	Hemiplegia, moderate or severe kidney disease, diabetes with end-organ damage, tumor, leukemia, lymphoma
3	Moderate or severe liver disease
6	Malignant tumor, metastasis, AIDS

Weighted scores are added, an additional point is added for every decade >40 years of age and calculated score is compared to table to determine probability of 1-year and 2-year survival. Adapted from Charlson, Mary E.; Pompei, Peter; Ales, Kathy L.; MacKenzie, C. Ronald (1987). "A new method of classifying prognostic comorbidity in longitudinal studies: Development and validation." *Journal of Chronic Diseases* **40** (5): 373–83.

The ability to accurately assess the burden of a patient's co-morbidities on their health status and its impact on the hospital course remains a challenge. Scales such as the Charlson Index (Table 19.2) can be used to evaluate the mortality rate due to the accumulative burden of co-morbidity and age. This index uses a point system to assess risk of dying with the presence of multiple diseases.[11] Evaluating the patient's co-morbidities pre- and post-ICU admission may help to predict outcome and quality of life, and better prepare the perioperative physician in discussing the risks and benefits of various treatment options with patients and their families.

Cognitive Impairment and Daily Functioning

Cognitive impairment and disability increase the risk of death and institutionalization in the elderly population and various scales are available to assess their impact on overall health status. Examples include: the Mini-Mental State Examination, the Montreal Cognitive Assessment, the Cognitive Abilities Screening Instrument, the Mini-Cog and Katz Index, and SHERPA scale.

The Mini-Mental State Examination (MMSE) is a 30-point questionnaire to measure cognitive impairment. The test is available for purchase online, and has been translated into various languages. A score >25 points out of 30 is considered normal, while a score of ≤9 points indicates severe, 10–18 points moderate and 19–23 points mild cognitive impairment.

The Katz Activities of Daily Living Scale is used to calculate a score that reflects the level of difficulty and need for assistance with bathing, dressing, getting in or out of bed or chairs, eating, walking and toileting.[12]

The SHERPA scale includes five factors: age, impairment in premorbid instrumental ADLs, falls in the year before hospitalization, cognitive impairment (MMSE below 15) and poor self-rated health. The sensitivity and specificity for predicting the risk of functional decline after hospitalization were 67.9% and 70.8%, respectively.[13] Low preadmission functioning and or a loss of function after discharge predict higher overall health resource utilization, higher rates of institutionalization and death.[14]

Cognitive function can also be assessed via the Cognitive Abilities Screening Instrument (CASI),[15] which is based on the MMSE, but has better translation to various languages and cultures. The Mini-Cog, testing word recall and clock drawing, is another assessment that is very short, easy to administer, free to use and easily accessed for clinical use. The Montreal Cognitive Assessment (MoCA) is another test available for download online, geared at first-line questioning in assessing dementia. These tests can identify cognitive dysfunction early and allow the perioperative physician to take action to mitigate insults that can lead to worsening cognitive decline during the acute care phase.

Assessment of the elderly patient's frailty, co-morbidities, cognitive impairment and daily functioning guide the perioperative physician in the triage, risk stratification and harm prevention in the geriatric patient being evaluated for admission to the ICU. The goal of ICU admission should aim to restore patients to their previous health status and navigate them through the period of acute critical illness.

Admission to the ICU

Given the cost and risk of admitting elderly patients to the ICU, physicians should give careful consideration to the question: who should be admitted? The answer is complex and depends on concepts such as resource allocation, potential benefit versus harm to the patient, and of course the patient's goals and wishes.

The Eldicus study demonstrated that physicians are more likely to deny elderly patients admission to the ICU. This practice likely originates from the thought that care may be futile, especially in the setting of a limited life expectancy. Surprisingly, the study uncovered a greater mortality benefit with ICU admission in older patients when compared to their younger counterparts. Investigators observed multiple ICU triage decisions with the primary outcome of mortality at both 28 days and 3 months. Results revealed that mortality was significantly lower in the group admitted to the ICU when compared to the group denied admission. These results offer the argument that admitting sick elderly patients to the ICU improves their chances of survival and may also be cost effective.

Ideally providers should make decisions on the allocation of care based on objective information; in the ICU setting this is particularly difficult. A recent survey of Eldicus investigators and other staff involved in ICU care and triage was performed to determine if there was a consensus on the Society of Critical Care Medicine statement on ICU triage. This cohort agreed upon almost all objective criteria, including number of beds available, the admission diagnosis, severity of disease, age and operative status. They did not agree, however, on criteria involving likelihood of survival. This survey demonstrated that there was no agreement on a survival cutoff for triage, not even for a chance of survival of 0.1%.[16]

Perhaps it is the poor record on prognostication that prevents physicians from denying care to the patient with little chance of survival. It has been suggested that the culture of large hospitals is to emphasize intervention and aim for a "cure" even if some of these interventions are at the cost of patient comfort, the underlying drive being that acceptance of death and transitioning to end-of-life care is difficult for the patient, family and even care providers.[17] It is the intensivist's responsibility to offer the patient and family reasonable expectations regarding prognosis. The goal should be to improve the patient's health and not prolong their suffering, while complying with patient and family wishes for end-of-life care. Multidisciplinary team involvement, including early involvement of palliative care teams, physical therapists and the patient's geriatrician or primary care physician, may help the intensivist arrive at an informed decision about triage, impact on survival and quality of life after discharge.

The scarcity of resources and rising costs mean that not every patient who might benefit from the ICU is able to receive ICU care. In general, patients with longer life expectancies are given more liberal access to the resources in the ICU. Thus, based on age alone, elderly patients are at risk of being denied this same level of care in addition to having worse outcomes. Experts agree that admission decisions should be based on objective criteria (i.e. illness severity and availability of useful interventions) and that providing futile care to one group of patients, regardless of age, may at the same time lead to delays and divert care from a group that may benefit.

The cost of the ICU resources must also be considered. The US spends a larger proportion of its wealth on health care than other nations, reaching 2.8 trillion dollars in 2012 (www.chcf.org). Traditionally, critical care has been viewed as a division of medicine that is high in cost. Multiple studies have been conducted to determine the cost per life saved and cost per life year saved in this cohort. Results demonstrate that costs fall as predicted mortality rises, suggesting that intensive care becomes more cost effective for patients with greater severity of illness.[16] This, along with data from the Eldicus study, makes a strong argument for admission of the very ill elderly.

Common Diagnoses of Critically Ill Geriatric Patients

Delirium

Delirium is defined as a syndrome with various symptoms, including impaired short-term memory, impaired attention, disorientation, acute onset, and a waxing and waning course.[18] The incidence of ICU delirium is thought to range from 30% to 87%, and effects mechanically ventilated patients at a higher proportion compared with nonventilated patients. Older age and dementia are both independent risk factors for the development of delirium in the critically ill patient, making it a very common diagnosis in the old and very old patient. Elderly patients are more likely to experience the hypoactive subtype of delirium. Hypoactive delirium manifests as lack of alertness, slowed or completely absent speech, hypokinesia and lethargy. This subtype is associated with worse prognosis among ICU patients of any age.

There are multiple validated tools for assessing delirium; the most extensively studied is the Confusion Assessment Method for the Intensive Care Unit (CAM-ICU) which is especially useful for ventilated patients since it is a nonverbal scoring system. It evaluates four main factors: acute onset, inattention, disorganized thinking and altered level of consciousness.[18]

Regardless of age, severity of illness and co-morbidity, delirium has been shown to be associated with a 3.2-fold increase in 6-month mortality and also an increase in hospital length of stay.[18] Mortality also increases with increased duration of delirium and leads to cognitive impairment up to 1 year after discharge. The latter complication can lead to decreased quality of life for both patients and their caregivers, and should be taken into consideration when discussing admission and discharge to the ICU.

Both pharmacological and nonpharmacological therapies exist for the treatment and prevention of delirium. Nonpharmacological therapies target risk factors for delirium such as dehydration, immobility, sleep deprivation, visual impairment and hearing

Table 19.3 Common medication therapy for delirium

Medication Class	Indication
Typical antipsychotic haloperidol	– First-line agent
Atypical antipsychotic risperidone, olanzapine, quetiapine	– Some come in sublingual form, similar side effect profile to haloperidol
Benzodiazepines	– Useful in delirium tremens – Associated with increased risk of delirium in elderly – Should not be abruptly discontinued in dependent patients

impairment.[19] Pharmacological treatments include typical and atypical antipsychotics; haloperidol, a first-generation drug, has also been shown to be preventative in a select group of patients. Benzodiazepines can be used for delirium associated with alcohol withdrawal, but should be avoided in other cases and especially with the elderly since there is evidence that these medications and others such as opioids may increase the risk of delirium.[18,20] Recognition, prevention and treatment of delirium – a common, under-diagnosed complication in the ICU – is the responsibility of all caregivers. Common drug therapies for delirium are listed in Table 19.3.

Sepsis

Sepsis carries a mortality rate of about 30% and is the second leading cause of death in the intensive care unit. Older patients are more prone to infection as a result of age-related changes in the immune system, frequent presence of co-morbidities and the iat-rogenic interventions associated with hospitalization.[4] Older patients may present with atypical presentations of infection or impending sepsis, such as altered mental status, delirium and falls, which may lead to a delay in diagnosis and an increase in morbidity. Elderly patients most commonly suffer from infections of the lung, followed by urinary tract and then abdomen. The increased mortality from sepsis is thought to be due to increased co-morbidity, increase in number of invasive procedures and problems associated with being in long-term care facilities and hospitalization. The risk of infection and propensity of acquiring hospital infections in the ICU also goes up with aging. Compromised immunity (failed antigen recognition) and impaired cytokine release may be the cause of the increased susceptibility to infections. Lack of adequate immune response to infection may also delay the recognition of infection in the old and very old population. Infection should be recognized and treated promptly with organism-specific antibiotics. Minimizing risk of hospital-acquired infection is also paramount, encouraging hand washing, proper use of precautions (contact, droplet, etc.) and judicious use of central access and bladder catheterization will help to limit the spread of infection.

For ICU sepsis and septic shock, data from the medical ICU revealed similar outcomes to those discussed in the previous section. In a recent study, age was found to be the only independent predictor of mortality in patients with sepsis. Other studies also found that severity of illness and consciousness impacted mortality and were independent risk factors.[21] The incidence of sepsis increases with age, as does mortality and the risk of dying when compared to younger patients. Delay in treatment of early sepsis may worsen the course in these patients, leading to greater need for invasive therapy such as lines and mechanical ventilation, which can have further adverse effects on prognosis.

Trauma

Over 33 billion dollars a year is spent treating trauma in patients >65 years of age (www.sccm.org). Geriatric patients are at a high risk for trauma, especially falls. The rate of falls is up to three times higher than for other age groups.[22] These patients have higher rates of admission after injury, longer length of stay, and higher morbidity and mortality, even with less severe injury, than their younger counterparts. Poor functional and nutritional status places them at an even greater risk of falls, motor vehicle and pedestrian versus motor vehicle accidents, which are the most common causes of injury in this group.

Though the management of the trauma patient is similar in all adults, special consideration should be taken to account for changes due to aging. The injuries may be less severe than those that would warrant ICU admission in a younger patient, but due to advanced age the complications may be disastrous.[23] Evaluation and proper resuscitation of the elderly trauma patient begins in the emergency department and should continue once admitted to the ICU. Elderly adults have a low tolerance for hemodynamic perturbations and may clinically deteriorate suddenly with little outward indication of impending instability. Low respiratory and cardiac reserve in elderly patients means that even minor injuries can have major complications of cardiac or respiratory failure. Pain, anemia and hypovolemia may result in myocardial ischemia due to underlying coronary artery disease.[24]

The reason why geriatric patients have worse outcomes, despite less severe injury, is multifactorial. Elderly patients cannot compensate for blood loss as well as younger adults. Decreased sensitivity to catecholamines in combination with a stiffened myocardium may result in the inability to increase cardiac output when under stress. Weaker respiratory muscles, less alveolar surface area for gas exchange and decreased chest wall and lung compliance may lead to earlier compromise, especially when faced with injuries such as rib fracture. Decreased cardiovascular and pulmonary reserve may require early initiation of supportive care (i.e. mechanical ventilation, vasopressors). Despite the adversity facing these patients upon admission, the data are promising. One multicenter retrospective study conducted at four level I trauma centers showed an overall mortality of 18%,[22] while another reported geriatric trauma survival rates approaching 85%. Another study demonstrated that admission to the ICU and use of invasive monitoring improved outcome in more severely injured geriatric patients. These patients were victims of blunt trauma, excluding minor falls and burns.[25] Literature suggests that recognition of the impact of even moderate trauma in the elderly is paramount. Triage to a level I trauma center and admission to the ICU with close monitoring can greatly impact outcome, improving the chance of survival.

Outcomes
Mortality of Critically Ill Elderly

In 2013, it was estimated that 1.4 million patients over the age of 65 were discharged from the hospital after ICU admission. Elderly adults are surviving illnesses that were previously considered fatal in this age group. At first glance this is a promising statistic, but long-term outcomes appear to be much more grim. One-third of elderly survivors of critical illness are sent to skilled nursing facilities, 50% are readmitted to the hospital and 25–65% die within 6 months of discharge. Baldwin et al.[26,27] derived a model to predict 6-month mortality in this cohort. They demonstrated that variables, which incorporate frailty, disability, the burden of co-morbidity and patient preferences regarding resuscitation during the hospitalization, have the most predictive power.

It is also known that older adults (over the age of 75) have poorer outcomes than younger patients for any given illness.[28] These patients have high short-term mortality and high rates of long-term disability. Current data suggest that older age compromises survival regardless of type of illness. Biston et al.[29] demonstrated that mortality rates increased with age for patients 75 years and older in the ICU, regardless of the type of shock. These patients are more likely to suffer from cardiogenic shock and equally likely to suffer from septic shock as their younger counterparts. Of very old patients (>85 years old) who were admitted with a diagnosis of sepsis and on at least one vasopressor, <1% were still alive at 1 year after discharge.

The data suggest that for elderly patients, fewer co-morbidities may be of benefit to their long-term survival. Reasonable estimations of prognosis should be discussed with elderly patients and their families early in the admission process. However, identifying the correct patients and providing the correct amount of care does improve chance of survival. Good patient selection is the key to improving outcomes for the elderly. But what happens to quality of life for geriatric patients after the ICU? As survival in the geriatric ICU population increases, this becomes a larger topic of consideration.

Quality of Life After ICU Admission

The World Health Organization defines quality of life as "an individual's perception of their position in life in the context of the culture and value systems in which they live and in relation to their goals, expectations, standards and concerns." In addition to taking into consideration the likelihood of survival, patients, families and physicians should consider the expected quality of life after discharge. Many issues such as disability, independence and cognitive status will affect the elderly patient upon discharge and may lead to changes in decision-making.

Cognitive decline is an important issue for geriatric patients and their caregivers to consider. There is evidence that critical illness may have an impact, in a dose-dependent fashion, on the incidence and severity of cognitive dysfunction.[30] Hypoxemia, delirium, blood glucose derangements, systemic inflammation and sedatives all may play a role in the decline of brain health, independent of stroke.

A large retrospective longitudinal study by Barnato et al.[31] showed worsened disability and dependence for elderly patients after survival of mechanical ventilation. The increase in disability after intervention was small but significant in that it was higher than predicted for given prehospitalization functional status. The investigators concluded that loss of ADLs was likely due to more than just the acute illness-related immobility and may have had a cognitive component as well.

Informing our patients of these and other possible sequelae of admission to the ICU may have an impact on their own personal goals of care. In older patients who have been demonstrated to have a higher 6-month mortality upon discharge from the ICU, the postacute care period may be the targeted time to initiate palliative care to improve access if this is indeed in line with their wishes.

Summary

Issues involved in the care of the critically ill elderly patient are numerous and complex. Thorough initial evaluation, careful patient selection for ICU admission and recognition of potential complications specific to the geriatric population can greatly increase the survival of the elderly critically ill patient. Expectations regarding prognosis and quality of life post ICU stay should be addressed with patients and their families as early as possible. The goal of the perioperative physician during acute critical illness should be to understand the fragile physiologic state of the geriatric patient and to provide care that benefits the patient, while protecting them from iatrogenic harm.

References

1. Luce JM, Rubenfeld GD. Can health care costs be reduced by limiting intensive care at the end of life. *Am J Respir Crit Care Med.* 2002; 165(6): 1–5.

2. Angus DC, Shorr AF, White A, *et al.* Critical care delivery in the United States: distribution of services and compliance with Leapfrog recommendations. *Crit Care Med.* 2006; 34(4):1016–1024.

3. Marik PE. The cost of inappropriate care at the end of life: implications for an aging population. *Am J Hosp Palliat Care.* 2015; 32(7):703–708.

4. Nasa P, Juneja D, Singh O, Dang R, Arora V. Severe sepsis and its impact on outcome in elderly and very elderly patients admitted in intensive care unit. *J Intensive Care Med.* 2011; 27:179–183.

5. Fried LP, Tangen CM, Walston J, *et al.* Frailty in older adults: evidence for a phenotype. *J Gerontol A Biol Sci Med Sci.* 2001; 56:M146–M156.

6. Sternberg SA, Schwartz AW, Karunananthan S, Bergman H, Mark Clarfield A. The identification of frailty: a systematic literature review. *J Am Geriatr Soc.* 2011; 59(11):2129–2138.

7. Bagshaw SM, Stelfox HT, McDermid RC, *et al.* Association between frailty and short- and long-term outcomes among critically ill patients: a multicentre prospective cohort study. *CMAJ.* 2014; 186(2):E95–E102.

8. Fairhall N, Sherrington C, Cameron ID. Effect of a multifactorial interdisciplinary intervention on mobility-related disability in frail older people: randomised controlled trial. *BMC Med.* 2012; 10:120.

9. Valderas JM, Starfield B, Sibbald B, Salisbury C, Roland M. Defining comorbidity: implications for understanding health and health services. *Ann Fam Med.* 2009; 7(4):357–363.

10. Baldwin MR, Narain WR, Wunsch H, *et al.* A prognostic model for 6-month mortality in elderly survivors of critical illness. *Chest.* 2013; 143(4):910–919.

11. Charlson ME, Pompei P, Ales KL, MacKenzie CR. A new method of classifying prognostic comorbidity in longitudinal studies: development and validation. *J Chronic Dis.* 1987; 40(5):373–383.

12. Schweickert WD, Pohlman MC, Pohlman AS, *et al.* Early physical and occupational therapy in mechanically ventilated, critically ill patients: a randomised controlled trial. *Lancet.* 2009; 373:1874–1882.

13. Cornette P, Swine C, Malhomme E, *et al.* Early evaluation of the risk of functional decline following hospitalization of older patients: development of a predictive tool. *Eur J Publ Health.* 2006; 16(2):203–208.

14. Covinsky KE, Justice AC, Rosenthal GE, *et al.* Measuring prognosis and case-mix in hospitalized elders: the importance of functional status. *J Gen Intern Med.* 1997; 12:203–208.

15. Teng EL, Hasegawa K, Homma A, *et al.* The Cognitive Abilities Screening Instrument (CASI): a practical test for cross-cultural epidemiological studies of dementia. *Int Psychogeriatr.* 1994; 6:45.

16. Sprung CL, Geber D, Eidelman LA, *et al.* Evaluation of triage decisions for intensive care admission. *Crit Care Med.* 1999; 27:1073–1079.

17. SUPPORT Principle Investigators. A controlled trial to improve care for seriously ill hospitalised patients: the study to understand prognoses and preferences for outcomes and risks of treatment. *JAMA.* 1995; 274:1591–1598.

18. Cavallazzi R, Saad M, Marik PE. Delirium in the ICU: an overview. *Ann Intensive Care.* 2012; 2:49.

19. Patel J, Baldwin J, Bunting P, Laha S. The effect of a multicomponent multidisciplinary bundle of interventions on sleep and delirium in medical and surgical intensive care patients. *Anaesthesia.* 2014; 9:540–549.

20. Clegg A, Young JB. Which medications to avoid in people at risk of delirium: a systematic review. *Age Ageing.* 2011; 40:23–9.

21. Vosylius S, Sipylaite J, Ivaskevicius J. Determinants of outcome in elderly patients admitted to the intensive care unit. *Age Ageing.* 2005; 34:157–162.

22. Tornetta P, Mostafavi H, Riina J, *et al.* Morbidity and mortality in elderly trauma patients. *J Trauma.* 1999; 46(4):702–706.

23. Meldon SW, Reilly M, Drew BL, Mancuso C, Fallon W. Trauma in the very elderly: a community-based study of outcomes at trauma and nontrauma centers. *J Trauma.* 2002; 52(1):79–84.

24. Mackersie R. Pitfalls in the evaluation and resuscitation of the trauma patient. *Emerg Med Clin North Am.* 2010; 28:1–27.

25. Scalea T, Simon H, Duncan A, *et al.* Geriatric blunt multiple trauma: improved survival with early invasive monitoring. *J Trauma.* 1990; 30:129–136.

26. Baldwin MR, Wunsch H, Reyfman PA. High burden of palliative needs among older intensive care unit survivors transferred to postacute care facilities: a single-center study. *Ann Am Thorac Soc.* 2013; 10(5):458–465.

27. Baldwin MR, Narain WR, Wunsch H, *et al.* A prognostic model for 6-month mortality in elderly survivors of critical illness. *Chest.* 2013; 143(4):910–919.

28. Fuchs L, Chronaki CE, Park S, *et al.* ICU admission characteristics and mortality rates among elderly and very elderly patients. *Intensive Care Med.* 2012; 38:1654–1661.

29. Biston P, Aldecoa C, Devriendt J, *et al.* Outcome of elderly patients with circulatory failure. *Intensive Care Med.* 2013; 40(1):50–56.

30. Jones C. Surviving the intensive care. *Thoracic Surg Clin North Am.* 2012; 22(4):509–516.

31. Barnato AE, Albert SM, Angus DC, Lave JR, Degenholtz HB. Disability among elderly survivors of mechanical ventilation. *Am J Respir Crit Care Med.* 2011; 183(8):1037–1042.

Chapter 20

Pain in the Elderly

Jason L. McKeown and Thomas R. Vetter

Key Points

- Multimodal analgesic regimens for older surgical patients permit lower doses of opioids and a reduction in serious side effects with more rapid return to baseline function.
- Acetaminophen is very well tolerated in the older adult with almost no side effects and is one of the most important components of multimodal analgesic regimens.
- Gabapentin and pregabalin are examples of opioid-sparing medications. The main risk of gabapentinoids in the elderly is dose-dependent sedation and reduction of starting doses is recommended.
- Local anesthetics possess greater opioid-sparing capacity than other multimodal agents.
- Regional anesthetic techniques are associated with superior pain control compared to systemic analgesics and should be used in older patients undergoing surgery as much as possible.
- Aging is associated with an increase in body fat, leading to increase in volume of distribution (and thus duration) for lipophilic analgesics drugs such as fentanyl and ketamine. Reduction in dosing by 25–50% and slow titration of drugs can help avoid exaggerated adverse effects.

Introduction

Due to declining fertility, improved overall health status and greater longevity, most of the world's population is now aging at an unprecedented rate.[1] For example, in the United States, the population who are age 65 years and older has increased 21% from 35.5 million in 2002 to 43.1 million in 2012. This number is projected to more than double to 92 million in 2060. Given advances in health care across the age spectrum, the 85 and older population in the United States is projected to increase by a remarkable 139% from 5.9 million in 2012 to 14.1 million in 2040.[2] At least in economically developed countries like the United States, this aging of the population will be accompanied by an increasing number of surgical operations on elderly patients, with attendant unprecedented health care workforce demands.[3]

Given their major past societal contribution, it can be cogently argued that equitable and compassionate health care for the elderly is a hallmark of a just, higher-order society.[4,5] It is thus quite problematic that the especially vulnerable geriatric population remains very prone to inadequate pain treatment across all care settings – even in developed, higher-income countries like the United States.[4,6] Notably, a gap still exists between best practice recommendations for perioperative pain management in older adults and current clinical practice.[6,7]

This chapter will initially define the Perioperative Surgical Home and specifically discuss its applicability in the geriatric population and its potential role in addressing the unique biopsychosocial pain-related needs of the older surgical patient. It will then use a case-based approach to review geriatric pain management across the perioperative continuum.

One Definition of the Perioperative Surgical Home

Surgical care currently accounts for an estimated 52% of hospital admission expenses in the US.[8] Factors contributing to excessive surgical expenditures include fragmentation and inefficiencies in delivery, defensive medicine, discordant incentives between the stakeholders who deliver versus pay for care and a lack of emphasis on value.[9,10] To address these and other factors, the Perioperative Surgical Home model has been developed using the guiding principles of the ideally aligned Patient-Centered Medical Home.[11,12]

The Perioperative Surgical Home is a highly patient-centered approach to the surgical patient, with a strong emphasis on standardization, coordination, transitions and value of care, throughout the perioperative continuum, including the postdischarge phase.[11-13]

The Perioperative Surgical Home is well positioned to achieve the Triple Aim of health care proposed by Berwick, Nolan and Whittington, and promulgated by the Institute for Healthcare Improvement.[12] This Triple Aim comprises three interdependent goals: (i) improving the individual experience of care, (ii) improving the health of populations, and (iii) reducing per capita costs of care.[14,15] Not surprisingly, many elderly surgical patients have major co-morbidity from chronic diseases.[16] They also often lack the social capital and the wherewithal needed to optimally navigate the complex health care system – especially when undergoing surgery. The older surgical patient is thus a logical and prime candidate for the Perioperative Surgical Home care model.

Role of the Perioperative Surgical Home in Geriatric Perioperative Pain Management

The Perioperative Surgical Home concept continues to evolve. There will very likely be multiple future variations and successive iterations of the Perioperative Surgical Home concept that may work effectively – depending on institutional infrastructure, priorities and resources, as well as internal and external political and economic forces. Nevertheless, there are several opportunities afforded by this new care model that are relevant to perioperative pain management:

- Comprehensive review of prescription and over-the-counter medications, as well as herbal supplements, for potential intraoperative and postoperative adverse reactions and interactions.
- Informing the patient and family members of the patient's right to effective postoperative pain control and the available and most appropriate analgesic options.
- Consenting the patient prior to the day of surgery for an indicated interventional pain modality.

- Educating the patient, family members and other caregivers about the need for close monitoring for postoperative medication-related side effects, so as to avoid over- or underutilization of analgesics, to reduce the risk of falls and to mitigate dose-dependent side effects (e.g. constipation, dysphoria).
- Postoperative, postdischarge care planning, including the need for transition planning, social support and a health care system "navigator."
- Diagnosis and treatment of psychological conditions like depression and anxiety that can exacerbate pain perception.
- Screening for baseline cognitive impairment and an increased risk of postoperative delirium that will obfuscate accurate assessment of pain intensity.

Case Presentation

Mrs. P is a 72-year-old female with history of low back pain and degenerative joint disease of the hips. Acetaminophen has controlled all of her pain symptoms until recently. She is widowed and takes paroxetine for depression. Her joint pain has increased to the point that she is less able to independently care for herself. Reluctantly she has begun relying more on family for shopping and cleaning, and she has stopped going to church because of pain with ambulation. Her primary care physician has prescribed hydrocodone, but she avoids taking it because it makes her dizzy and sleepy. She wants to avoid surgery because she has not had anesthesia in 20 years and she has heard of many people her age who "were never the same afterwards." Unfortunately her orthopedic surgeon says she needs the surgery and there is no other alternative. She consults with an anesthesiologist in preparation for hip replacement surgery.

Mrs. P Presents for Surgery

On the day of surgery the anesthesiologist visits with Mrs. P and her family in the preoperative holding area. She reviews the preoperative assessment and the home medications that the patient was advised to take. Mrs. P's cognitive screening is included in the preoperative notes. The anesthesiologist comforts and reassures her and offers her a nerve block and a preoperative regimen of multimodal analgesic medications to help with pain control.

Multimodal Analgesia

Nonopioid adjuvant analgesics have found a central role in the practice of modern acute pain medicine. Opioids are not unsafe in elders, but the utmost care is required to avoid complications. Combining a range of opioid-sparing adjuvants for preventive analgesia is a wise practice, especially because of the unique sensitivities of the elderly patient.

Acetaminophen

Acetaminophen is very well tolerated in the older adult and has a long history of safe use. It acts as a central cyclo-oxygenase inhibitor with analgesic and antipyretic effects. Besides being a first-line drug for chronic pain treatment in the elderly, acetaminophen has become one of the most important components of multimodal analgesic regimens.[17,18] It provides opioid-sparing analgesia for surgical pain. Side effects are very rare. It is not associated with GI disturbance. It has very low risk for toxicity, except in patients with heavy alcohol consumption or severely impaired liver function. Hypovolemic surgical patients and malnourished patients are also at higher risk for liver damage.

Hepatic toxicity is a serious concern as many over-the-counter cold remedies contain acetaminophen. Patients discharged after surgery on acetaminophen or combination analgesics containing it should be reminded not to exceed the maximum dose of 4000 mg a day. For ease of adherence to a prescribed regimen it may be best to avoid combination analgesics altogether and instead use a stand-alone analgesic like oxycodone; acetaminophen can then be added as a separate dose, e.g. acetaminophen 650 mg every 6 hours. In malnourished adults (>50 kg) with depressed hepatic or renal function, the maximum recommended daily dose is lowered to 2000 mg.

Nonsteroidal Anti-Inflammatory Drugs (NSAIDs)

NSAIDs inhibit cyclo-oxygenase enzymes which mediate inflammation in postsurgical pain. These drugs have a strong role in postoperative pain treatment, especially in orthopedic procedures where peripheral inflammation is a primary pain mechanism. NSAIDs are quite effective analgesics, but are sometimes not tolerated well in the elderly. Gastrointestinal bleeding and ulceration are more common in older adults. Anticoagulants, antiplatelet drugs and glucocorticoid steroids increase gastric risks. The COX-2-selective drugs like celocoxib are less associated with bleeding complications, but the protective effect is over-ridden with concurrent use of aspirin. All NSAIDs may cause fluid retention and hypernatremia, which may be dangerous in patients with CHF. Acute kidney injury is a risk that is increased in anemic or hypovolemic patients. Concomitant use of ACE inhibitors and diuretics increases renal risk as well. Given the physiologic decline in renal function with aging, glomerular filtration rate is the most sensitive lab value to guide the use of NSAIDs. Serum creatinine is sometimes misleading because of decreased muscle mass in older adults. The vasoconstrictive effect of NSAIDs in patients with coronary or cerebrovascular disease is unlikely to have clinical significance when used short-term for acute postsurgical pain. NSAIDs occasionally may cause confusion in the frail elder.

Gabapentinoids

Gabapentin and pregabalin have an excellent history of efficacy in chronic neuropathic pain. Analgesia is produced by binding to the $\alpha_2\delta$ subunit of neuronal calcium channels. Gabapentinoids have been extensively studied for a variety of surgical procedures like hysterectomy, orthopedics and spine. The opioid-sparing effect of this class of drugs is well documented.[19,20] Reduction in pain scores has been shown to extend to 24 hours after surgery with a single preoperative dose. The main risk of gabapentinoids in the elderly is dose-dependent sedation. Reduced dosing is advisable, especially in patients who are naïve to this class of drugs. Single preoperative oral doses of gabapentin 300–400 mg are reasonable. Gabapentinoids undergo no hepatic metabolism and are excreted completely by the kidney. Therefore patients with compromised renal function are at particular risk for adverse effects. Other side effects pertinent to the elderly are dizziness and cognitive complaints. Lower extremity swelling and visual disturbances are more common when used long term for chronic pain. Pregabalin may cause fewer side effects, including sedation. It is more potent and bioavailable than gabapentin. Gabapentin has been studied as a medication preventive against postoperative delirium; its opioid-sparing effects were thought to be protective.[21]

Tramadol

Tramadol is a weak opioid agonist, but its lower potency and properties similar to antidepressants have led to its inclusion in some multimodal plans as a substitute for stronger opioids. Its analgesic efficacy is comparable to codeine, roughly one-tenth the potency of morphine. Also similar to codeine is its dependence on CYP 2D6 for production of its active metabolite, O-desmethyl-tramadol. Tramadol is useful because of lower respiratory risk, but unfortunately it is linked to delirium in older patients. Because of its inhibitory effects on serotonin and norepinephrine reuptake it must be used with caution in patients taking other antidepressants. Drug–drug interactions such as serotonin syndrome are possible. Tramadol is also contraindicated in patients with seizures or compromised renal function, which can lead to accumulation of epileptogenic metabolites.

Regional Analgesic Techniques

Local anesthetics possess greater opioid-sparing capacity than other multimodal agents. Regional anesthetic techniques are associated with superior pain control compared to systemic analgesics and have many other positive benefits in the postoperative period. Aspects of enhanced recovery include earlier hospital discharge time, shorter intensive care stays, earlier ambulation, earlier return of bowel function and improved mental status, and lower mortality rate.[22,23]

Perineural Blocks

Regional anesthesia has become irreplaceably important in the treatment of pain after joint replacement and many other types of surgery. Common techniques are single-dose perineural injections and indwelling catheter insertion for continuous infusion of local anesthetics. The use of disposable infusion pumps and even newer sustained-release liposomal local anesthetics are expanding the limits of ambulatory surgery. Inpatient stays are shortened as well, and the effectiveness of physical therapy is enhanced. Other considerations make perineural blocks preferable when compared to neuraxial interventions. There are fewer serious risks associated with hemorrhage at the catheter site. Perineural catheters can be placed and removed without monitoring specific lab values. Perineural blocks have minimal effects on hemodynamics. Another important advantage for ambulatory surgery is the elimination of the need for a urinary catheter. The elimination of parenteral opioids by regional analgesia also helps to avoid urinary retention that may be caused by opioids.

Perineural injection techniques are safe in the elderly, but the risk of local anesthetic toxicity deserves special attention in frail patients. Lower serum protein levels lead to higher concentrations of unbound local anesthetic in the plasma. Older adults with end-organ disease, particularly cardiac, hepatic and renal, are at greatest risk for harm. Levoisomer drugs like ropivacaine have less risk for cardiac and CNS toxicity, but an important practice no matter what anesthetic is used is to administer the smallest volume and lowest concentration of drug appropriate for a specific block.[24] If multiple perineural catheters are used, the total volume of local anesthetic infused should be reduced accordingly.

Older patients may present technical challenges for regional interventionalists. Patients who present with acute trauma can be difficult to position. The risks of procedural sedation in the elderly such as delirium and respiratory depression must be considered. Small doses of fentanyl and propofol, and avoidance of benzodiazepines are best during positioning. Low-dose ketamine or dexmedetomidine also offer potent but short-duration analgesia, while helping to maintain spontaneous ventilation. Ultrasound guidance and nerve stimulation techniques both may be complicated in older patients. Loss of muscle mass and poor tissue echogenicity may cause poor visualization. Obesity challenges the identification of surface landmarks and increases the depth of needle placement when a stimulator approach is used.

Other unique considerations affect the elderly with cognitive impairment. When such individuals are discharged home with blocks and indwelling catheters, caregivers should be aware of increased fall risk and should be vigilant toward the risk of the patient pulling and dislodging indwelling catheters. Leakage of fluid at the catheter site can cause premature migration and failure of the catheter. Wetness and skin irritation could be a source of agitation and confusion in cognitively impaired patients. Bedbound patients should have attentive monitoring for skin breakdown at catheter and dressing sites.

In all patients a step-down plan to oral analgesics should be prescribed in advance for when a single-dose block wears off or when a catheter is removed. In elderly patients and especially those with cognitive impairment, caregivers should be thoroughly educated on this plan.

Neuraxial Techniques

Epidural analgesia has been shown to provide superior pain control in the postoperative period compared to systemic opioids. Other benefits from regional anesthesia like the sparing of opioids and mitigation of the surgical stress response may benefit elderly patients who are sicker with multiple co-morbidities. Outcomes that are very beneficial to older patients are related to earlier normalization of bowel function and earlier ambulation.[25,26] Effects on bowel motility are limited to thoracic-level epidurals through which local anesthetics cause a sympathectomy to the gut. Local anesthetics, not opioids, alter the surgical stress response.[27] Technical difficulties, the use of anticoagulant drugs and complexities of postoperative catheter management often prevent older patients from receiving epidural analgesia.

Epidural analgesia with opioid, local anesthetic or a combination of both provides superior analgesia for dynamic or rest pain compared to systemic opioids.[28] A combined low-dose infusion of opioid and local anesthetic is most appropriate for limiting the toxic effects of each drug. Older adults are more sensitive to systemic and epidural opioids compared to younger patients. Surprisingly dilute opioid epidural infusions produce profound analgesia. Elderly patients are also more sensitive to the effects of local anesthetics within the epidural space. Age-related central and foraminal stenosis reduce the capacity of the epidural space and lead to wider spread of injected volume. The risk of greater cephalocaudal spread is a more pronounced sympathectomy and subsequent hypotension. Bolus doses must be reduced accordingly. Catheter placement at the spinal level that corresponds to the surgical dermatome will help limit the volume required to cover incisional pain.

PACU Stay

Mrs. P decides against regional analgesia because of concern over the risk of persistent nerve deficit after the block. She undergoes an uncomplicated general anesthetic. She receives fentanyl and ketamine during the case. She is extubated and transferred to the

PACU. Ninety minutes after arrival she remains drowsy. She rouses to voice, is moderately confused and is oriented only to person. She complains of no pain, but moans and calls for her deceased husband.

Concerns with Regional Anesthesia

Elders with co-morbidities such as diabetes-related and other peripheral neuropathies may be at higher risk for persistent neural deficits after regional blockade. Nevertheless a complete risk versus benefits discussion should be presented to older patients not as a way to minimize the risk of nerve injury (2 in 10,000 blocks), but to candidly present the risks of systemic opioid medication in postoperative pain treatment. The advantageous qualities of the regional anesthetic techniques described above need to be stressed. If appropriate for the surgical procedure and in the absence of contraindications like coagulopathy, or aortic stenosis, older patients should always be offered the option of regional anesthesia. Preoperative counseling should also sensitively allay fears of regional techniques that are based on misconceptions. When elders quickly refuse it is wise to ask specifically what their greatest concern is. It is also important to address any hearing loss or other communication barrier the patient may have. If cognitive impairment is present, having a spouse or family member participate during counseling is valuable.

Pharmacokinetic Changes

The aging adult's body composition differs from that of a younger adult with the loss of muscle mass and the replacement of muscle with adipose. Due to this pharmacokinetic change in volumes of drug distribution the older patient becomes vulnerable in two ways. Water-soluble drugs like morphine exert greater toxic effects per unit dose. This underlies the old adage "Start low and go slow." Reduction in dosing by 25–50% and slow titration of drugs helps to avoid exaggerated adverse effects. More significant in the case of Mrs. P is the increase in fat volume of distribution. Lipophilic drugs commonly used during surgery like fentanyl and ketamine are more widely distributed and have longer half-lives as a consequence. This can contribute to prolonged emergence, postoperative delirium and the need for continued airway support.

Postoperative delirium can have many causes in the elderly patient, especially the patient with cognitive dysfunction. All possible causes must be explored, but a very common cause is uncontrolled pain. While overdosing of some analgesics can promote delirium, in some cases more proactive opioid dosing actually decreases risk for some patients, such as those with dementia.[29] It is important for the clinician to recognize patient and surgical factors and plan in advance how measured an approach to use.

Pain Perception and Pain Behavior

Elderly patients are at greater risk for undertreatment of pain compared to younger counterparts. Different presentations of pain like traumatic, headache or abdominal may also bias towards undertreatment.[30] Cognitively impaired individuals are at greater risk than intact patients. Pain perception thresholds have been shown in lab models to be normally maintained in older patients, including those with cognitive impairment.[31] Although thresholds are normal, pain stimuli are processed differently at the cortical level. Central neurodegenerative changes alter the way in which pain is expressed by the patient, especially the affective component of pain. A patient's affect and pain behavior strongly influence a clinician's objective assessment. Thus it is not surprising that pain in the cognitively impaired patient could be underestimated. In the patient with cognitive impairment or altered mental status the direct observation of pain behaviors like grimacing, resistance to movement, vocalization and restlessness inform the clinician of uncontrolled pain.

Measurement of Pain

In all patients the experience of pain is a unique experience subject to factors that may lead to difficult interpretation of scores. Such factors include level of education, depression, vision or hearing loss and cognitive dysfunction. But pain scoring instruments are available and have been tested successfully in patients with all sorts of limitations. Most older patients can report pain and give a numeric score or can respond to another pain scale. The Numeric Pain Scale using 0–10 scoring and the Verbal Descriptor Scale with "mild, moderate, severe" responses are validated, preferred tools, even in patients who have mild to moderate cognitive decline. The Visual Analog Scale is a type of tool used in patients with speech or hearing impairment. Doloplus-2 and Pain Assessment Checklist for Seniors with Limited Ability to Communicate are useful for patients with severe dementia.[32,33]

Postoperative Course

Mrs. P is discharged to a step-down ICU for monitoring of her delirium, which begins to resolve as her pain is successfully controlled, and her family is present at her bedside to comfort and reorient her.

Treatment of Postoperative Pain with Opioids

Even though opioids by intravenous route carry the highest risk of adverse events in older patients, in the case of major surgery opioids are still first-line agents. Elders are physiologically more sensitive to analgesics. A general rule of thumb is to reduce the starting dose by half compared to a younger patient.[34] Intravenous PCA is an effective way in most patients to allow self-titration to comfort with a lowered cumulative dose. It can safely be used in some patients with cognitive impairment.[35] If oral opioids are used, an effective practice is to routinely schedule low doses to be given as "offer may refuse" instead of "as needed." This is appropriate in patients with cognitive impairment.

Selection of opioid analgesics should be influenced by patient factors such as renal or hepatic impairment, as well as frailty. The specific metabolism of various opioids must be considered. In the acute setting with typical dosing, opioid metabolites pose little risk to patients, but opioids with active metabolites have a greater risk of harm in susceptible patients. The conjugates, morphine-6-glucuronide and morphine-3-glucuronide, have longer half-lives than native morphine and can accumulate in patients with renal insufficiency causing respiratory depression and delirium. Normeperidine, the abundant product of meperidine metabolism presents a threat for seizure in patients with age-related physiologic renal decline. Glomerular filtration rate is the most accurate indicator of renal status considering decline in muscle mass and serum creatinine. Hydromorphone and fentanyl are the most efficacious opioid analgesics for intravenous acute pain relief that are devoid of potentially harmful metabolites.

Opioid-Related Adverse Effects

Elderly patients are physiologically more sensitive to all effects of analgesic drugs, including the harmful effects. Patients with other co-morbidities and those with polypharmacy risk must be carefully managed. The sedative effect of opioids pose a much greater risk in patients with obstructive sleep apnea, which is common in older patients. Increased vigilance with monitoring of pulse oximetry and end-tidal capnography are recommended when patients at high risk for airway obstruction are receiving moderate doses of opioids. Drugs used to treat side effects in younger patients are often potentially harmful to older patients. Diphenhydramine to treat pruritus and scopolamine for nausea should not be used in the elderly. Both drugs can precipitate delirium. Finally, older patients should always be prescribed a bowel regimen when opioid therapy is begun. Constipation can lead to confusion and agitation. Docusate combined with stimulant laxatives such as sennosides or bisacodyl are effective.

Discharge Concerns

Five days after surgery Mrs. P is not sleeping well. During the day she is irritable but alert. While participating with physical therapy she does not appear uncomfortable, but when questioned about her pain she complains tearfully of how horrible it is. She is fearful she will never have her life back and that her family will abandon her.

The similarity in neurophysiology between depression, anxiety and chronic pain underlies the common co-existence of these states. Across all ages of adult chronic pain patients the rate of co-morbid depression is similar.[36] Elders with chronic pain report fewer anxiety symptoms than younger patients.[37] Pre-existing co-morbid mood disorders should be identified preoperatively and managed proactively because pain intensity is amplified in these patients and analgesic consumption is increased.[38,39] Subclinical psychiatric disease can certainly be unmasked during the stressful postoperative period. It is critically important to resume any preoperative medications for mood disorders as soon as possible in the postoperative phase.

Clinicians must also be mindful of the biopsychosocial framework of pain and that all pain reported from a physical source may not be. True organic pain may be augmented by social or spiritual suffering; distress from these domains may also mimic physical pain. When a patient's reported level of pain seems out of proportion to the objective findings and other sources (infection, compartment syndrome, neuralgia) of postoperative pain are ruled out, interdisciplinary specialties like family support, psychology and pastoral care should be consulted. These specialists can sensitively explore and treat areas of suffering that may be contributing to uncontrolled pain.

Summary

Undergoing a major surgical procedure is undoubtedly one the most stressful events in an individual's life. An otherwise independent, well-informed and proactive person can become a dependent, passive and bewildered patient – in the very foreign and often ironically hostile health care environment. Thus a very appropriate question posed by many surgical patients is "What can I do to improve the outcomes that are most important to me?" Assuring that patients and their families can answer this key question not only optimizes clinical outcomes, but also the patient experience. Effective yet safe pain treatment is an important outcome for patients, their family members and their health care providers. Perioperative medicine naturally encompasses robust pain management. Bridging the gap that still exists between best practices for perioperative pain management in older adults and current clinical practice will entail a more personalized approach to care and allow for more consistently positive outcomes.

References

1. Kinsella K, He W. *An Aging World: 2008, International Population Reports, P95/09-1.* Suitland, MD, US Census Bureau, 2009.

2. Administration on Aging. *A Profile of Older Americans: 2013*. Washington, DC, US Department of Health and Human Services, 2014.

3. Dall TM, Gallo PD, Chakrabarti R, et al. An aging population and growing disease burden will require a large and specialized health care workforce by 2025. *Health Affairs (Project Hope)*. 2013; 32(11):2013–2020.

4. Vetter TR. Healthcare policy in pain management. In: Benzon HT, Rathmell JP, Wu CL, Turk DC, Argoff CE, Hurley RW, eds., *Raj's Practical Management of Pain, 5th edn*. New York, Elsevier, 2013; 47–55.

5. Levine MA, Wynia MK, Schyve PM, et al. Improving access to health care: a consensus ethical framework to guide proposals for reform. *Hastings Center Report* 2007; 37(5):14–19.

6. Herr K. Pain in the older adult: an imperative across all health care settings. *Pain Manag Nurs*. 2010; 11(2 Suppl):S1–S10.

7. Schofield PA. The assessment and management of peri-operative pain in older adults. *Anaesthesia*. 2014; 69 (Suppl 1):54–60.

8. Health Care Cost Institute. Health care cost and utlization report: 2011/2012. 2013. Available from: www.healthcostinstitute.org/files/HCCI_HCCUR2011.pdf (Accessed July 18, 2017).

9. Cormier JN, Cromwell KD, Pollock RE. Value-based health care: a surgical oncologist's perspective. *Surg Oncol Clin North Am*. 2012; 21(3):497–506.

10. Fry DE, Pine M, Jones BL, Meimban RJ. The impact of ineffective and inefficient care on the excess costs of elective surgical procedures. *J Am Coll Surg*. 2011; 212(5):779–786.

11. Vetter TR, Goeddel LA, Boudreaux AM, et al. The Perioperative Surgical Home: how can it make the case so everyone wins? *BMC Anesth*. 2013; 13:6.

12. Vetter TR, Boudreaux AM, Jones KA, Hunter JM Jr., Pittet JF. The Perioperative Surgical Home: how anesthesiology can collaboratively achieve and leverage the Triple Aim in health care. *Anesth Analg*. 2014; 118(5):1131–1316.

13. Vetter TR, Ivankova NV, Goeddel LA, McGwin G Jr., Pittet JF. An analysis of methodologies that can be used to validate if a Perioperative Surgical Home improves the patient-centeredness, evidence-based practice, quality, safety, and value of patient care. *Anesthesiology*. 2013; 119(6):1261–1274.

14. Berwick DM, Nolan TW, Whittington J. The Triple Aim: care, health, and cost. *Health Affairs*. 2008; 27(3):759–769.

15. Stiefel M, Nolan K. A guide to measuring the Triple Aim: population health, experience of care, and per capita cost. IHI Innovation Series White Paper. Cambridge, MA, Institute for Healthcare Improvement, 2012. Available from: www.IHI.org (Accessed July 18, 2017).

16. Turrentine FE, Wang H, Simpson VB, Jones RS. Surgical risk factors, morbidity, and mortality in elderly patients. *J Am Coll Surg*. 2006; 203(6):865–877.

17. Moon YE, Lee YK, Lee J, Moon DE. The effects of preoperative intravenous acetaminophen in patients undergoing abdominal hysterectomy. *Arch Gynecol Obstetr*. 2011; 284(6):1455–1460.

18. Toms L, McQuay HJ, Derry S, Moore RA. Single dose oral paracetamol (acetaminophen) for postoperative pain

in adults. *Cochrane Database Syst Rev.* 2008(4):CD004602.

19. Chang CY, Challa CK, Shah J, Eloy JD. Gabapentin in acute postoperative pain management. *Biomed Res Int.* 2014; 2014:631756.

20. Kong VK, Irwin MG. Gabapentin: a multimodal perioperative drug? *Br J Anaesth.* 2007; 99(6):775–786.

21. Leung JM, Sands LP, Rico M, *et al.* Pilot clinical trial of gabapentin to decrease postoperative delirium in older patients. *Neurology.* 2006; 67(7):1251–1253.

22. Pasero C, Rakel B, McCaffery M. Postoperative pain management in the older adult. In: Gibson SJ, Weiner DK, eds., *Pain in Older Persons.* Progress in Pain Research and Management. Vol. 35. Seattle, IASP Press, 2005; 377–395.

23. Bulka CM, Shotwell MS, Gupta RK, Sandberg WS, Ehrenfeld JM. Regional anesthesia, time to hospital discharge, and in-hospital mortality: a propensity score matched analysis. *Reg Anesth Pain Med.* 2014; 39(5):381–386.

24. Rosenberg PH, Veering BT, Urmey WF. Maximum recommended doses of local anesthetics: a multifactorial concept. *Reg Anesth Pain Med.* 2004; 29(6):564–575; discussion 24.

25. Park WY, Thompson JS, Lee KK. Effect of epidural anesthesia and analgesia on perioperative outcome: a randomized, controlled Veterans Affairs cooperative study. *Ann Surg.* 2001; 234(4):560–569; discussion 9–71.

26. Moraca RJ, Sheldon DG, Thirlby RC. The role of epidural anesthesia and analgesia in surgical practice. *Ann Surg.* 2003; 238(5):663–673.

27. Kehlet H, Holte K. Effect of postoperative analgesia on surgical outcome. *Br J Anaesth.* 2001; 87(1):62–72.

28. Block BM, Liu SS, Rowlingson AJ, *et al.* Efficacy of postoperative epidural analgesia: a meta-analysis. *JAMA.* 2003; 290(18):2455–2463.

29. Morrison RS, Magaziner J, Gilbert M, *et al.* Relationship between pain and

opioid analgesics on the development of delirium following hip fracture. *J Gerontol Ser A, Biol Sci Med Sci.* 2003; 58(1):76–81.

30. Hwang U, Belland LK, Handel DA, *et al.* Is all pain is treated equally? A multicenter evaluation of acute pain care by age. *Pain.* 2014; 155(12):2568–2574.

31. Scherder E, Oosterman J, Swaab D, *et al.* Recent developments in pain in dementia. *BMJ (Clinical research ed).* 2005; 330(7489):461–464.

32. Falzone E, Hoffmann C, Keita H. Postoperative analgesia in elderly patients. *Drugs Aging.* 2013; 30(2):81–90.

33. Gagliese L, Katz J. Age differences in postoperative pain are scale dependent: a comparison of measures of pain intensity and quality in younger and older surgical patients. *Pain.* 2003; 103(1–2):11–20.

34. Pasero CL, McCaffery M. Managing postoperative pain in the elderly. *Am J Nurs.* 1996; 96(10):38–45; quiz 6.

35. Licht E, Siegler EL, Reid MC. Can the cognitively impaired safely use patient-controlled analgesia? *J Opioid Manag.* 2009; 5(5):307–312.

36. Herr KA, Mobily PR, Smith C. Depression and the experience of chronic back pain: a study of related variables and age differences. *Clin J Pain.* 1993; 9(2):104–114.

37. Corran TM GS, Farrell MJ, Helme RD. Comparison of chronic pain experience between young and elderly patients. In: Gebhart GF, Hammond D, Jensen TS, eds., *Proceedings of the 7th World Congress on Pain.* Seattle, IASP Press, 1994:895–906.

38. De Cosmo G, Congedo E, Lai C, Primieri P, Dottarelli A, Aceto P. Preoperative psychologic and demographic predictors of pain perception and tramadol consumption using intravenous patient-controlled analgesia. *Clin J Pain.* 2008; 24(5):399–405.

39. Taenzer P, Melzack R, Jeans ME. Influence of psychological factors on postoperative pain, mood and analgesic requirements. *Pain.* 1986; 24(3):331–342.

Chapter 21

Palliative Care

Mary K. Buss and Ellen P. McCarthy

Key Points

- Palliative care is specialized medical care for people living with serious illness. It focuses on providing relief from the symptoms and stress of a serious illness. The goal is to improve quality of life.
- Despite increased mortality and morbidity associated with surgery in older patients, 18% of Medicare beneficiaries have surgery during their last month and 8% had surgery during the last week of life.
- Palliative care can be divided into three major domains: symptom management, psychosocial-spiritual support and decision-making.
- Hospice is an important component of palliative care that provides care focused on comfort and symptom relief, without a curative intent. To qualify for hospice care, patients must have a life expectancy of 6 months or less.
- Palliative care is appropriate for various patient populations, such as older adults with limited life expectancy, patients with serious illness, patients with multimorbidity, heavy symptom burden, or frailty, or other geriatric syndromes.
- Palliative care teams can be especially valuable for patients undergoing surgery, help patients manage postoperative symptoms, adapt to new limits and facilitate decision-making if complications or frailty limit postoperative functional status.

Introduction

Surgery is common among older patients with chronic illnesses. Approximately one in three Medicare beneficiaries have surgery during their last year of life.[1] Despite increased mortality[2] and morbidity[3–5] associated with surgery in older patients, 18% of Medicare beneficiaries had surgery during their last month and 8% had surgery during the last week of life.[6] Older patients who received surgery have more hospitalizations, longer stays in the hospital and in intensive care units[6] compared to hospitalized patients who did not undergo surgery. The number of frail elders who undergo surgery is also notable, with prevalence estimates of 4–50% across various older surgical populations.[7] Studies suggest that surgery performed on frail elders has little capacity to increase survival or allow individuals to return to their prior level of function or quality of life[8,9] and is associated with poor postoperative outcomes and institutionalization postdischarge.

Patient preferences alone do not explain the trends in increased surgical intensity at the end of life. A survey of Medicare beneficiaries found that most respondents expressed preferences for less intensive care. For example, fewer than 10% wanted to die in a hospital, 17% wanted potentially life-saving drugs that would make them feel worse all the time and only 21% would want mechanical ventilation to extend their life by 1 month; conversely, more than 75% wanted medication to make them feel better, even if it shortened their life.[10] Despite preferences for improved quality of life and functional status over prolongation of life, when faced with the decision to undergo a high-risk surgical intervention, many elders will choose surgery.[11] The reasons for this choice are manifold, but inadequate understanding of the long-term consequences related to surgery and perceptions that failure to undergo surgery is choosing to die play a substantial role in this choice. Moreover, up to half of elders do not have advanced care planning prior to surgery despite the high rates of morbidity and mortality related to surgery.[12] An improved appreciation and understanding of the role of palliative care may help elders make more informed decisions about surgical interventions that are more consistent with their overall preferences and goals of care.

What is Palliative Care?

The field of palliative care has grown tremendously in the last two decades. Starting in 2006, Hospice and Palliative Medicine became an official subspecialty of the American Board of Medical Specialties (ABMS) and was recognized by the American Osteopathic Association (AOA) the following year. Despite its growth, many do not understand what "palliative care" entails or have misconceptions about the field. A recent survey of Americans found that 70% were "not at all knowledgeable" about palliative care. Ideally this knowledge gap creates an opportunity for clinicians to clarify the intent of palliative care and how it can help patients and their families. Practically, however, the same survey found that most health care professionals equate palliative care with end-of-life care.[13] This common misconception deprives patients, families and other providers of opportunities to integrate palliative care into medical care earlier in the course of illness. Simply defined:

> "Palliative care, [also known as] palliative medicine, is specialized medical care for people living with serious illness. It focuses on providing relief from the symptoms and stress of a serious illness – whatever the diagnosis. The goal is to improve quality of life for both the patient and the family." (www.capc.org/about/palliative-care/)

Palliative care is a comprehensive approach to medical care, which embraces needs of patients and their families and requires an interdisciplinary team. Physicians and nurses work side by side with other specialists, such as social workers, chaplains, pharmacists, psychologists and dieticians to address physical as well as psychosocial and spiritual needs of patients and families.

The components of palliative care fall into three major domains: symptom management, psychosocial-spiritual support and decision-making (see Figure 21.1). Assessment and management of pain, nausea, delirium, anorexia, fatigue and dyspnea are common reasons to involve a palliative care subspecialty team in the care of a patient. Often symptoms can be improved with an approach that focuses solely on the physical aspects, but complex or refractory symptoms frequently heighten anxiety or depression and can impact a person's ability to fulfill key social roles, such as successful small business owner, family breadwinner, supportive spouse or loving parent. In such circumstances, the role

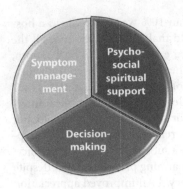

Figure 21.1 Components of palliative care.

of the chaplain, social worker or psychologist is key to finding ways for the individual to adapt and cope, even if physical limitations remain. Palliative care is devoted to helping patients find value and make meaning, even in a time of serious illness or limited prognosis. Supportive care can extend to family caregivers, during active caregiving and into bereavement, when appropriate.

Finally, palliative care teams take an active role in helping patients and families with difficult medical choices. If patients know they have less than a year to live, they often elect to eschew more aggressive care.[14] However, many patients overestimate their prognosis and have unrealistic ideas about what medical treatments can accomplish.[15] Palliative care providers work closely with the patient's other specialists to ensure that patients and families have a clear understanding of their prognosis so they can make decisions grounded in realistic expectations that also align with their personal values and goals. Patients and families sometimes have differing opinions about whether the patient should pursue a particular intervention. Palliative care teams work with families to understand individual perspectives and reconcile differences. Palliative care teams also advocate that patients choose a health care proxy and complete advance directives, so that their wishes regarding medical care are honored if they become too sick to speak for themselves.

When is Palliative Care Appropriate?

The common misconception that palliative care is equivalent to end-of-life care denies patients and families access to palliative care until very late in the illness trajectory. There is emerging evidence indicating the benefits of early integration of palliative care. A randomized controlled trial of patients with stage IV non-small-cell lung cancer (median survival: 9–12 months) comparing early, integrated palliative care to standard of care found that patients who received early palliative care had an improvement in quality of life, reduced depression and were less likely to receive aggressive care at the end of life, such as visits to the emergency room and time in the intensive care unit.[16] Despite less aggressive care, patients receiving early palliative care also lived 2.7 months longer than those in the standard arm, a difference that was statistically significant (11.6 versus 8.9 months; p = 0.02). This sentinel study has been instrumental in helping promote the benefits of early palliative care and dispel myths that palliative care is appropriate only at the end of life. Additionally, this study, which is now joined by several other high quality studies,[17–20]

(a)

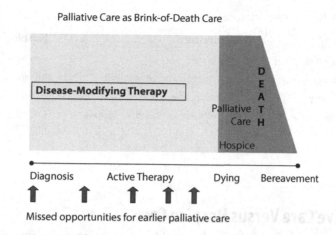

(b)

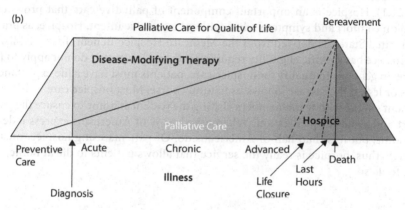

Figure 21.2 (a) Palliative care: delayed integration model. (b) Palliative care: early integration model.

argues strongly against an inherent and unspoken concern of many patients and providers that a palliative approach to care might shorten survival. There is no evidence that early integration of palliative care decreases survival.

The scientific evidence does demonstrate that palliative care improves patient quality of life, enhances patient and caregiver satisfaction, reduces symptom burden and decreases health care utilization at the end of life.[21,22] The benefits of palliative care for patients with serious illnesses being maximized through integration early in the trajectory of illnesses are evident and health care professionals should utilize opportunities created by decision points (such as surgery) to educate patients and their families on the benefits afforded by an integrated palliative care approach. By conceiving of palliative care more narrowly as "end-of-life" care, one risks palliative care becoming "brink-of-death" care and deprives patients and families of the benefits to quality of life seen with earlier integration (see Figure 21.2). Determining how best to identify the patients and the point of entry for palliative care for diagnoses beyond lung cancer and other solid tumors is an active area of research.

Table 21.1 Palliative Care ≠ Hospice

	Palliative care	Hospice
Philosophy/goals	Quality of life	Comfort
Life expectancy	Serious illness; no prognostic limits	<6 months
Primary delivery	Consultation; co-management	Home-based nursing
Approach to disease	WITH treatment for underlying disease	EXCLUDES disease-directed treatment

Palliative Care Versus Hospice Care

Palliative care is often mistakenly considered to be synonymous with hospice care (Table 21.1). Hospice is an important component of palliative care that provides care focused on comfort and symptom relief, without a curative intent. Hospice, as practiced in the United States, is derived from the Medicare Hospice Benefit, first established in 1983. Hospice has specific eligibility requirements and limits that do not apply to palliative care, in general. To qualify for hospice care, patients must have a life expectancy of 6 months or less, if the disease follows its natural course. Most hospice care is delivered in the patient's home with team members visiting the patient at home to ensure the patient's comfort and avoid hospitalization. When asked, 80% of Americans express a desire to die at home, but less than half of Americans do. Of patients using hospice, most died at home.[23] Thus, hospice is really the service that allows patients to die at home, if they choose to do so.

Hospice Services

When patients and families elect to use their hospice benefit, they receive pain and symptom management from an interdisciplinary team, comprising a nurse, a social worker, home health aides, chaplain, volunteers and a hospice medical director. The patient chooses a primary physician of record, usually their primary care physician, though patients seen primarily by a specialist, such as an oncologist or cardiologist, may elect the specialist to be the doctor of record for hospice. Team members visit the patient and family at the patient's residence to assess symptoms, adjust medications to alleviate or mitigate symptoms, and provide comfort and support to the patient and the family. Durable medical equipment, such as a hospital bed, commode and supplemental oxygen are delivered to the home. Hospice also covers the cost of all medications related to the hospice diagnosis, including schedule II opioid analgesics. Patients on hospice have access to a hospice provider 24 hours a day/7 days a week. For example, patients with worsening symptoms, can call or page the on-call nurse and receive guidance over the phone. When needed or appropriate, the hospice provider will come to the patient's home. Facilitating access to a provider and their expertise is an enormous source of comfort to family members, who provide the bulk of care to patients and is what allows patients to stay in their own home at this critical time.

Limitations of Hospice

Hospice care has specific limitations related to the Medicare Hospice Benefit. First, a physician must certify that the patient is expected to die within the next 6 months if the disease follows its natural course.[24] Notably, patients can live longer than 6 months while receiving hospice care and physicians can recertify patients, if this criterion remains true. Should patients make an unexpected recovery, they would no longer qualify for hospice and would disenroll from hospice and resume their prior medical care. Similarly, patients can revert to prior medical care if they decide to pursue care with curative intent. Physician uncertainty in prognosticating often defers early access to hospice care.[25]

Perhaps, a more important limitation relates to the current reimbursement structure. Hospice provides *only* comfort-focused care, meaning that most patients need to forgo disease-modifying care, such as chemotherapy, even if the intent of the disease-modifying treatment is palliative and not curative. This creates a false dichotomy in care that forces patients to choose comfort-focused care over disease-modifying care that leads to later hospice referrals for patients and providers who anticipate benefit from continuing disease-modifying treatments.

Myths of Hospice

Myth 1: Hospice is Only for the Final Days

Many patients and providers have a personal experience with hospice in which a patient lived only a few days after enrolling. Such individuals may assume that starting hospice means one is just days away from dying. In fact, patients enrolled in hospice for under 3 days do not reap the benefits of hospice, and enrollment of less than 7 days is considered a poor quality metric.[26,27] Providers wishing to discuss the benefits of hospice must anticipate this common misconception and be prepared to educate patients and allay related fears.

Myth 2: Hospice Shortens Survival

Even among those who understand hospice is best when used before the final days, there remains a common, often unspoken belief that choosing hospice is paramount to agreeing to shorten one's life. No evidence supports this belief. In contrast, care focused on comfort and quality may allow patients to live both better and even a little longer. A study comparing two cohorts of patients with a terminal diagnosis found that patients who chose hospice lived an average of 29 days longer than comparable patients who died without hospice.[28]

Myth 3: A Do Not Resuscitate (DNR) Order is Required

While a choice to forgo attempts at cardiopulmonary resuscitation (CPR) is appropriate and consistent with the goals and philosophy of hospice, it is not required. Patients who wish comfort-focused care, but, for some reason, may still want the option for resuscitation, can be enrolled in hospice. The hospice team will continue to address the issue of code status with the patient and family after enrollment.

Clinical Issues that Warrant Consideration of Palliative Care

When is palliative care appropriate? What message am I sending patients when recommending palliative care? These are important questions that many health care providers struggle to answer, and often hinder early access to palliative care. Palliative care is appropriate for various patient populations, such as older adults with limited life expectancy, patients with serious illness, patients with multimorbidity, heavy symptom burden, or frailty, or other geriatric syndromes. Patients with diseases that have prompted multiple emergency room visits, hospitalizations or an intensive care unit stay in the past year can all benefit. Palliative care is not solely appropriate for patients with life-limiting illness or poor prognoses; it is not limited to the final days, weeks or months of life. Health professionals need to begin to consider palliative care earlier in the disease trajectory, and move beyond personal concerns that a palliative care referral may send patients and their loved one's a message that equates to death and find ways to articulate the value of palliative care.

Consideration of surgery is a particularly valuable opportunity to initiate palliative care for elders. The palliative care team can work alongside the surgical team to help to clarify patients' goals in the context of their values and thereby help patients understand their illness and make informed decisions about the risks and benefits of surgery. Palliative care can be a positive alternative for those who choose to forgo surgery. For those who undergo surgery, palliative care teams can help manage postoperative symptoms, help patients adapt to new limits and facilitate decision-making if complications or frailty limit postoperative functional status.

When patients are facing the end of life, they frequently have clear priorities. Comfort, in the form of pain and other symptom management, is among them. Alleviating sources of physical distress is a priority for patients nearing the end of life, but should not be done in exclusion of other patient goals, which may include avoiding being a burden to loved ones and the ability to close or strengthen relationships.[29,30] Multidisciplinary palliative care and hospice teams have expertise in assessing and managing, not only physical symptoms, but also psychosocial, spiritual and existential distress of both the patient and the family. However, all clinicians should have proficiency in managing common symptoms faced by patients at the end of life and address the concerns of their families.

Common Symptoms at the End of Life

While each patient's trajectory of illness differs, the following physical symptoms are common among patients in the final days to weeks of life. Expertise in assessing and managing these symptoms is an essential component of high-quality care at the end of life. Depending on the clinical context, a diagnostic workup to ascertain an underlying, potentially reversible cause should be undertaken. *The focus here is on palliating these common symptoms.*

Pain

Many patients fear dying in pain and unfortunately, pain is highly prevalent and frequently undertreated in elderly patients.[31,32] When comfort is the goal, pain can be well managed in nearly all patients. In assessing pain, scales asking patients to rate their pain from mild, moderate to severe, or 0 to 10, are helpful adjuncts to eliciting pain history. However, accurate pain assessment in elderly patients, especially those with any cognitive impairment, can pose challenges. Stoicism and fears of becoming addicted to pain medications may lead patients to under-report and undertreat pain. Providers need to anticipate such issues when devising a treatment plan for pain. Lack of knowledge about managing pain and exaggerated fears of addiction among physicians remain barriers to pain control.[33-35] Opioid medications remain the mainstay of analgesia for patients at EOL with many patients requiring long-acting and short-acting formulations to address both their chronic pain and episodic flares. Frequent availability (as often as every 1–3 hours) of "as-needed" short-acting opioids and adequate dosing (10–20% of the total daily opioid consumption) are important components of a pain treatment plan.

Dyspnea

Dyspnea, the sensation of breathlessness, is also a common symptom for patients with advanced illness.[36] The inability to breathe is among the most anxiety-provoking of symptoms. Because patients are often not symptomatic at rest, dyspnea may be overlooked by providers. Dyspnea related to poor oxygenation can be treated with supplemental oxygen, but in patients who are not hypoxic, oxygen has no proven benefit over supplemental air and may be overused.[37] Fans may help. Opioids are the mainstay of pharmacologic management and can be dosed similarly to how they are dosed for pain.[38] Anxiolytics, especially benzodiazepines, are commonly used, with little evidence supporting their use.[39]

Delirium

Delirium, an alteration of consciousness and inability to focus one's attention, frequently accompanied by disorientation, delusions and paranoid ideation, occurs in up to 90% of patients before they die.[40] For family caregivers, delirium is among the most distressing symptoms, as it often results in a loved one being "lost" before they actually die.[41] A patient's mental status can change over the course of the day. This unpredictability causes additional distress for family caregivers and can negatively effect bereavement.[42] Educating caregivers that such behavior is common and not a reflection of the patient's true self can reassure family members.

Constipation

A slowing of the bowels is very common in patients nearing the end of life.[43] Reduced physical activity and decreased oral intake of both food and fluids lead to less stool production. Opioids, often used to manage other symptoms, cause constipation. Increased fluids are recommended, but often not feasible nor adequate to relieve constipation. All patients on chronic opioids should be on chronic laxative regimen, such as senna, bismuth salicyclates or lactulose.[44] Patients with opioid-induced constipation may benefit from methynaltrexone, a quartenary amine opioid antagonist administered subcutaneously. It reverses the effect of opioids on the bowels, without impairing their analgesic effect.[45]

Anorexia-Cachexia

Decreased appetite is nearly ubiquitous as patients approach the end of life. While research has elucidated the multifactorial aspects of this syndrome, few patients benefit from treatment. Progestational agents, such as megesterol acetate, can increase weight and appetite, but not nutritional status or quality of life. Risks include venous thrombosis and adrenal insufficiency.[46] Corticosteroids, such as dexamethasone, are commonly prescribed for appetite stimulation and may also combat fatigue.[47] Side effects of long-term use usually limit the use of corticosteroids. Medicinal uses of marijuana and other cannabinoids have received increasing attention in the lay press with few high-quality studies to support their use.[48] Dronabinol, which is FDA-approved for weight loss associated with AIDS, is commonly prescribed for the purpose of stimulating appetite.[49] Understanding the mechanism of anorexia-cachexia and finding effective agents to treat it are active areas of research. Loss of appetite and/or weight can distress families as much or even more than patients. Educating family members that the disease has taken the patient's appetite is critical, as many patients cannot tolerate regular meals. Contrary to many caregivers' fears, patients rarely report hunger and do not "starve to death." Explaining that patients' cannot process nutrition appropriately due to the nature of their illness can be critical when addressing patients' or families' questions about the use of artificial nutrition or hydration. Only in rare circumstances does artificial nutrition (e.g. gastric tube feeding or parenteral nutrition) extend survival or improve quality of life for patients with a terminal diagnosis. Use of artificial nutrition at the end of life is generally considered ineffective and burdensome.

Syndrome of Imminently Dying Patient

While clinicians are notoriously poor at predicting a patient's prognosis, accuracy increases in the final days of life. For patients with an advanced illness for whom the goal of medical care is comfort, not prolongation of life, the following clinical findings generally indicate that a patient is "actively dying," meaning within the final 24–72 hours of life. These findings include: decreased interaction with loved ones, decreased level of consciousness with reduced (sometimes no) periods of wakefulness, irregular breathing patterns (Cheynes–Stokes respirations), noisy, often sonorous respirations (aka the "death rattle"), temperature fluctuations, cool, mottled extremities and decreased urine output. Preparing families for these symptoms can be a source of comfort.

Summary

In the current American health care system, surgery in the perioperative period is often a missed opportunity to benefit from palliative care. Despite increased morbidity[3-5] and mortality[2] associated with surgery in older patients, it continues to be an increasingly common component of the care that individuals receive as they age and even as they approach the end of life.[1] However, as the prevalence of progressive, chronic illnesses increases, the medical community has begun to recognize the need to acknowledge to themselves, as well as with patients, the inevitability of death. The medical community continues to evolve in its approach to patients facing the end of life. The expansion of palliative care in the health care system will further address issues of symptoms and quality of life. The development of new models of integrated palliative care will allow patients and families to consider their own personal goals and quality of life when making choices about the direction of their medical care, including whether or not to pursue surgical interventions. When attuned to patients' personal values, providers can help individuals find meaning and joy when living with limited function and/or limited life expectancy.

References

1. Barnato AE, McClellan MB, Kagay CR, Garber AM. Trends in inpatient treatment intensity among Medicare beneficiaries at the end of life. *Health Serv Res.* 2004; 39(2):363–375.

2. Leung JM, Dzankic S. Relative importance of preoperative health status versus intraoperative factors in predicting postoperative adverse outcomes in geriatric surgical patients. *J Am Geriatr Soc.* 2001; 49(8):1080–1085.

3. Makary MA, Segev DL, Pronovost PJ, et al. Frailty as a predictor of surgical outcomes in older patients. *J Am Coll Surg.* 2010; 210(6):901–908.

4. Dasgupta M, Rolfson DB, Stolee P, Borrie MJ, Speechley M. Frailty is associated with postoperative complications in older adults with medical problems. *Arch Gerontol Geriatr.* 2009; 48(1):78–83.

5. Garibaldi RA, Britt MR, Coleman ML, Reading JC, Pace NL. Risk factors for postoperative pneumonia. *Am J Med.* 1981; 70(3):677–680.

6. Kwok AC, Semel ME, Lipsitz SR, et al. The intensity and variation of surgical care at the end of life: a retrospective cohort study. *Lancet.* 2011; 378(9800):1408–1413.

7. Partridge JS, Harari D, Dhesi JK. Frailty in the older surgical patient: a review. *Age Ageing.* 2012; 41(2):142–147.

8. Finlayson E, Fan Z, Birkmeyer JD. Outcomes in octogenarians undergoing high-risk cancer operation: a national study. *J Am Coll Surg.* 2007; 205(6):729–734.

9. Finlayson E, Zhao S, Boscardin WJ, et al. Functional status after colon cancer surgery in elderly nursing home residents. *J Am Geriatr Soc.* 2012; 60(5):967–973.

10. Barnato AE, Kahn JM, Rubenfeld GD, et al. Prioritizing the organization and management of intensive care services in the United States: the PrOMIS Conference. *Crit Care Med.* 2007; 35(4):1003–1011.

11. Nabozny MJ, Kruser JM, Steffens NM, et al. Constructing high-stakes surgical decisions: it is better to die trying. *Ann Surg.* 2016; 263(1):64–70.

12. Barnet CS, Arriaga AF, Hepner DL, et al. Surgery at the end of life: a pilot study comparing decedents and survivors at a tertiary care center. *Anesthesiology.* 2013; 119(4):796–801.

13. Parikh RB, Temel JS. Early specialty palliative care. *N Engl J Med.* 2014; 370(11):1075–1076.

14. Weeks JC, Cook EF, O'Day SJ, et al. Relationship between cancer patients' predictions of prognosis and their treatment preferences. *JAMA.* 1998; 279(21):1709–1714.

15. Temel JS, Greer JA, Admane S, et al. Longitudinal perceptions of prognosis and goals of therapy in patients with metastatic non-small-cell lung cancer: results of a randomized study of early palliative care. *J Clin Oncol.* 2011; 29(17):2319–2326.

16. Temel JS, Greer JA, Muzikansky A, et al. Early palliative care for patients with metastatic non-small cell lung cancer. *N Engl J Med.* 2010; 363(8):733–742.

17. Zimmermann C, Swami N, Krzyzanowska M, et al. Early palliative care for patients with advanced cancer: a cluster-randomised controlled trial. *Lancet.* 2014; 383(9930):1721–1730.

18. Bakitas M, Lyons KD, Hegel MT, et al. Effects of a palliative care intervention on clinical outcomes in patients with advanced cancer: the Project ENABLE II randomized controlled trial. *JAMA.* 2009; 302(7):741–749.

19. Bakitas MA, Tosteson TD, Li Z, et al. Early versus delayed initiation of concurrent palliative oncology care: patient outcomes in the ENABLE III randomized controlled trial. *J Clin Oncol.* 2015; 33(13):1438–1445.

20. Dionne-Odom JN, Azuero A, Lyons KD, et al. Benefits of early versus delayed palliative care to informal family

caregivers of patients with advanced cancer: outcomes from the ENABLE III randomized controlled trial. *J Clin Oncol.* 2015; 33(13):1446–1452.

21. Von Roenn JH, Temel J. The integration of palliative care and oncology: the evidence. *Oncology (Williston Park).* 2011; 25(13):1258–1260, 1262, 1264–1265.

22. El-Jawahri A, Greer JA, Temel JS. Does palliative care improve outcomes for patients with incurable illness? A review of the evidence. *J Support Oncol.* 2011; 9(3):87–94.

23. National Hospice and Palliative Care Organization. 2005. www.nhpco.org/ sites/default/files/public/Statistics_ Research/2015_Facts_Figures.pdf (Accessed July 27, 2017).

24. US Department of Health and Human Services. Medicaid CfMa. 2015. www .cms.gov/Regulations-and-Guidance/ Guidance/Manuals/downloads/ bp102c09.pdf (Accessed October 2017).

25. Christakis NA, Lamont EB. Extent and determinants of error in doctors' prognoses in terminally ill patients: prospective cohort study. *BMJ.* 2000; 320(7233):469–472.

26. Smith AK, Earle CC, McCarthy EP. Racial and ethnic differences in end-of-life care in fee-for-service Medicare beneficiaries with advanced cancer. *J Am Geriatr Soc.* 2009; 57(1):153–158.

27. McCarthy EP, Burns RB, Ngo-Metzger Q, Davis RB, Phillips RS. Hospice use among Medicare managed care and fee-for-service patients dying with cancer. *JAMA.* 2003; 289(17):2238–2245.

28. Connor SR, Pyenson B, Fitch K, Spence C, Iwasaki K. Comparing hospice and nonhospice patient survival among patients who die within a three-year window. *J Pain Symptom Manage.* 2007; 33(3):238–246.

29. Singer PA, Martin DK, Kelner M. Quality end-of-life care: patients' perspectives. *JAMA.* 1999; 281(2):163–168.

30. Steinhauser KE, Christakis NA, Clipp EC, *et al.* Factors considered important at the end of life by patients, family, physicians,

and other care providers. *JAMA.* 2000; 284(19):2476–2482.

31. Breidung R. [Incidence of pain in elderly patients. A questionnaire survey of healthy members of a senior citizen meeting]. *Fortschr Med.* 1996; 114(13):153–156.

32. Achterberg WP, Gambassi G, Finne-Soveri H, *et al.* Pain in European long-term care facilities: cross-national study in Finland, Italy and The Netherlands. *Pain* 2010; 148(1):70–74.

33. Breuer B, Chang VT, Von Roenn JH, *et al.* How well do medical oncologists manage chronic cancer pain? A national survey. *Oncologist.* 2015; 20(2):202–209.

34. Brown JA, Von Roenn JH. Symptom management in the older adult. *Clin Geriatr Med.* 2004; 20(4):621–640, v–vi.

35. Buss MK, Lessen DS, Sullivan AM, *et al.* Hematology/oncology fellows' training in palliative care: results of a national survey. *Cancer.* 2011; 117(18):4304–4311.

36. Currow DC, Plummer JL, Crockett A, Abernethy AP. A community population survey of prevalence and severity of dyspnea in adults. *J Pain Symptom Manage.* 2009; 38(4):533–545.

37. Abernethy AP, McDonald CF, Frith PA, *et al.* Effect of palliative oxygen versus room air in relief of breathlessness in patients with refractory dyspnoea: a double-blind, randomised controlled trial. *Lancet.* 2010; 376(9743):784–793.

38. Abernethy AP, Currow DC, Frith P, *et al.* Randomised, double-blind, placebo-controlled crossover trial of sustained release morphine for the management of refractory dyspnoea. *BMJ.* 2003; 327(7414):523–528.

39. Currow DC, Abernethy AP. Potential opioid-sparing effect of regular benzodiazepines in dyspnea: longer duration of studies needed. *J Pain Symptom Manage.* 2010; 40(5):e1–e2; author reply e-4.

40. Bush SH, Bruera E, Lawlor PG, *et al.* Clinical practice guidelines for delirium management: potential application in

palliative care. *J Pain Symptom Manage.* 2014; 48(2):249–258.

41. Breitbart W, Gibson C, Tremblay A. The delirium experience: delirium recall and delirium-related distress in hospitalized patients with cancer, their spouses/caregivers, and their nurses. *Psychosomatics.* 2002; 43(3):183–194.

42. Morita T, Akechi T, Ikenaga M, *et al.* Terminal delirium: recommendations from bereaved families' experiences. *J Pain Symptom Manage.* 2007; 34(6):579–589.

43. Brown E, Henderson A, McDonagh A. Exploring the causes, assessment and management of constipation in palliative care. *Int J Palliat Nurs.* 2009; 15(2):58–64.

44. Kumar L, Barker C, Emmanuel A. Opioid-induced constipation: pathophysiology, clinical consequences, and management. *Gastroenterol Res Pract.* 2014; 2014:141737.

45. Thomas J, Karver S, Cooney GA, *et al.* Methylnaltrexone for opioid-induced constipation in advanced illness. *N Engl J Med.* 2008; 358(22):2332–2343.

46. Berenstein EG, Ortiz Z. Megestrol acetate for the treatment of anorexia-cachexia syndrome. *Cochrane Database Syst Rev.* 2005(2):CD004310.

47. Yennurajalingam S, Frisbee-Hume S, Palmer JL, *et al.* Reduction of cancer-related fatigue with dexamethasone: a double-blind, randomized, placebo-controlled trial in patients with advanced cancer. *J Clin Oncol.* 2013; 31(25):3076–3082.

48. Belendiuk KA, Baldini LL, Bonn-Miller MO. Narrative review of the safety and efficacy of marijuana for the treatment of commonly state-approved medical and psychiatric disorders. *Addict Sci Clin Pract.* 2015; 10(1):10.

49. Marinol New Drug Application. www.fda .gov/ohrms/dockets/dockets/05n0479/ 05N-0479-emc0004-04.pdf (Accessed July 18, 2017).

Chapter 22

Quality Assessment and Improvement in the Elderly

Marissa Wagner Mery

Key Points

- Improving perioperative care for the elderly requires customizing the systems and metrics used to deliver and measure age-appropriate care.
- Measuring performance improves perioperative outcomes.
- Readmission rates and patient satisfaction following surgery are two examples of outcomes that are particularly relevant to surgical patients of all ages.
- Process measures are a type of outcome measurement that are frequently used in quality improvement initiatives. They often promote the adoption of guidelines or desired practices and can lead to decreased variability among providers; however, process measures have significant limitations.
- Elderly-specific quality measures are limited, but should include measures that reflect what is important to this population, such as postoperative functional and cognitive status.
- The care of older patients will be best served by a team-based approach, with collaborative decision-making and responsibility for patient outcomes.

Introduction

Elderly patients (aged 65 and older) are expected to comprise almost 75% of the surgical caseload by 2020, with adults older than 80 years of age being surgery's fastest growing population segment.[1,2] Assessing and improving the quality of surgical services delivered to this population is essential, as elderly patients' baseline complexity and co-morbidities increase the likelihood of developing perioperative complications and functional decline. Furthermore, the personal and financial costs of these complications are indefensible to our patients, their families and our health care system.

Quality of care and patient safety entered the public spotlight following the Institute of Medicine's (IOM) 1999 publication *To Err is Human*, which revealed that preventable medical errors generate up to 98,000 annual deaths.[3] This and the IOM's subsequent report, *Crossing the Quality Chasm*, rebuked any antecedent assumptions that US patients reliably received care that was safe or efficient, and made quality improvement a national priority.[3,4]

The IOM highlighted perioperative locations such as operating rooms, ICUs and emergency departments as especially dangerous for patients, as these sites not only had high error rates, but also errors likely to precipitate severe clinical consequences.[3] These locations are also notable for significant over-representation by the elderly, many of whom have complex co-morbidities that independently elevate their risk for complications following a hospital admission. As the number and proportion of elderly patients undergoing surgery is expected to rise, there is increased urgency to raise the quality of care for this complex population by not only minimizing errors, but also generating care delivery models that acknowledge the older population's unique needs.[1,2]

The incentive for boosting quality of care extends beyond a moral prerogative. The Department of Health and Human Services (DHHS) and other major health payers are increasingly tying remuneration for health care to clinical performance metrics. For example, the DHHS recently announced a goal that 90% of Medicare's fee-for-service payments be tied to quality or value by 2018.[5]

Improving perioperative care for the elderly requires customizing the systems and metrics used to deliver and measure care for this population. Similar to the recognition that pediatric patients are not simply smaller adults, improving perioperative outcomes for the elderly necessitates a new paradigm of team-based care delivery and quality assessment altogether.

Defining a Framework for Quality of Care

While the public focus on quality and its assessment may be recent, individual institutions have long employed these methods to improve the efficacy of their own clinical practices and decision-making. As early as the 1930s, E.A. Codman, a physician at the Massachusetts General Hospital, advocated "the common sense notion that every hospital should follow every patient it treats, long enough to determine whether or not the treatment has been successful, and then to inquire, 'If not, why not?' with a view to preventing similar failures in the future."[6] In recent years, internal auditing systems have been augmented or even supplanted by government and discipline-specific data registries such as the Center for Medicare and Medicaid's (CMS) Physician Quality Reporting System (PQRS) and the National Anesthesia Clinical Outcomes Registry (NACOR). Started for quality improvement, these registries are increasingly employed for public reporting, allowing patients to compare process adherence and clinical outcomes across institutions.

Outcomes Measurement

Evidence supports the intuition that measuring performance improves perioperative outcomes. In 1989 the New York State Department of Health (NYSDH) started collecting data on patients undergoing coronary artery bypass grafting (CABG) to identify clinical risk factors for poor outcomes and providers with higher-than-predicted complications.[7] Following data compilation and analysis, the NYSDH delivered feedback in the form of risk-adjusted outcomes to all providers and instructed those with the worst outcomes on best practices.[8] Three years following the program's inception, post-CABG risk-adjusted mortality fell by 41%. Publishing rates of central-line-associated bloodstream infections (CLABSI) yielded similar results, a 53% reduction in 5 years.[9] However, an unintended consequence of public reporting is that providers may avoid high-risk patients, including the elderly, and although risk-adjustment attempts to mitigate this, models are currently imperfect.[10,11]

Two categories of outcome measurement especially applicable to surgical patients are readmission rates and patient satisfaction.[12,13] For medical conditions, readmission rates have not been correlated with improved mortality and unfairly penalize teaching and safety-net hospitals.[14,15] For surgical admissions, however, quality appears correlated with readmission rates. Hospitals with the lowest postoperative mortality have significantly lower rates of postoperative readmissions than those with higher mortality.[12] Similarly, hospitals with the highest quartile patient satisfaction scores had lower postoperative readmissions, length of stay and postoperative mortality when compared to hospitals in the lowest quartile of patient satisfaction.[13]

Process Measurement

In addition to assessing outcomes, quality improvement initiatives often measure adherence to "best practice" processes. Process measurement accelerates adoption of guidelines or desired practices and diminishes variability among providers.[10,16] For example, beta-blockers were found to confer a survival benefit to MI survivors in 1982, but in the mid-1990s only 34–38% of eligible patients received them.[17,18] In 2002 still fewer than 50% received them, but in 2004 the Joint Commission (JCAHO) began publicly reporting hospitals' rates.[16] By 2009 over 96% of hospitals reported post-MI administration rates of greater than 90%.[16]

Their lack of a need for risk-adjustment is another appealing quality of process measures. Patient eligibility is determined by predefined inclusion and exclusion criteria, simplifying reporting and measure interpretation. Finally, individual institutions can study associations between their processes and outcomes for internal innovation.

Process measurement has limitations. Foremost, adherence to specified processes has not always guaranteed anticipated outcome benefits because clinical results are the product of numerous patient and provider factors.[19] Moreover, many of the guidelines and processes whose adherence is being measured are based on expert recommendations or committee-determined standards, as opposed to evidence.[20] Finally, providers can "game" process measures and receive credit for guideline adherence even if its implementation is incorrect or unsafe.[11,21] Data for patients with non-ST-segment elevation acute coronary syndrome were reviewed for both *adherence* to guidelines recommending antithrombotic administration as well as *safety*, the proportion of patients receiving ACC/AHA recommended dosing of the antithrombotic.[21] Adherence was 85%, whereas safe dosing occurred only 53% of the time.[21] Hospitals with low adherence and safety (<median) as well as those with mixed performance had higher risk-adjusted mortality than those with both high adherence and safety.[21] Adherence-based process metrics alone are likely insufficient to improve outcomes or mark a provider as high or low quality, but they are a powerful tool to incentivize behavior as part of a broader quality improvement program.

Current Quality Measures in Elderly Perioperative Care

Elderly-Specific Quality Indicators

The elderly (≥65 years) account for 60% of surgical patients and can present with complex co-morbidities, including cardiopulmonary disease, cognitive impairment and frailty.[1] Morbidity and mortality rates following major surgery increase with age, and diminished functional status or cognitive capability is not uncommon.[22] The elderly are also more likely to value quality over quantity of life, and a majority would prefer to die at home when the time arrives.[23] Thus, while they are the most likely to receive a diagnosis amenable to surgical intervention, the risks to their physical well-being and personal autonomy complicate perioperative decision-making.

Quality assessment data are most robust for mortality, discharge location, readmission and traditional morbidity measures such as MI, pneumonia, CLABSI and reoperation. For all hospitalizations, older age increases average length of stay and diminishes one's chance of being discharged home.[24] Fewer than half of patients over age 85 are discharged home, and mortality per admission is 6%.[24] However, these general statistics mask the heterogeneous courses perioperative patients face. For VA patients undergoing noncardiac surgery, the overall 30-day mortality for patients over age 80 was 8%, but less than 2% following common operations such as carotid endarterectomy, knee replacement and vertebral disc surgery.[22] Postoperative complications were a harbinger of death, elevating the 30-day mortality rate to 26% from 4%.[22] And age was not the strongest predictor of mortality, with other risk factors, including ASA score, functional status, BUN and weight loss, more heavily influencing the odds of death.[22]

Improving care for the elderly necessitates measuring processes and outcomes customized to their needs and goals. RAND's Assessing Care of Vulnerable Elders (ACOVE) project developed process metrics for surgical patients in addition to indicators for surgical diseases including breast and colorectal cancer.[25,26] In a separate effort, McGory *et al.* engaged a multidisciplinary team to define processes of care for elderly patients undergoing major abdominal surgery (Table 22.1), and the American College of Surgeons (ACS)

Table 22.1 Process measures more applicable to the elderly undergoing operations versus perioperative care items universal to all surgical patients

Domain of care	Process measures more applicable to elderly undergoing operations	Process measures universal to all surgical patients
Co-morbidity assessment	• Complete standardized cardiovascular risk evaluation per ACC/AHA guidelines • Estimation of creatinine clearance	• Standardized preoperative lab panel • Pulmonary physical exam/review of systems • Obtain history of diabetes • Assess use of tobacco/alcohol • Smoking cessation
Evaluation of elderly issues	• Screen for nutrition, cognition, delirium risk, pressure ulcer risk • Assess functional status including ambulation, vision/hearing impairment and ADLs/IADLs • Referral for additional evaluation for impaired cognition or functional status, high risk for delirium, or polypharmacy	• Not applicable
Medication use	• Indications for inpatient bowel preparation • Evaluation of medication regimen and polypharmacy • Avoid delirium-triggering medications and other potentially inappropriate medications (e.g. Beers criteria)	• Instruction on preoperative medication management • Perioperative β-blockade • Intravenous antibiotic prophylaxis • Endocarditis prophylaxis • Deep venous thrombosis prophylaxis

(cont.)

Table 22.1 (cont.)

Domain of care	Process measures more applicable to elderly undergoing operations	Process measures universal to all surgical patients
Patient-to-provider discussions	• Assess patient's decision-making capacity • Specific discussion on expected functional outcomes, life-sustaining preferences, and surrogate decision maker	• Informed consent about treatment options and risks-to-benefits of operation • Treatment preferences (e.g. do not resuscitate) should be followed
Intraoperative care	• Not applicable	• Prevent hypothermia • Proper positioning
Postoperative management	• Prevent malnutrition, delirium, deconditioning, pressure ulcers • Daily screen for postoperative delirium and standardized workup for delirium episode • Make staff aware if hearing/vision impairment • Patient access to glasses, hearing aid, dentures • Consider home health care for assistance for ostomy care • Infection prevention with daily assessment of central line and indication for use, early Foley catheter removal, and standardized fever workup	• Appropriate restraint use • Measure daily input/output • Aspiration precautions • Use of incentive spirometer • Use of translator or interpreted materials for deaf or non-English speaking • Education about ostomy self-care • Pain assessment with each set of vital signs
Discharge planning	• A discussion with the patient or caretaker about purpose of drug, how to take it, and expected side effects/adverse effects for all medications prescribed for outpatient use • Assess social support and need for home health care prior to operation • Assess nutrition, cognition, ambulation and ADLs prior to discharge	• A complete list of medications and dosages to continue on discharge from the hospital • Assess need for medical equipment, home health care, skilled nursing facility prior to discharge • Written and oral discharge instructions • Discharge summary to indicate followup labs, tests, appointments • Followup visit within 6 weeks • Communication to primary care doctor

ACC/AHA, American College of Cardiology/American Heart Association; ADL, activities of daily living; IADL, instrumental activities of daily living.
Source: Reprinted with permission from McGory ML, Shekelle PG, Rubenstein LZ, Fink A, Ko CY. Developing quality indicators for elderly patients undergoing abdominal operations. *Journal of the American College of Surgeons.* 2005;201(6):870–883. Copyright Elsevier 2005.

Table 22.2 New variables collected by the ACS NSQIP Geriatric Surgery Pilot Project

Preoperative variables	Intent of variable (definition)
Origin from home with support	To determine baseline functional status (lives alone at home, lives with support in home, origin status not from home)
Use of mobility aid	To quantify baseline mobility (uses a walking aid—yes/no)
History of prior falls	To define the presence of a geriatric syndrome prior to admission (prior fall—yes/no)
History of dementia	To determine baseline cognition (history of dementia—yes/no)
Competency status on admission	To define significant cognitive impairment (consent signed by patient or by surrogate—yes/no)
Palliative care on admission	To identify patients admitted from palliative care or hospice (from palliative care/hospice—yes/no)

Postoperative occurrences	Intent of variable (definition)
Postoperative pressure ulcer	To define the presence of a geriatric syndrome at discharge (a pressure ulcer is present at discharge; did it occur during the hospital stay—yes/no)
Postoperative delirium	To define the presence of a geriatric syndrome during the hospital stay (delirium is present if there are one or more episodes of acute confusion during hospitalization—yes/no)
Do not resuscitate (DNR) order during hospitalization	To capture changes in DNR status during the hospital stay (was there a new DNR order during hospitalization—yes/no)
Palliative care consult	To understand treatment goals of patients with short life expectancy (palliative care consult obtained during hospitalization or patient made comfort care—yes/no)
Discharge functional health status	To determine functional status at discharge (ability to perform activities of daily living at discharge—independent/partially dependent/dependent)
Fall risk on discharge	To quantify mobility at discharge (define fall risk at time of discharge—high/low)
Need of mobility aid on discharge	To understand a patient's mobility at discharge (new use of mobility aid walker/cane at time of discharge—yes/no)
Discharge with/without services	To capture care needs at discharge (home alone with self-care, home alone with skilled care, home with support and self-care, home with support and skilled care)

Source: Reprinted with permission from Robinson TN, Rosenthal RA. The ACS NSQIP Geriatric Surgery Pilot Project: Improving care for older surgical patients. *Bulletin of the American College of Surgeons.* 2014;99(10):21. Copyright American College of Surgeons 2014.

is piloting preoperative risk variables as well as outcome measures for elderly patients (Table 22.2).[27,28]

Preoperative Assessment and Consent

The ASA does not endorse specific guidelines for elderly preoperative assessment, and preoperative quality indicators are absent from the Anesthesia Quality Institute's (AQI) NACOR registry. The American College of Surgeons (ACS) National Surgical Quality Improvement Program (NSQIP) is piloting a set of preoperative variables for elderly

Table 22.3 Checklist for the *Optimal Preoperative Assessment of the Geriatric Surgical Patient*

In addition to conducting a complete and thorough history and physical examination of the patient, the following assessments are strongly recommended:
- ☐ Assess the patient's cognitive ability and capacity to understand the anticipated surgery.
- ☐ Screen the patient for depression.
- ☐ Identify the patient's risk factors for developing postoperative delirium.
- ☐ Screen for alcohol and other substance abuse/dependence.
- ☐ Perform a preoperative cardiac evaluation according to the American College of Cardiology/American Heart Association (ACC/AHA) algorithm for patients undergoing noncardiac surgery.
- ☐ Identify the patient's risk factors for postoperative pulmonary complications and implement appropriate strategies for prevention.
- ☐ Document functional status and history of falls.
- ☐ Determine baseline frailty score.
- ☐ Assess patient's nutritional status and consider preoperative interventions if the patient is at severe nutritional risk.
- ☐ Take an accurate and detailed medication history and consider appropriate perioperative adjustments. Monitor for polypharmacy.
- ☐ Determine the patient's treatment goals and expectations in the context of the possible treatment outcomes.
- ☐ Determine patient's family and social support system.
- ☐ Order appropriate preoperative diagnostic tests focused on elderly patients.

Source: Reference 29.

---

patients (Table 22.2), and while the ACS recommends a preoperative checklist (Table 22.3), its utilization is undetermined.[29] What little we do know regarding compliance with elderly preoperative testing guidelines comes from cataract surgery, where multiple specialty societies have opposed routine preoperative testing since 2002. However, more than a third of ophthalmologists still order preoperative tests on greater than 75% of patients, and testing is more strongly correlated with physician practice patterns than patient characteristics, suggesting the guidelines are not followed.[30]

Research into preoperative optimization and risk assessment has proliferated; however, the work is not implemented on a national scale, and no metrics incentivize its use. Popular risk-assessment tools include ASA score, frailty indices, the ACS NSQIP Surgical Risk Calculator and the Revised Cardiac Risk Index[31]; yet evidence suggests that customized models perform better. Kwok *et al.* created a mortality risk prediction score for elderly patients undergoing an emergent colectomy.[32] It utilized preoperative predictors identified from the NSQIP database and predicted 30-day mortality with greater accuracy than either the ACS Colorectal Surgery Risk Calculator or the ASA score and Surgical Risk Scale.[32]

Neither the ASA preoperative practice guidelines nor ACS *Optimal Preoperative Assessment of the Geriatric Surgical Patient* explicitly recommend advance directives (AD) prior to surgery.[29,33] They are not routinely used for high-risk patients despite evidence that dying patients with ADs received care strongly aligned with their stated preferences.[34,35] In one tertiary center's anesthesia preoperative testing facility, only 54% of those who died within 1 year of surgery had an AD at the time of their procedure.[35]

Intraoperative Care

Little is known regarding intraoperative management and practice variability in the geriatric population beyond JCAHO Surgical Care Improvement Project measures and mortality. Yet we know that intraoperative management influences postoperative events. In 2007 a surgical APGAR score was created to rate a patient's condition at the end of an operation and predict major complications and mortality.[36] This simple 10-point score determined by estimated blood loss, lowest heart rate and lowest mean arterial pressure during a procedure was significantly associated with major complications, ICU admission and 30-day mortality for general and vascular surgery procedures.[36] If a score consisting of three measurements can predict complications, advances in physiologic monitoring and predictive analytics should be engaged to better anticipate and improve short- and long-term outcomes.

Postoperative cognitive dysfunction, functional capacity decline, MI and pneumonia are prevalent postoperative events. Our ability to minimize their incidence is stymied by a lack of knowledge regarding intraoperative practices. Even for well-studied topics such as lung protective ventilation, the rate of intraoperative implementation is unknown.

Postoperative Care

The elderly have unique postoperative needs to reduce in-hospital complications and readmissions. They are more likely to experience cardiac, pulmonary and urologic complications with no relative increase in rates of surgical site infections, reoperation or postoperative bleeding.[37] Age and complications are independently associated with discharge to skilled care facilities, which is in turn associated with a fourfold risk of death at 1 year.[38]

Elders are less likely to receive recommended care for conditions that primarily affect them than conditions ubiquitous to the larger population.[39] A single-institution study looked at adherence to 15 perioperative desired processes, 5 of which were specific to the elderly.[26,40] No elderly-specific processes had greater than 53% adherence, and three (postoperative delirium screening, cognition/function assessment at discharge and level of care documentation) had less than 5% adherence.[39] While these are recommended by the ACS best practice guidelines for geriatric surgical patients, there is no evidence to suggest they are routinely integrated into perioperative care.

Continuity of Care: Readmissions and Functional Status

Readmission rates are included in many quality assessment programs, and the Hospital Readmissions Reduction Program (HRRP) has begun including surgical procedures, starting with hip and knee replacements.[41] Hospitals with the lowest mortality rates have significantly lower rates of postoperative readmissions among Medicare beneficiaries, and surgical readmissions are therefore considered indicative of quality care.[12] However, the three most common etiologies for postoperative readmission, surgical site infection, ileus and bleeding, are not themselves felt to be easily preventable.[42]

Outcome metrics have traditionally ignored other postdischarge co-morbidities, including functional and cognitive status, but these are especially meaningful to elderly patients. Potential cognitive sequelae of anesthesia and surgery, including postoperative cognitive dysfunction (POCD) are of increasing concern as the elderly undergo more procedures.[43] However, outcome metrics are limited to what we can measure, and the current set-up of most perioperative systems is not amenable to long-term neurologic and functional tracking.

Improving Perioperative Quality and Its Assessment for the Elderly

Proposed General Tenets

Designing quality metrics and interventions for the elderly is challenging because they represent a very heterogeneous population with respect to preoperative risks and postoperative goals. *A first principle for improving care in this population is recognizing its unique attributes and the need to revamp provider education, training and patient management strategies accordingly.* As children are not young adults, the elderly are not simply older adults.

A second is to measure outcomes important to the elderly, and consider doing so on an extended time scale and across a broader range of complications. The impact of a surgical procedure continues beyond 30 days. Improvement in health care processes and decision-making require feedback that short-term metrics do not provide, especially for a population where long-term function may outweigh 30-day mortality. At present, the infrastructure for such measurement does not exist. Clinical data acquisition is extremely expensive, and tracking patients is difficult under current practice models. However, it is not difficult to believe that changes in health delivery (Accountable Care Organizations, medical and surgical homes), telemedicine models and advances in passive data collection will make this possible and affordable at scale in the near future. Furthermore, intraoperative anesthetic management needs to be measured. Intuitively, intraoperative care must bear some significance for postoperative outcomes, and this needs to be better understood.

Third, measured outcomes should serve as a platform to develop quality improvement interventions for the elderly. From preoperative assessments to readmissions reduction, interventions should be hypothesized, studied and analyzed for effectiveness across a broad range of elderly patients and procedures. Such interventions could include structural changes such as special wards designed to reduce delirium or processes such as postoperative medication algorithms designed to curtail polypharmacy.

Fourth, AD and informed consent processes should be overhauled. Elderly-tailored risk profiles should be utilized to guide consent for emergent and elective procedures. Risk models should be expanded to include mortality beyond 30 days, common complications, postoperative functional status and discharge location. Having data behind the consent process empowers patients to make decisions aligned with their goals. Similarly, while there is concern that the rigidity of traditional ADs renders them inappropriate for the perioperative period, documented formal discussions can elucidate a patient's wishes under a number of circumstances. The limitation here is that more than half of surgeons reported they would decline to operate on patients with an AD limiting postoperative life-supporting therapy.[44] An unintended consequence of using 30-day mortality as a quality benchmark is the conflict of interest it creates for physicians and interference with patients' autonomy. This will need to be addressed to adequately care for palliative or elderly patients.

Finally, the care of these patients will be best served by a team-based approach, with collaborative decision-making and responsibility for patient outcomes. These teams could be comprised of surgeons, anesthesiologists, geriatricians, social workers, nurses, rehab specialists and ideally with input from a patient's primary physician. Not every member is necessarily involved with every patient, but this approach has the potential to provide care that is patient-centered as opposed to provider-centered. Teams would collabora-tively plan care for high-risk patients, similar to tumor boards, in addition to developing practice models and processes for routine elderly care.[45] Not only would patient decisions be team-based, but also the accountability for outcomes. Shared accountability requires a significant cultural shift and does not decrease a surgeon's role or responsibility, but acknowledges the impact other providers have on the long-term outcomes for complex patients.[45] Team-based care could be part of a surgical home, analogous to the Agency for Healthcare Research and Quality's (AHRQ) medical home, and a potential subspecialty model for the ASA's Perioperative Surgical Home.[45]

Potential Pathway

How would the general guiding principles be applied to a particular patient? A potential pathway for an elderly patient considering major surgical intervention could include the following.

Preoperative

- Thorough preoperative screening utilizing the ACS *Optimal Preoperative Assessment of the Geriatric Surgical Patient* checklist.
- Medical optimization and prehabilitation to improve baseline functional status.[46]
- Customized informed consent (for patient's age, frailty, co-morbidities and procedure) that involves discussion of less invasive alternatives and AD discussion specific to postoperative complications and life-sustaining intervention preferences.
- Monitor adherence to these processes via institutional metrics, so as to foster innovation in processes and quality improvement.
- Record preoperative status via variables such as those from the ACS NSQIP Geriatric Surgery Pilot Project for future risk stratification.

Intraoperative

- Surgical safety checklist and time out prior to incision, including discussion regarding special equipment, blood availability (if applicable) and planned discharge location.
- Immediately available crisis safety checklists.[47]
- Anesthetic plan accounting for age-related physiologic changes, baseline co-morbidities and procedural risks.
- Postoperative debriefing including review of surgical APGAR (or other preferred risk model) score and appropriate handoff to PACU/ICU.
- Report anesthetic case data and PQRS measures to NACOR.
- Longer term tracking of anesthetic delivery, medication choices and physiologic data for research related to data mining and predictive analytics.

Postoperative

- Process measurement for tracking adherence to recommended postoperative pathways for common clinical complications.
- Pain management to maximize function and mobility while limiting polypharmacy and side effects of narcotics.

- Assessment of functional and cognitive status, compared to preoperative state.
- Extensive discharge planning with patient and support system, postdischarge follow-up if elevated predicted readmission rate.
- Report anesthesia-specific postoperative quality indicators to NACOR, consider implementing ACS Geriatric Surgery Pilot outcomes indicators.
- If readmitted, perioperative team representative to review for team feedback.
- As technology and resources allow, follow-up for functional and cognitive status and other complications at 6 month or 1 year mark.

While these recommendations focus on improving quality assessment and care for the elderly, they have broader applications. A patient-centered model of care emphasizing performance measurement and continual improvement is pertinent to all surgical patients.

References

1. Etzioni DA, Liu JH, Maggard MA, Ko CY. The aging population and its impact on the surgery workforce. *Ann Surgery*. 2003; 238(2):170–177.

2. Etzioni DA, Liu JH, O'Connell JB, Maggard MA, Ko CY. Elderly patients in surgical workloads: a population-based analysis. *Am Surg*. 2003; 69(11):961–965.

3. Institute of Medicine (US) Committee on Quality of Health Care in America; Kohn LT, Corrigan JM, Donaldson MS, eds. *To Err is Human: Building a Safer Health System*. Washington, DC, National Academy of Sciences, 2000.

4. Institute of Medicine (US) Committee on Quality of Health Care in America. *Crossing the Quality Chasm: A New Health System for the 21st Century*. Washington, DC, National Academy of Sciences, 2001.

5. Burwell SM. Setting value-based payment goals: HHS efforts to improve U.S. health care. *N Engl J Med*. 2015; 372(10):897–899.

6. Codman EA. *The Shoulder: Rupture of the Supraspinatus Tendon and Other Lesions in or about the Subacromial Bursa*. Boston, MA, T. Todd Company, 1934.

7. Hannan EL, Kilburn H Jr. O'Donnell JF, Lukacik G, Shields EP. Adult open heart surgery in New York State: an analysis of risk factors and hospital mortality rates. *JAMA*. 1990; 264(21):2768–2774.

8. Hannan EL, Kilburn H Jr., Racz M, Shields E, Chassin MR. Improving the outcomes of coronary artery bypass surgery in New York State. *JAMA*. 1994; 271(10):761–766.

9. New York State Department of Health. *Hospital-Acquired Infections: New York State 2012*. Albany, NY, New York State Department of Health, 2013.

10. Glance LG, Neuman M, Martinez EA, Pauker KY, Dutton RP. Performance measurement at a "tipping point." *Anesth Analg*. 2011; 112(4):958–966.

11. Moscucci M. Public reporting of percutaneous coronary intervention outcomes: harm or benefit? *J Am Coll Cardiol*. 2015; 65(11):1127–1129.

12. Tsai TC, Joynt KE, Orav EJ, Gawande AA, Jha AK. Variation in surgical-readmission rates and quality of hospital care. *N Engl J Med*. 2013; 369(12):1134–1142.

13. Tsai TC, Orav EJ, Jha AK. Patient satisfaction and quality of surgical care in US hospitals. *Ann Surg*. 2015; 261(1):2–8.

14. Joynt KE, Jha AK. Characteristics of hospitals receiving penalties under the Hospital Readmissions Reduction Program. *JAMA*. 2013; 309(4):342–343.

15. Krumholz HM, Lin Z, Keenan PS, et al. Relationship between hospital readmission and mortality rates for patients hospitalized with acute myocardial infarction, heart failure, or pneumonia. *JAMA*. 2013; 309(6):587–593.

16. Chassin MR, Loeb JM, Schmaltz SP, Wachter RM. Accountability

measures–using measurement to promote quality improvement. *N Engl J Med*. 2010; 363(7):683–688.

17. [No authors listed] A randomized trial of propranolol in patients with acute myocardial infarction. I. Mortality results. *JAMA*. 1982; 247(12):1707–1714.

18. Gottlieb SS, McCarter RJ, Vogel RA. Effect of beta-blockade on mortality among high-risk and low-risk patients after myocardial infarction. *N Engl J Med*. 1998; 339(8):489–497.

19. Werner RM, Bradlow ET. Relationship between Medicare's hospital compare performance measures and mortality rates. *JAMA*. 2006; 296(22):2694–2702.

20. Shaneyfelt TM, Centor RM. Reassessment of clinical practice guidelines: go gently into that good night. *JAMA*. 2009; 301(8):868–869.

21. Mehta RH, Chen AY, Alexander KP, *et al.* Doing the right things and doing them the right way: the association between hospital guideline adherence, dosing safety, and outcomes among patients with acute coronary syndrome. *Circulation*. 2015; 131(11):980–987.

22. Hamel MB, Henderson WG, Khuri SF, Daley J. Surgical outcomes for patients aged 80 and older: morbidity and mortality from major noncardiac surgery. *J Am Geriatr Soc*. 2005; 53(3):424–429.

23. Fried TR, Bradley EH, Towle VR, Allore H. Understanding the treatment preferences of seriously ill patients. *N Engl J Med*. 2002; 346(14):1061–1066.

24. Levant S, Chari K, DeFrances CJ. Hospitalizations for patients aged 85 and over in the United States, 2000–2010. *NCHS Data Brief*. 2015; 182:1–8.

25. Arora VM, Johnson M, Olson J, *et al.* Using assessing care of vulnerable elders quality indicators to measure quality of hospital care for vulnerable elders. *J Am Geriatr Soc*. 2007; 55(11):1705–1711.

26. Wenger NS, Roth CP, Shekelle P, Investigators A. Introduction to the assessing care of vulnerable elders-3 quality indicator measurement set. *J Am Geriatr Soc*. 2007; 55(Suppl 2):S247–S252.

27. McGory ML, Shekelle PG, Rubenstein LZ, Fink A, Ko CY. Developing quality indicators for elderly patients undergoing abdominal operations. *J Am Coll Surg*. 2005; 201(6):870–883.

28. Robinson TN, Rosenthal RA. The ACS NSQIP Geriatric Surgery Pilot Project: improving care for older surgical patients. *Bull Am Coll Surg*. 2014; 99(10):21.

29. Chow WB, Rosenthal RA, Merkow RP, *et al.*; American College of Surgeons National Surgical Quality Improvement Program. Optimal preoperative assessment of the geriatric surgical patient: a best practices guideline from the American College of Surgeons National Surgical Quality Improvement Program and the American Geriatrics Society. *J Am Coll Surg*. 2012; 215(4):453–466.

30. Chen CL, Lin GA, Bardach NS, *et al.* Preoperative medical testing in Medicare patients undergoing cataract surgery. *N Engl J Med*. 2015; 372(16):1530–1538.

31. Makary MA, Segev DL, Pronovost PJ, *et al.* Frailty as a predictor of surgical outcomes in older patients. *J Am Coll Surg*. 2010; 210(6):901–908.

32. Kwok AC, Lipsitz SR, Bader AM, Gawande AA. Are targeted preoperative risk prediction tools more powerful? A test of models for emergency colon surgery in the very elderly. *J Am Coll Surg*. 2011; 213(2):220–225.

33. Committee on Standards and Practise Parameters; Apfelbaum JL, Connis RT, Nickinovich DG, *et al.* Practice advisory for preanesthesia evaluation: an updated report by the American Society of Anesthesiologists Task Force on Preanesthesia Evaluation. *Anesthesiology*. 2012; 116(3):522–538.

34. Silveira MJ, Kim SY, Langa KM. Advance directives and outcomes of surrogate decision making before death. *N Engl J Med*. 2010; 362(13):1211–1218.

35. Barnet CS, Arriaga AF, Hepner DL, *et al.* Surgery at the end of life: a pilot study comparing decedents and survivors at a tertiary care center. *Anesthesiology*. 2013; 119(4):796–801.

36. Gawande AA, Kwaan MR, Regenbogen SE, Lipsitz SA, Zinner MJ. An Apgar score for surgery. *J Am Coll Surg.* 2007; 204(2):201–208.

37. Bentrem DJ, Cohen ME, Hynes DM, Ko CY, Bilimoria KY. Identification of specific quality improvement opportunities for the elderly undergoing gastrointestinal surgery. *Arch Surg.* 2009; 144(11):1013–1020.

38. Legner VJ, Massarweh NN, Symons RG, McCormick WC, Flum DR. The significance of discharge to skilled care after abdominopelvic surgery in older adults. *Ann Surg.* 2009; 249(2):250–255.

39. Bergman S, Martelli V, Monette M, *et al.* Identification of quality of care deficiencies in elderly surgical patients by measuring adherence to process-based quality indicators. *J Am Coll Surg.* 2013; 217(5):858–866.

40. McGory ML, Kao KK, Shekelle PG, *et al.* Developing quality indicators for elderly surgical patients. *Ann Surg.* 2009; 250(2):338–347.

41. Boccuti C, Casillas G. *Aiming for Fewer Hospital U-turns: The Medicare Hospital Readmission Reduction Program.* Menlo Park, CA, The Henry J. Kaiser Family Foundation, 2015.

42. Merkow RP, Ju MH, Chung JW, *et al.* Underlying reasons associated with hospital readmission following surgery in the United States. *JAMA.* 2015; 313(5):483–495.

43. Newman S, Stygall J, Hirani S, Shaefi S, Maze M. Postoperative cognitive dysfunction after noncardiac surgery: a systematic review. *Anesthesiology.* 2007; 106(3):572–590.

44. Redmann AJ, Brasel KJ, Alexander CG, Schwarze ML. Use of advance directives for high-risk operations: a national survey of surgeons. *Ann Surg.* 2012; 255(3):418–423.

45. Glance LG, Osler TM, Neuman MD. Redesigning surgical decision making for high-risk patients. *N Engl J Med.* 2014; 370(15):1379–1381.

46. Carli F, Scheede-Bergdahl C. Prehabilitation to enhance perioperative care. *Anesthesiol Clin.* 2015; 33(1): 17–33.

47. Ziewacz JE, Arriaga AF, Bader AM, *et al.* Crisis checklists for the operating room: development and pilot testing. *J Am Coll Surg.* 2011; 213(2):212–217.e10.

Index

Locators in **bold** refer to tables; those in *italics* to figures

Printed in the United States
by Baker & Taylor Publisher Services

Printed in the United States
by Baker & Taylor Publisher Services